Intelligent Data Analytics for Bioinformatics and Biomedical Systems

Scrivener Publishing
100 Cummings Center, Suite 541J
Beverly, MA 01915-6106

Sustainable Computing and Optimization

Series Editors: Prasenjit Chatterjee, Morteza Yazdani and Dilbagh Panchal
Email: dr.prasenjitchatterjee6@gmail.com

The objective of Sustainable Computing and Optimization series is to bring together the global research scholars, experts, and scientists in the research areas of sustainable computing and optimization from all over the world to share their knowledge and experiences on current research achievements in these fields. The series aims to provide a golden opportunity for global research community to share their novel research results, findings, and innovations to a wide range of readers, present globally. Data is everywhere and continuing to grow massively, which has created a huge demand for qualified experts who can uncover valuable insights from data. The series will promote sustainable computing and optimization methodologies in order to solve real life problems mainly from engineering and management systems domains. The series will mainly focus on the real life problems, which can suitably be handled through these paradigms.

Publishers at Scrivener
Martin Scrivener (martin@scrivenerpublishing.com)
Phillip Carmical (pcarmical@scrivenerpublishing.com)

Intelligent Data Analytics for Bioinformatics and Biomedical Systems

Edited by

Neha Sharma

Chitkara University Institute of Engineering and Technology, Chitkara University, Rajpura, Punjab, India

Korhan Cengiz

Department of Information Technologies, Faculty of Informatics and Management, University of Hradec Kralove, Kralove, Czech Republic

and

Prasenjit Chatterjee

Department of Mechanical Engineering, MCKV Institute of Engineering, West Bengal, India

Scrivener Publishing

WILEY

This edition first published 2024 by John Wiley & Sons, Inc., 111 River Street, Hoboken, NJ 07030, USA and Scrivener Publishing LLC, 100 Cummings Center, Suite 541J, Beverly, MA 01915, USA

For more information about Scrivener publications please visit www.scrivenerpublishing.com.

Wiley Global Headquarters
111 River Street, Hoboken, NJ 07030, USA

For details of our global editorial offices, customer services, and more information about Wiley products visit us at www.wiley.com.

Library of Congress Cataloging-in-Publication Data

ISBN 978-1-394-27088-0

Cover image: Pixabay.com
Cover design by Russell Richardson

Set in size of 11pt and Minion Pro by Manila Typesetting Company, Makati, Philippines

Printed in the USA

10 9 8 7 6 5 4 3 2 1

The Editors would like to dedicate this book to their parents, life partners, children, students, scholars, friends, and colleagues.

Contents

Preface

The combination of intelligent data analytics with the intricacies of biological data has become a crucial factor for innovation and growth in the fast-changing field of bioinformatics and biomedical systems. At the convergence of biology, medicine, and computational science, there is an urgent need for advanced analytical methods to interpret biological data.

The book explores the complex field of biological data analysis. It offers a thorough examination of advanced techniques, methodologies, and applications that utilize intelligence to solve biological puzzles and improve healthcare results. The introduction of high-throughput technology has resulted in a large amount of biological data, which has presented both unique issues and opportunities. The field of biological information is rapidly expanding, encompassing genomics, proteomics, clinical data, and medical imaging. This growth provides a rich environment for computational methods to uncover hidden patterns, trends, and insights within the data.

Chapter 1 delves into the progress of machine learning algorithms for analyzing biological data. The convergence of machine learning and biological data analysis has ushered in a new era of scientific exploration. This chapter examines state-of-the-art machine learning methods used with different forms of biological data, emphasizing their contribution to understanding intricate biological processes. The fusion of artificial intelligence and biology demonstrates how these methods improve our comprehension of genomes, proteomics, metabolomics, and medical uses. By providing vivid examples, this section illustrates the potential of machine learning to revolutionize biological research by pushing its limits.

Chapter 2 examines the application of predictive analytics in clinical diagnosis, and its impact on customers, healthcare professionals, and the healthcare system. Predictive analytics utilizes information, statistical formulae, and artificial intelligence to forecast and analyze disease hazards. The initial stage involves delineating the data sources, preprocessing techniques, and predictive modeling approaches employed in healthcare predictive analytics. This book demonstrates the significance of predictive analytics in the diagnosis of ailments, evaluation of risks, and provision of personalized treatment recommendations through the use of compelling application examples. In addition to image analysis, the technology offers medical practitioners accurate insights through the interpretation of pictures, making it an essential analytical tool.

Chapter 3 classifies the various categories of skin diseases. The fields of dermatology and dermoscopy present distinct difficulties due to their intrinsic intricacy and the elevated level of proficiency necessary for precise diagnosis. To tackle these difficulties, this chapter suggests a computerized method that utilizes advanced techniques in deep learning and machine learning to diagnose skin problems based on images. The goal is to surpass the constraints of traditional diagnostic procedures by utilizing cutting-edge computational technologies.

To start, simpler approaches that combined conventional machine learning models with image processing techniques were analyzed. This entailed utilizing techniques such as Histogram of Oriented Gradients (HOG) and Fast Fourier Transform (FFT) to extract features, along with image augmentation methods. The collected features were subsequently employed to train different conventional machine learning models for the categorization of skin conditions. Next, the field of deep learning is explored with training conducted on models such as ResNet18, ResNet50, EfficientNet, and InceptionNet. Compared to human procedures, these deep learning models demonstrated superior accuracy and efficiency, indicating the promise of a more dependable and efficient diagnostic system.

Chapter 4 investigates computer-aided polyp detection via a tailored Convolutional Neural Network (CNN) architecture. Identifying polyp frames manually is a time-consuming task, especially for gastroenterologists who specialize in this area. Utilizing deep learning algorithms for the automatic detection of polyps can potentially optimize the efficiency of gastroenterologists by reducing the time required for diagnosis. This chapter presents an automated approach for polyp detection with a customized CNN architecture. The development process involved significant tweaking of several parameters, including optimizers, filter size, color space, image dimension, and kernel initializers. The efficacy of the suggested design was assessed using systematic ablation research, test set evaluation, and feature mapping. The system attained optimal outcomes with increased accuracy in polyp detection, together with decreases in execution time and number of trainable parameters.

Chapter 5 delves into the modern healthcare risks that stem from computational intelligence. AI with IoT is transforming every aspect of this field, from remote patient data collection, electronic health record storage, drug delivery, research-based drug trials, pathological results synthesis or implementation, and patient and doctor functionality.

While providing great benefits, IoT with AI also poses major challenges and risks for patients and doctors in areas such as the protection of sensitive data, patient consent and EULA implementation, compliance with security standards for preserving data integrity at transit or storage, the handling the socio-economics-based digital divide in remote areas, discrepancies in multiple vendor agreements, and hierarchical implementation. This chapter lists all the important AI-based risk studies in medical IoT devices.

Chapter 6 discusses a hybrid deep learning architecture to identify and classify sleep apnea from single-channel ECG signals into four classifications. ECG waveforms were preprocessed with a discrete wavelet transform to remove noise and undesired signals. After filtering the signals, a suggested relational autoencoder compressed the information into a lower-dimensional representation to automatically extract the most relevant characteristics. The trained feature set for sleep apnea diagnosis is presented using a bidirectional long short-term memory network. The chapter compares the proposed sleep apnea diagnosis performance measurements to show efficacy.

Chapter 7 proposes Wireless Capsule Endoscopy (WCE) images for deep ensemble feature extraction-based bleeding region classification. WCE is a minimally invasive medical imaging method that provides real-time visual information about the digestive tract to diagnose gastrointestinal problems. It provides digestive system health insights with minimum discomfort and invasiveness compared to traditional endoscopic procedures. Due to illumination, artifacts, and bleeding patches, the classification in normal WCE photos can be difficult. This chapter presents an ensemble feature extraction method that uses ResNet 50, VGG 16, and Inception V3 neural networks for classification instead.

Image processing, augmentation, data pretreatment, and feature extraction can improve classification accuracy in the framework. In addition, an autoencoder reconstructs retrieved features and a Support Vector Machine (SVM) classifier helps for more accurate identification. Readers will see that our experimental results had 99% accuracy and 99.5% precision, and see how WCE imaging helps to diagnose and treat gastrointestinal diseases faster.

Chapter 8 reviews advances in brain tumor classification and localization. Medical imaging technologies like MRI and CT scans provide comprehensive tumor features, while K-means and CNNs improve detection and localization. This chapter shows the effectiveness of SVM classification and the promise of Fractional Harley transformation, It also explains how multi-CNN designs improve accuracy, whereas K-means and Fuzzy K-means improve segmentation.

CNN routinely identify brain tumors well, and deep learning, especially CNNs, performs better but can be complicated and stretch resources. This chapter highlights the evolving landscape of brain tumor detection and localization, while showcasing the power of deep learning to improve diagnostics and treatment planning.

Chapter 9 integrates the Apriori algorithm with data mining classification to improve primary tumor prediction. To improve the prediction accuracy of primary tumors based on pertinent medical variables, classification approaches are combined with the Apriori algorithm, which is known for its association rule mining capabilities. When mining frequent item sets and finding correlations in enormous datasets, the Apriori method performs exceptionally well. Through the use of identified association rules, this hybrid strategy improves prediction performance by enriching the feature set intended for categorization.

Chapter 10 deals with deep learning techniques for neurodevelopmental disorders, personalized medicine, and genomics. For illness curation, patient aggregates with more unusual treatment reactions or unique medical care needs are identified using prediction medication procedures. By using contemporary computation, artificial intelligence generates a reservoir of information that enables the framework to learn and engage in clinical work with increased insight. A combination of genomic and nongenomic variables, in addition to patient-side effects, clinical history, and lifestyle data, would facilitate personalized medicine analysis and prognosis. This chapter investigates the drug combinations that will help the most challenging difficulties in personalized medicine.

Chapter 11 discusses advanced methods of efficiently managing the data from biological investigations, such as biological databases, big data methodologies, software, and computational tools. NGS technology generates big data, or extremely huge volumes of data collected by various biological studies, which are essential to genomic and biomedical research. New computer algorithms must be developed for the NGS experiment to meet high-performance computing analysis requirements.

The healthcare sector produces a large amount of data for a variety of uses, including clinical operations, medicine development and research, patient profile analysis, and patient care. This chapter reviews the academics to understand the importance of big data technology in the field.

Chapter 12 explores the transformative impact of wearable devices and the synergy of big data and AI in enhancing remote patient care, fostering early detection of health issues, and ultimately improving overall patient outcomes. With the use of these technologies, people can have a variety of physiological and behavioral data continuously and instantly collected, which gives medical professionals the ability to remotely monitor their health. Vital signs, physical activity, sleep patterns, and other data can be tracked via wearable technology, which includes smartwatches, fitness trackers, and medical sensors. The combination of wearable technology, big data, and AI empowers people to take an active role in their health management while also giving medical professionals the information they need to make wise decisions, spot abnormalities, and act quickly.

Chapter 13 explores how the integration of biomarker discovery and big data analytics has become a key strategy in the quest to improve disease diagnosis, prognosis, and treatment. An overview of the complex interactions between the identification of illness biomarkers and the application of large-scale data analysis tools is provided. This chapter addresses ethical issues and highlights the critical role that machine learning plays in interpreting multi-omics data. It also sheds light on obstacles, approaches, and case studies. Furthermore, this chapter highlights the potential to reveal new insights by analyzing the combination of heterogeneous omics data, which is revolutionizing healthcare with customized medicine paradigms.

Patients with epilepsy are always vulnerable to an attack. Unpredictable epileptic events can inflict irreversible harm, and when they occur in high-risk situations, patients may pass away. To lower the dangers for patients, it is essential to recognize epileptic events before they happen. Chapter 14 delves into blockchain-based systems for real-time epilepsy monitoring and alerting that use IoT devices and machine learning techniques. Using cutting-edge technology like blockchain, machine learning, and the Internet of Things, this chapter suggests an intelligent alarm system. The proposed mechanism reduces the psychological and physical effects of epileptic seizures by predicting them to a large degree. Additionally, it uses the HLF blockchain to secure any communication process, which should greatly allay worries about communication process security.

Chapter 15 illustrates the use of quantum computing in bioinformatics and biomedical research. This convergence has the potential to release enormous computational power and groundbreaking methods, transforming biological data processing and interpretation while accelerating the rate of life sciences discovery. This chapter provides an overview of the basic ideas of quantum computing and highlights its potential. It also provides a brief explanation of the current state of quantum computing in bioinformatics and medicinal research.

Chapter 16 discusses the future perspectives and emerging trends in Computational Intelligence (CI). CI blends biological disciplines to solve the hardest disease understanding and healthcare problems. The chapter covers bioinformatics, which has advanced genetic analysis prediction, protein structure prediction, and cell network decoding; and it discusses Neural Networks (NN), Deep Learning (DL), Evolutionary Algorithms, and Machine Learning (ML) that combine to synchronize CI approaches.

The Editors

Acknowledgment

The editors wish to express their warm thanks and deep appreciation to those who provided valuable inputs, support, constructive suggestions, and assistance in the editing and proofreading of this book.

The editors would like to thank all the authors for their valuable contributions in enriching the scholarly content of the book.

Mere words cannot express the editors' deep gratitude to the entire editorial and production teams of Scrivener Publishing, particularly Martin Scrivener and Linda Mohr for their great support, encouragement, and guidance all through the publication process. This book would not have been possible without their significant contributions.

The editors would like to sincerely thank the reviewers who kindly volunteered their time and expertise for shaping such a high-quality book on a very timely topic.

The editors wish to acknowledge the love, understanding, and support of their family members during the book's preparation.

Finally, the editors use this opportunity to thank all the readers and expect that this book will continue to inspire and guide them for their future endeavors.

The Editors

1

Advancements in Machine Learning Techniques for Biological Data Analysis

S. Kanakaprabha[1*], G. Ganesh Kumar[2], Y. Padma[3], Gangavarapu[4] and Venkata Nagaraju Thatha[5]

[1]Department of CSE, Rathinam Technical Campus, Coimbatore, TN, India
[2]Department of IT, Hindusthan Institute of Technology, Coimbatore, TN, India
[3]Department of IT, Department of Information Technology, Vijayawada, India
[4]Department of IT, PVP Siddhartha Institute of Technology, Vijayawada, Andhra Pradesh, India
[5]Department of IT, MLR Institute of Technology Hyderabad, Telangana, India

Abstract
The intersection of machine learning and biological data analysis is accompanied by a new period of scientific discovery. This chapter explores cutting-edge machine learning techniques applied to various biological data types, highlighting their role in unraveling complex biological processes. We delve into the integration of artificial intelligence and biology, showing how these techniques enhance our understanding of genomics, proteomics, metabolomics, and medical applications. Through illustrative examples, we establish the transformative possibility of machine learning to push the boundaries of biological research.

***Keywords*:** Machine learning, biological data analysis, genomics, proteomics, multi-omics integration, disease diagnostics, biomarker discovery, personalized medicine

1.1 Introduction

The realm of biological sciences has undergone profound metamorphosis with the introduction of machine learning techniques into data analysis. This introductory section sets the stage for a comprehensive exploration

**Corresponding author*: skanakaprabha@gmail.com

Neha Sharma, Korhan Cengiz and Prasenjit Chatterjee (eds.) Intelligent Data Analytics for Bioinformatics and Biomedical Systems, (1–26) © 2024 Scrivener Publishing LLC

of how machine learning is revolutionizing the study of biological data, unraveling intricate patterns. and empowering researchers to unlock the mysteries of life. In the intricate tapestry of life sciences, a revolutionary convergence has emerged between the realms of machine learning and biology. The union of these two disciplines has given rise to a transformative era in scientific inquiry, opening new doors to unravel the mysteries encrypted in biological data. As we embark on this journey, we delve into the profound implications of advanced data analysis techniques, underpinned by the prowess of machine learning, within the field of biology. The symbiotic connection between machine learning and biology epitomizes a paradigm shift in scientific exploration. Similar to the genetic code orchestrating the formation of life, machine learning algorithms encode patterns and relationships within complex biological datasets. These algorithms possess the uncanny ability to decipher intricacies that elude conventional analysis methods. From genomic sequences to protein structures, the partnership between artificial intelligence and biology has forged an alliance capable of unveiling insights concealed by the sheer complexity of biological systems.

1.1.1 Significance of Advanced Data Analysis in Biology

In the ever-evolving field of biological research, the significance of advanced data analysis cannot be overstated. Traditional methods, while invaluable, often fail to comprehensively capture the multifaceted nature of biological processes. Herein lies the crux of the matter: the intricate interplay of genes, proteins, and cellular pathways necessitates a new dimension of analysis that is not confined by human limitations. Advanced data analysis, empowered by machine learning techniques, transcends these barriers by discerning hidden correlations, identifying novel biomarkers, and predicting intricate molecular interactions.

By wielding the power of machine learning, scientists can extract invaluable insights from vast datasets, paving the way for breakthroughs in modified medicine, disease diagnosis, drug discovery, and ecology. This convergence marks a pivotal moment in the annals of scientific progress, enabling us to navigate uncharted waters and redefine the boundaries of our understanding (see Figure 1.1).

In the subsequent chapters of this exploration, we embark on a captivating journey through the frontiers of machine learning techniques applied to biological data analysis. As we traverse the landscapes of genomics, proteomics, and beyond, we shall uncover the innovations that reshape the contours of biological discovery and revolutionize the way we perceive life itself.

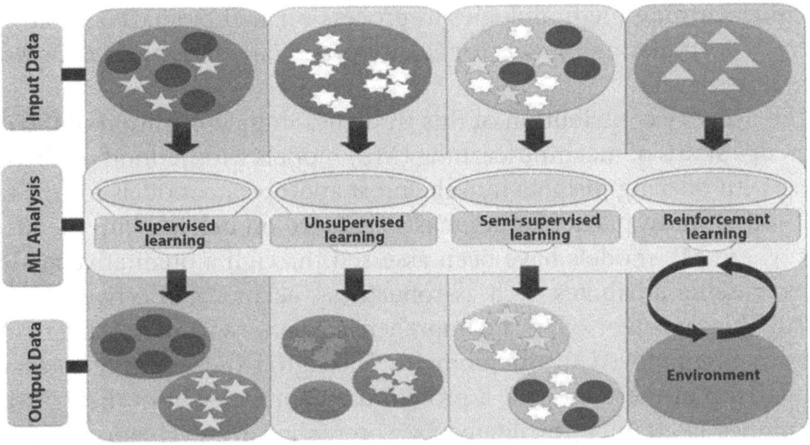

Figure 1.1 A new prospect in multi-omics data analysis of cancer.

1.2 Literature Survey

Employing a narrative methodology coupled with a systematic search strategy [1], this literature review meticulously examined the contemporary landscape of intellectual property analytics through an assessment of 57 recent scholarly articles. By meticulously analyzing the bibliographic particulars of these articles, we subsequently delved into a comprehensive discourse categorized into four principal domains: knowledge management, technology management, economic valuation, and extraction coupled with proficient administration of information. This review aims to provide a valuable resource for both academic researchers and industrial practitioners, serving as a guiding compass for navigating the most current endeavors in the realm of intellectual property analytics.

Wearable sensors have exhibited potential as non-intrusive avenues for amassing biomarkers, which could potentially correlate with heightened stress levels [2]. Stressors trigger a range of living reactions, and these physical responses can be gauged using biomarkers such as Heart Rate Variability (HRV), Electrodermal Activity (EDA), and Heart Rate (HR). These biomarkers signify the stress response stemming from the Hypothalamic–Pituitary–Adrenal (HPA) block, the Autonomic Nervous System (ANS), and resistant system. Although the magnitude of cortisol response remains the conventional benchmark for evaluating stress [1], recent strides in wearable technologies have yielded various consumer devices with the capacity to capture biomarkers such as HRV, EDA, and HR, along with additional signals. Concurrently, investigators have harnessed machine learning methodologies to process verified biomarkers, with the intent of formulating models capable of potentially prognosticating escalated stress levels.

The primary contribution of this study lies in its illustration of the cutting-edge status of machine learning (ML) models within flood prediction, along with offering insights into the most appropriate models for the task [3]. In this study, particular emphasis is placed on delving into the literature where ML models have been assessed through a qualitative analysis encompassing attributes such as robustness, accuracy, effectiveness, and speed. This endeavor offers a comprehensive panorama of the diverse ML algorithms employed in this domain. Through a thorough performance comparison of these models, a profound comprehension of their distinct techniques is attained, facilitated by comprehensive evaluation and discourse. Consequently, this study introduces the most promising predictive approach suitable for both extended and immediate flood predictions. Moreover, this study delves into noteworthy trends aimed at attracting the caliber of flood prediction models. Notably, strategies such as hybridization, data decomposition, algorithm ensemble, and model optimization have emerged as the most efficacious avenues for bolstering ML methods. This survey is a valuable reference for hydrologists and climate scientists in selecting the most appropriate ML approach aligned with their specific prediction tasks.

The role of agriculture in sustaining global activities remains pivotal, confronting significant challenges such as overpopulation and resource competition that imperil planetary food security [4]. To combat the escalating complexities of agricultural production, the progression of smart farming and precision agriculture presents indispensable solutions for tackling sustainability issues in this domain. Data analytics is a critical instrument for ensuring food security, preserving food safety, and upholding ecological equilibrium. Revolutionary information and communication technologies, including machine learning, big data analytics, cloud computing, and blockchain, can address a spectrum of concerns, encompassing augmented productivity, enhanced yields, judicious water usage, safeguarding soil and plant well-being, and amplifying environmental stewardship.

In recent years, digital twinning has emerged as a prominent technology trend, with substantial relevance in the industrial landscape [5]. The convergence of big data analytics and artificial intelligence/machine learning (AI-ML) methodologies with digital twinning amplifies its importance, unlocking fresh avenues and presenting distinctive obstacles for exploration. Although numerous scientific models pertaining to this dynamic domain have been formulated and executed, a comprehensive review encompassing the interplay of numerical twinning, AI-ML, and big data is lacking. This dearth underscores the need for an organized examination that directs both academia and industry towards forthcoming advancements in this arena.

Analyzing systematically gathered molecular outlines from patient tumor examples in conjunction with clinical metadata enables the identification of patterns that can guide tailored treatments and effectively manage cancer patients who share similar molecular subtypes. Addressing the existing gap [6], there is a pressing need to develop computational algorithms for cancer diagnosis, prognosis, and therapeutic guidance, which can discern intricate patterns and facilitate classifications rooted in the abundance of developing cancer research findings within the communal domain. Machine learning, a facet of artificial intelligence, presents substantial promise for deciphering concealed patterns within intricate cancer datasets, as evidenced by recent surveys in the literature. This review focuses on the present landscape of machine learning claims in cancer research, accentuating trends and dissecting notable accomplishments, obstacles, and challenges that stand in the way of its clinical implementation.

In this review, executed deep learning (DL) architectures are thoroughly examined, along with a comprehensive assessment of the extensively employed assessment metrics, attributes, and databases [7]. The classification of UAV livestock monitoring systems employing DL techniques can be categorized into three main groups: detection, classification, and localization. Consequently, the forthcoming advantages and limitations of these DL-centered Precision Livestock Farming (PLF) approaches utilizing UAV imagery are discussed in this study. Furthermore, alternative methodologies utilized to alleviate the challenges of PLF are discussed. The core intention of this endeavor is to offer insights into the most pertinent investigations concerning the advancement of UAV-based PLF systems, with a specific emphasis on deep neural network-based methodologies [8–10].

1.3 Machine Learning Fundamentals

Machine learning serves as the cornerstone of modern data analysis and provides tools for unlocking insights from complex datasets. At its core, machine learning involves the use of algorithms that enable computers to learn from data, recognize patterns, and make informed decisions without explicit programming. This fundamental approach has proven invaluable for removing expressive information from biological data [11].

1.3.1 Supervised, Unsupervised, and Semi-Supervised Learning

Supervised Learning: In supervised learning [12], models are proficient in labeled data, where each statistical point is associated with a known consequence or label. The algorithm maps the input features to the correct output, allowing it to make forecasts or classifications of new, unseen data.

Unsupervised Learning: Unsupervised learning [13] operates on unlabeled data, seeking to uncover inherent patterns, groupings, or constructions within the data. Clustering and dimensionality reduction are common tasks in this group, aiding the detection of hidden relationships within life datasets, as shown in Figure 1.2.
Semi-Supervised Learning: This hybrid approach combines the basics of both supervised and unsupervised learning. It influences a small amount of labeled data alongside a larger pool of unlabeled data to enhance model recital, especially when acquiring labeled data is challenging or costly [14].

1.3.2 Feature Engineering and Selection

Feature engineering involves the formation and selection of relevant input variables (features) to enhance the presentation of machine learning models. In the context of biological information, this process entails the identification of biomarkers, genetic attributes, or molecular properties that carry essential information. Effective feature engineering can significantly improve the model accuracy and efficiency, enabling the extraction of biologically meaningful insights.

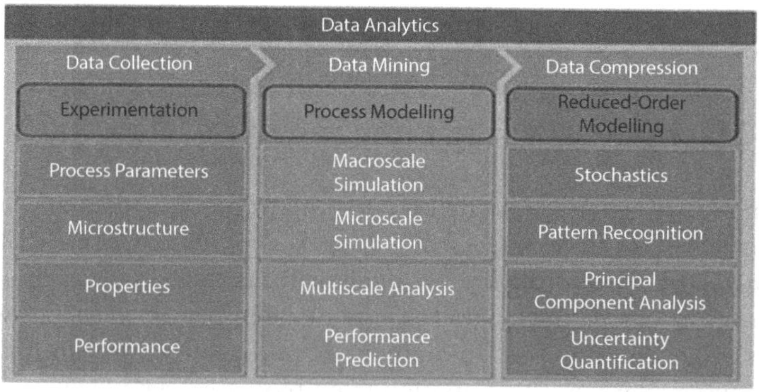

Figure 1.2 Machine learning and data mining approaches in continuum materials.

1.3.3 Deep Learning Architectures for Biological Data

Deep learning, a subset of machine learning, employs intricate neural network architectures to procedure and analyze data. Inspired by the interconnected neurons of the human brain, these architectures excel at capturing intricate patterns and hierarchies in complex datasets. In the realm of biological data, deep learning models such as convolutional neural networks (CNNs) [15] and recurrent neural networks (RNNs) [16] have proven to be adept at tasks such as image analysis, sequence prediction, and molecular structure analysis. These architectures have revolutionized the ability to gain insights from diverse biological datasets ranging from medical images to genomic sequences.

In the subsequent sections, we investigate deeper into the practical application of these machine learning fundamentals, elucidating their role in advancing the examination of biological data and propelling us towards a more comprehensive understanding of life's intricacies.

1.4 Genomic Sequence Analysis

Genomic sequence analysis stands is a testament to the transformative power of machine learning in deciphering the intricate blueprint of life encoded within DNA. Through advanced algorithms and computational techniques, machine learning (Figure 1.3) has enabled us to unlock

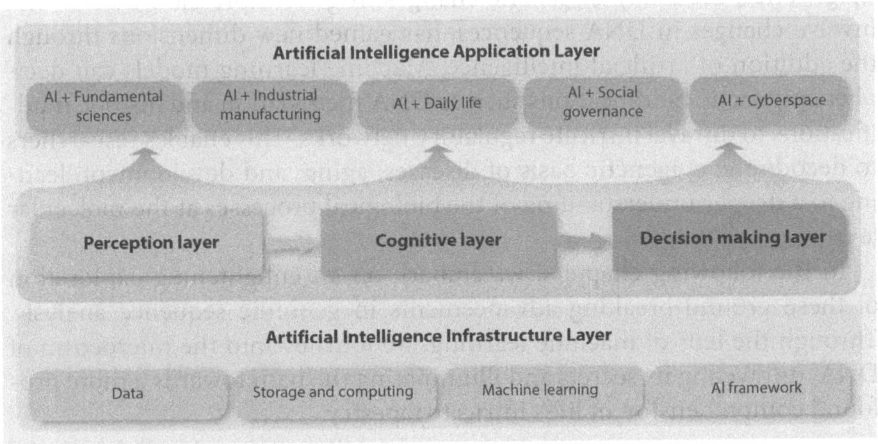

Figure 1.3 Artificial intelligence example for methodical study.

unprecedented insights from genomic data, paving the way for breakthroughs in personalized medicine, genetic disorders, and evolutionary studies.

1.4.1 DNA Sequence Classification and Prediction

Machine learning algorithms have transformed the classification and prediction of DNA sequences. By training models on vast datasets of annotated sequences, these algorithms can distinguish between different genetic elements such as enciphering regions, supervisory elements, and non-coding regions. This ability holds immense promise for identifying disease-associated mutations, annotating genomes, and unraveling the complexities of gene regulation.

1.4.2 Genomic Variant Analysis with Machine Learning

The analysis of genomic variants, including single-nucleotide polymorphisms (SNPs) and structural variations, has been dramatically accelerated by machine learning. These algorithms can detect subtle genetic variations related to diseases and traits, helping identify genetic risk factors and potential therapeutic targets. Machine learning-driven variant prioritization has the potential to streamline the interpretation of genomic data, making personalized medicine a tangible reality [17].

1.4.3 Enhancing Epigenetic Studies through AI

Epigenetics, the study of genetic changes in gene expression that do not involve changes in DNA sequences, has gained new dimensions through the addition of artificial intelligence. Machine learning models can decipher epigenetic modifications such as DNA methylation and histone modifications to unravel intricate regulatory networks. This enables researchers to decode the epigenetic basis of diseases, aging, and development, leading to a deeper understanding of the biological processes at the molecular level.

In the following chapters, we embark on an enlightening exploration of these ground-breaking advancements in genomic sequence analysis. Through the lens of machine learning, we journey into the microcosm of DNA, unraveling its secrets and illuminating the path towards a more profound comprehension of life's intricate tapestry.

1.5 Proteomic Profiling and Structural Prediction

Proteomic Profiling

1. **Deep Learning for Spectral Analysis:** Deep learning techniques, such as convolutional neural networks (CNNs) and recurrent neural networks (RNNs), have been applied to mass spectrometry data for proteomic profiling. These models can routinely learn shapes and features from complex spectral data, aiding protein identification and quantification.
2. **Transfer Learning:** Transfer learning has been used to influence pretrained mock-ups on large-scale proteomic datasets. Researchers perfect these models in specific experiments, reducing the need for extensive labeled data and improving the accuracy of protein identification [18].
3. **Multi-Omics Integration:** Machine learning has enabled the mixing of proteomic data with other omics data such as genomics and transcriptomics. This holistic approach provides a complete understanding of life processes and illness devices.
4. **Feature Selection and Dimensionality Reduction:** Advanced feature selection and dimensionality reduction techniques, such as autoencoders and t-distributed stochastic neighbor implanting (t-SNE), help to identify relevant features from high-dimensional proteomic data and enhance data visualization and analysis.

Structural Prediction:

1. **AlphaFold and Protein Folding:** AlphaFold, developed by DeepMind, has made significant strides in accurately predicting protein structures. Using deep learning and attention mechanisms, AlphaFold has achieved remarkable success in the Critical Calculation of Structure Prediction (CASP) struggle, contributing to our understanding of protein folding.
2. **Template-Based and Template-Free Methods:** Advances have been made in template-based modeling (comparative modeling), using available experimental structures as templates. Template-free methods, as shown in Figure 1.4, which

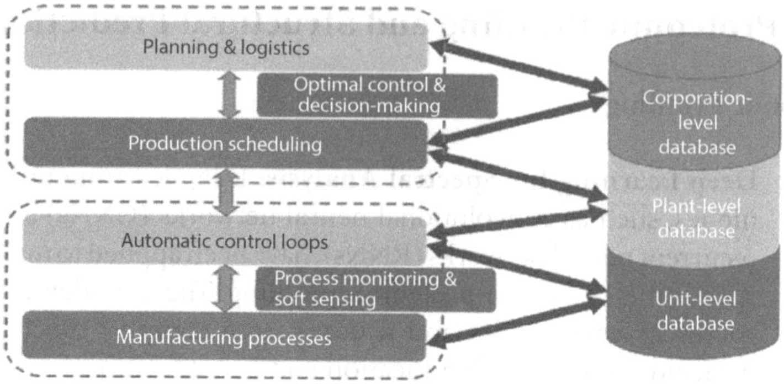

Figure 1.4 Data analytics and machine learning for smart process manufacturing.

predict structures without relying on known templates, have also been improved, contributing to the modeling of novel proteins.

3. **Integrating Evolutionary Information:** Machine learning techniques have been used to extract and integrate evolutionary information from protein sequences, thereby enhancing the accuracy of structural prediction methods.
4. **Ensemble Approaches:** Ensemble methods that combine predictions from multiple algorithms have shown improved prediction accuracy by leveraging the strengths of different techniques.
5. **Incorporating Physicochemical Principles:** Machine learning models have been developed to incorporate the physical and chemical principles governing protein folding, aiding in more accurate structural predictions.

1.5.1 Protein Structure Prediction Using Deep Learning

Predicting the three-dimensional structure of proteins is a fundamental problem in bioinformatics with applications in drug discovery, disease understanding, etc. Deep learning techniques such as neural networks have shown potential for improving the accuracy of protein structure prediction. Advances in this area include the following:

Alpha Fold: Developed by DeepMind, AlphaFold is a deep learning model that has confirmed remarkable accuracy in forecasting protein structures. It leverages a variant of a neural network called a "transformer" to model the complex relationships within protein sequences and their structures.

Improved Representations: Deep-learning techniques have enabled the development of more expressive and biologically meaningful representations of protein sequences and structures, leading to better predictions.
Transfer Learning: Transfer learning approaches allow models pre-trained on large datasets to be fine-tuned for exact tasks, thereby enhancing the accuracy of protein structure prediction [19].

1.5.2 Peptide and Protein Identification via Machine Learning

Mass spectrometry is a widely used technique for identifying peptides and proteins in complex biological samples. Machine learning methods have been used to improve the accuracy and speed of identification of peptides and proteins:

Spectral Analysis: Machine learning algorithms can analyze mass spectra to classify peptide sequences and match them to protein databases, aiding in protein identification.
Feature Selection: ML techniques help in selecting relevant features from high-dimensional mass spectrometry data, reducing noise, and improving identification accuracy.
Classification Algorithms: Support Vector Machines (SVMs), Random Forests, and neural networks were employed to classify mass spectra and identify peptides and proteins.

1.5.3 Functional Annotation of Proteins

Assigning functions to newly discovered proteins is a crucial task in proteomics (Figure 1.5). Machine learning approaches have been instrumental in forecasting protein functions based on numerous data sources:

Sequence Analysis: ML models can predict protein functions based on arrangement homology, motif identification, and domain analysis.
Network Analysis: Functional interaction networks can be analyzed using machine learning to infer protein functions based on their network neighbors.

These advancements in machine learning techniques have significantly accelerated proteomic research, enabling more accurate prediction of protein structures, faster identification of peptides and proteins, and improved functional annotation of proteins. As machine learning continues to

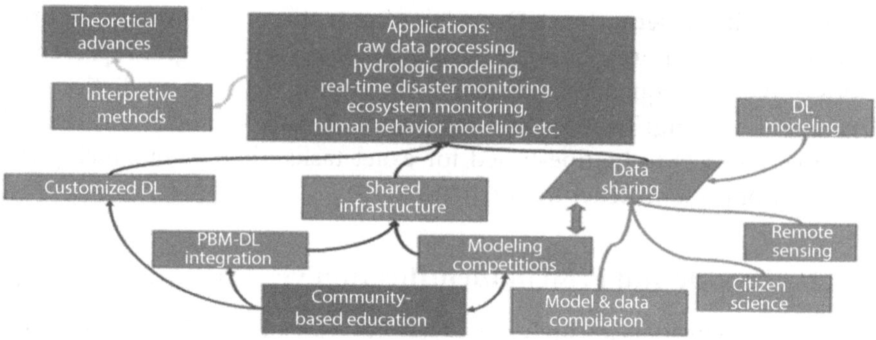

Figure 1.5 Deep-learning hydrologic science developments as a public.

evolve, further breakthroughs will likely be achieved in understanding the complexities of biological systems.

1.6 Metabolomics and Pathway Analysis

1. **Feature Selection and Dimensionality Reduction:** High-dimensional metabolomics data can be challenging to analyze. Advanced feature selection and dimensionality reduction techniques, such as LASSO (Least Absolute Shrinkage and Selection Operator) and PCA (Principal Component Analysis), help identify relevant metabolites and reduce noise in the data.
2. **Metabolite Identification Using Spectral Libraries:** Machine learning algorithms have been used to develop spectral libraries that aid in the identification of metabolites based on mass spectrometry data. These libraries enable more accurate and efficient metabolite annotation.
3. **Deep Learning for Metabolite Identification:** Deep learning architectures including convolutional neural networks (CNNs) and recurrent neural networks (RNNs) have been applied to spectral data for metabolite identification. These models can capture complex patterns in the spectra, thereby improving the identification accuracy.
4. **Metabolic Pathway Prediction and Reconstruction:** Machine learning techniques such as graph-based methods and constraint-based modeling have been utilized to

predict and reconstruct metabolic pathways. These methods help understand the flow of metabolites and interactions between enzymes.

5. **Metabolic Flux Analysis:** Machine learning algorithms were integrated with the experimental data to estimate metabolic fluxes within cellular pathways. This aids in quantifying the rate of metabolite flow in understanding metabolic regulation.
6. **Biomarker Discovery:** Machine learning plays a vital role in identifying biomarkers for various diseases and situations. Algorithms can distinguish between healthy and diseased states based on metabolite profiles, thereby contributing to early diagnosis and personalized medicine.
7. **Network Analysis and Integration:** Mixing metabolomics data with other omics data using network-based approaches allows for a holistic view of organic systems. Machine learning helps construct and analyze metabolic networks, uncovering functional relationships and regulatory mechanisms.
8. **Time-Series Analysis:** Longitudinal metabolomics data can reveal dynamic changes in metabolic pathways over time. Machine learning models, such as unseen Markov models (HMMs) and active Bayesian networks, help to capture temporal patterns and transitions.
9. **Metabolomics Data Integration with Clinical Data:** Machine learning permits the integration of metabolomics data with clinical and phenotypic information. This facilitates the discovery of associations between the metabolite profiles and patient outcomes.
10. **Transfer Learning in Metabolomics:** Transfer learning techniques leverage knowledge from one metabolomics dataset to improve the analysis of a related dataset with limited samples. This method is particularly useful when dealing with small or diverse datasets.

These advancements reflect ongoing efforts to elucidate the influence of machine learning on metabolomics and pathway analysis. As the field continues to evolve, researchers are likely to develop more sophisticated models and techniques to enhance sympathetic metabolism and its suggestions for health and disease as illustrated in Figure 1.6.

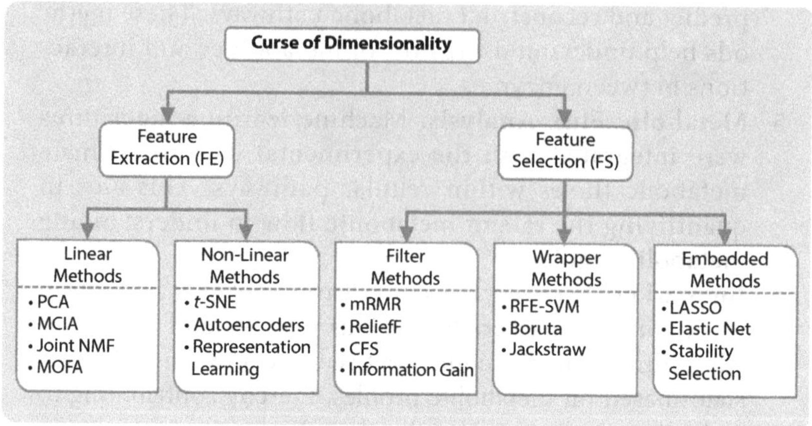

Figure 1.6 Machine learning and integrative analysis of biomedical big data.

1.6.1 Metabolite Identification and Quantification

Spectral Annotation with Deep Learning: Deep learning models, such as convolutional neural networks (CNNs) and recurrent neural networks (RNNs), have been applied to mass spectrometry data for metabolite identification and quantification. These models can learn multifaceted spectral patterns and improve the accuracy of metabolite annotations.

Isotope Pattern Analysis: Machine learning algorithms have been used to analyze isotope patterns in mass spectrometry data, aiding accurate metabolite identification by considering isotopic peaks.

1.6.2 Metabolic Pathway Reconstruction Using AI

Constraint-Based Modeling with Machine Learning: Machine learning techniques have been integrated with constraint-based modeling to predict the metabolic pathways and flux distributions. These methods enhance our understanding of cellular metabolism and enable the prediction of metabolic responses under different conditions.

Graph-Based Approaches: Graph-based machine learning techniques are used to model metabolic networks and predict metabolic pathways. These methods capture complex interactions between metabolites and enzymes, thereby aiding pathway reconstruction.

1.6.3 Integrative Analysis of Multi-Omics Data

Multi-Omics Data Fusion: Machine learning enables the mixing of metabolomics data with other omics data such as genomics, transcriptomics, and proteomics. Integrated analysis provides insights into the functional relationships between different molecular layers and helps to identify key regulatory mechanisms.
Network Inference: Machine learning algorithms are used to infer regulatory networks that connect metabolites to genes, proteins, and other molecules. This assists in elucidating how metabolic pathways are controlled and coordinated.
Deep Learning for Multi-Omics Integration: Deep learning models, such as autoencoders and variational autoencoders are applied to mix and interpret multi-omics data. These models capture compound interactions and dependencies within and between omics datasets, respectively.

The fields of bioinformatics and computational biology are dynamic, and new techniques and approaches are continually emerging. Researchers are pushing the boundaries of machine learning to gain deeper insights into biological processes, improve the accuracy of data analysis, and enable more precise predictions in metabolomics and pathway analysis. To stay updated on the latest advancements, it is recommended to explore recent research papers, attend conferences, and follow the developments in the field.

1.7 Medical Applications

1.7.1 Disease Diagnosis and Biomarker Discovery

Deep Learning for Image Analysis: Convolutional Neural Networks (CNNs) and other deep learning architectures have established remarkable potential in diagnosing diseases from medical images, such as detecting diabetic retinopathy from retinal images or identifying cancerous regions in histopathology slides.
Multi-omics Data Integration: Machine learning models integrate and analyze various types of omics data (genomics, proteomics, metabolomics) to identify disease-related biomarkers and gain a deeper understanding of complex diseases.

Transfer Learning in Medical Imaging: Pretrained models from general image domains (e.g., ImageNet) are fine-tuned on medical images, allowing for effective feature extraction and transfer of knowledge [20].

1.7.2 Personalized Treatment and Drug Discovery

Genomic Medicine: Machine learning is employed to analyze genetic data and recognize genetic variants associated with disease defenselessness and drug replies, enabling personalized treatment strategies (Figure 1.7).
Drug Target Identification: Machine learning models predict potential drug targets by analyzing biological pathways, protein interactions, and genetic data, thereby accelerating the drug discovery process.
Virtual Screening: Machine learning algorithms help identify potential drug candidates by screening large molecular databases and predicting their binding affinities to target proteins.

1.7.3 Predictive Modeling for Clinical Outcomes

Electronic Health Record (EHR) Analysis: Machine learning is used to analyze EHR data to predict patient outcomes, hospital readmissions, and disease progression. This helps clinicians make informed decisions and effectively allocate resources.

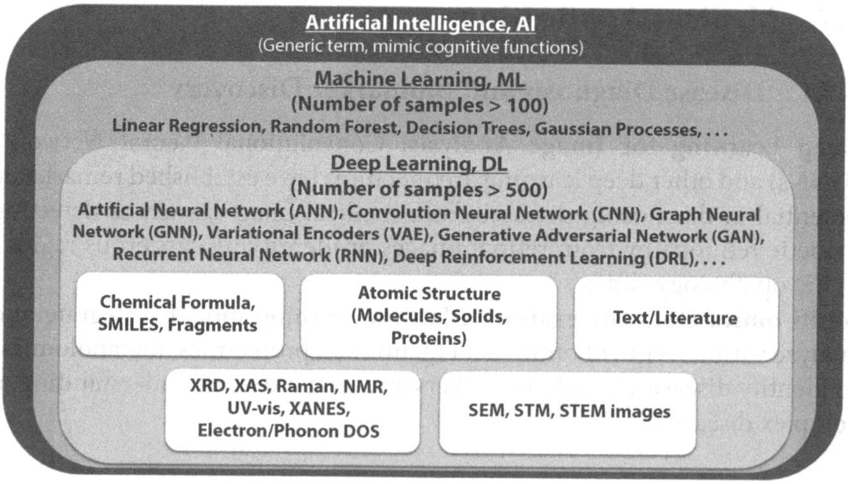

Figure 1.7 Advances and applications of deep learning methods in materials science.

Early Warning Systems: Machine learning models can continuously monitor patient data and provide early warnings for deteriorating health conditions, thereby allowing timely interventions.
Patient Stratification: By analyzing patient data, machine learning can identify subpopulations with similar characteristics, aid in tailoring treatment plans, and improve patient outcomes.

1.7.4 Drug Repurposing and Adverse Event Prediction

Drug Repurposing: Machine learning algorithms analyze current drug records and molecular data to identify possible new uses for existing drugs, speeding up the process of finding treatments for different diseases.
Adverse Event Prediction: Machine learning models analyze patient data to predict and prevent adverse reactions to medications, thereby enhancing patient safety.

1.7.5 Neuroinformatics and Brain Disorders

Connectomics Analysis: Machine learning techniques are useful for analyzing brain connectivity data (fMRI and DTI) to better understand neurological disorders and predict disease progression.
Neuroimaging Pattern Recognition: Machine learning helps identify specific patterns in brain images associated with conditions, such as Alzheimer's disease and schizophrenia.

These advancements demonstrate the growing role of machine learning in revolutionizing medical applications from early disease detection and personalized treatment to drug discovery and improving patient care. As technology and data availability continue to expand, machine learning is expected to play an even larger role in advancing medical investigation and healthcare.

1.8 Challenges and Future Directions

Challenges:

1. **Interpretable Machine Learning in Biology:**
   - **Challenge:** Complex machine learning models such as deep neural networks can be problematic to interpret, limiting their usefulness in providing actionable

insights and understanding the underlying biological mechanisms.
- **Impact:** Lack of interpretability hinders the adoption of machine learning models in critical medical decision-making processes.

2. **Addressing Data Privacy and Ethics:**
   - **Challenge:** Medical data are sensitive and must be handled with utmost maintenance to safeguard patient privacy and comply with ethical regulations.
   - **Impact:** Privacy concerns can hinder data sharing and collaboration, limiting the amount of available data for training robust models, and impeding progress in medical research.

3. **Advancing Quantum Computing in Biological Data Analysis:**
   - **Challenge:** Quantum computing is in its infancy, and its practical applications in biological data analysis are still under development.
   - **Impact:** Despite potential advantages in solving complex biological problems, the practical realization of the potential of quantum computing remains uncertain.

4. **Handling Heterogeneous and Multi-Modal Data:**
   - **Challenge:** Integrating diverse data types (e.g., genomics, imaging, and clinical data) is challenging due to the differences in data formats, quality, and scale.
   - **Impact:** Incomplete or inaccurate data integration can lead to biased or incomplete analyses, thus limiting the ability to derive comprehensive insights.

5. **Small Data and Imbalanced Datasets:**
   - **Challenge:** Limited availability of labeled data, especially in medical applications, can lead to overfitting and poor generalization (Figure 1.8).
   - **Impact:** Insufficient data can hamper the development of accurate and reliable machine learning models, particularly in rare disease cases.

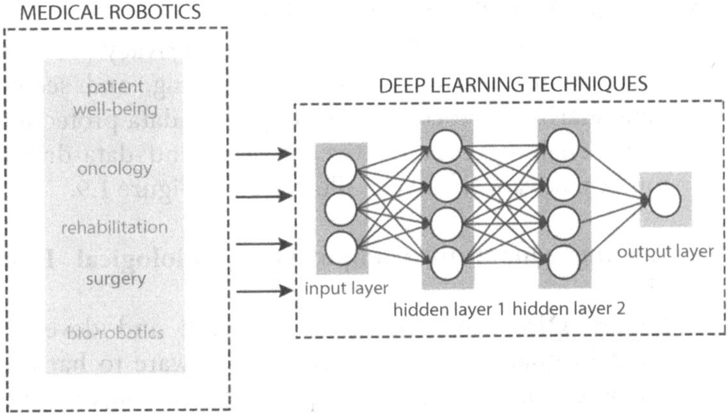

Figure 1.8 Biomedical and health informatics.

6. **Clinical Adoption and Validation:**
   - **Challenge**: Transitioning from research to clinical rehearsal requires rigorous validation, regulatory approval, and mixing with current healthcare workflows.
   - **Impact**: Lack of robust clinical validation can lead to unreliable or unsafe applications in medical settings, undermining trust in machine learning solutions.

7. **Ethical and Societal Implications:**
   - **Challenge:** The use of machine learning in healthcare raises ethical anxiety related to algorithmic bias, accountability, and potential job shifts.
   - **Impact:** Unaddressed ethical dilemmas can erode public trust and hinder the responsible and equitable deployment of machine learning technologies.

Future Directions:

1. **Interpretable Machine Learning in Biology:**
   - **Future Direction:** Research on developing interpretable machine learning techniques, such as model explanations and feature importance visualization, to enable a better understanding of complex models and facilitate their acceptance in medical applications.

2. **Addressing Data Privacy and Ethics:**
   - **Future Direction:** Advancements in privacy-preserving machine learning, federated learning, and secure data-sharing protocols to ensure patient data protection while enabling collaborative research and data-driven medical advancements, as illustrated in Figure 1.9.

3. **Advancing Quantum Computing in Biological Data Analysis:**
   - **Future Direction:** Continued research and development in quantum algorithms and hardware to harness the potential of quantum computing for solving complex biological problems such as drug discovery and molecular simulations.

4. **Handling Heterogeneous and Multi-modal Data:**
   Future Direction: Development of robust and scalable techniques for integrating and analyzing diverse data types, allowing for comprehensive insights and accurate predictions in complex biological systems.

5. **Small Data and Imbalanced Datasets:**
   Future Direction: Exploration of handover learning, active learning, and data augmentation strategies tailored to medical applications, enabling effective model training even with limited data.

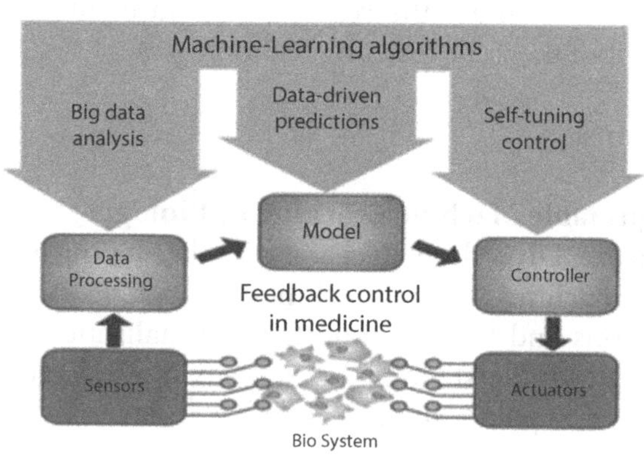

Figure 1.9 Machine learning in advancing exactness medication with feedback control.

6. **Clinical Adoption and Validation:**
   - **Future Direction:** Collaborative efforts between machine learning researchers, clinicians, and regulatory bodies to establish rigorous validation protocols, safety guidelines, and integration strategies for machine learning applications in medical practice.

7. **Ethical and Societal Implications:**
   - **Future Direction:** Development of ethical guidelines, regulations, and frameworks for responsible AI deployment in healthcare, considering fairness, transparency, and societal impacts.

By addressing these challenges and pursuing future directions, the field of machine learning for biological data analysis can overcome obstacles and continue to drive transformative advancements in medical applications, ultimately benefiting patient care and advancing our understanding of complex biological processes.

1.8.1 Interpretable Machine Learning in Biology

- **Challenge:** Complex machine learning models such as deep neural networks often lack interpretability, making it difficult to understand the underlying biological insights and decisions they provide.
- **Future Direction:** Research on developing more interpretable models and techniques, such as attention mechanisms, feature visualization, and rule-based explanations, will be crucial for gaining trust and understanding in medical decision-making.

1.8.2 Addressing Data Privacy and Ethics

- **Challenge:** Medical data are sensitive and highly regulated, raising concerns about patient privacy, data security, and potential biases in algorithmic decision making.
- **Future Direction:** Advancements in privacy-preserving machine learning, federated learning, and differential privacy are essential for ensuring patient data protection while enabling collaborative research. Ethical considerations and

transparent practices in the design and deployment of algorithms are also important.

1.8.3 Advancing Quantum Computing in Biological Data Analysis

- **Challenge:** Quantum computing is in its nascent stages, but holds promise for solving complex biological problems that are computationally intensive, such as simulating molecular interactions and optimizing drug discovery processes.
- **Future Direction:** Continued research on quantum algorithms and hardware development will potentially lead to breakthroughs in efficiently solving large-scale biological and medical problems, paving the way for transformative advancements.

1.8.4 Handling Heterogeneous and Multi-Modal Data

- **Challenge:** Integrating diverse data types (genomics, imaging, and clinical data) from various sources is challenging due to differences in data formats, quality, and scale.
- **Future Direction:** Developing robust and scalable machine learning techniques to effectively handle and integrate heterogeneous data is critical for comprehensive biological insights and accurate predictions.

1.8.5 Small Data and Imbalanced Datasets

- **Challenge:** Obtaining large labeled datasets in many medical applications can be challenging, leading to issues of overfitting and poor generalization, particularly when dealing with rare diseases or imbalanced classes.
- **Future Direction:** Investigating transfer learning, semi-supervised learning, and data augmentation techniques tailored to medical scenarios will help mitigate the limitations of small and imbalanced datasets (Figure 1.10).

1.8.6 Clinical Adoption and Validation

- **Challenge:** Transitioning from research to clinical practice requires rigorous validation, regulatory approval, and integration into existing healthcare workflows.

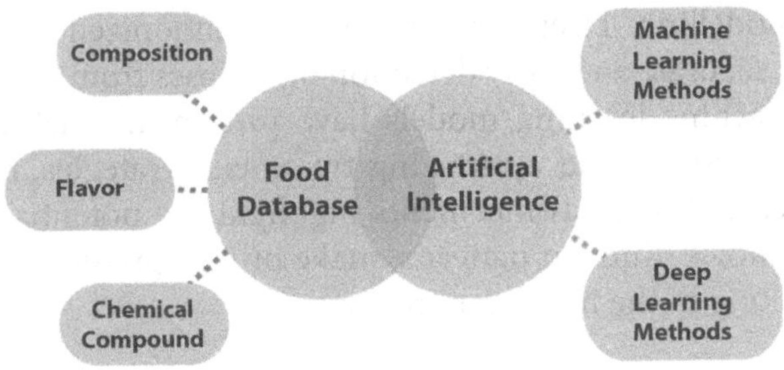

Figure 1.10 Machine learning and deep learning come to the big data in food chemistry.

- **Future Direction:** Collaborative efforts between machine learning researchers, clinicians, and regulatory bodies will be crucial for establishing the safety, efficacy, and real-world utility of machine learning applications in medical settings.

1.8.7 Ethical and Societal Implications

- **Challenge:** The use of machine learning in healthcare raises ethical dilemmas such as algorithmic biases, accountability for decisions, and potential job displacement.
- **Future Direction:** Ongoing discussions, regulations, and guidelines are needed to ensure fairness, transparency, and responsible deployment of machine learning technologies, while also considering broader societal implications.

As the field of machine learning continues to advance, addressing these challenges and pursuing future directions will play a vital role in harnessing the full potential of biological data analysis for medical applications, ultimately leading to improved patient care, enhanced disease understanding, and transformative healthcare innovations.

1.9 Conclusion

1.9.1 Synthesis of Key Contributions and Insights

The application of machine learning techniques to biological data analysis has ushered in a new era of medical discovery and innovation. By harnessing the power of advanced algorithms, researchers have made significant strides in disease diagnosis, personalized treatment, drug discovery, and predictive modelling. Deep learning has revolutionized image analysis, enabling the accurate and early detection of diseases from medical images. Moreover, machine learning models have proven invaluable in predicting clinical outcomes and optimizing treatment strategies, thus improving patient care. These advancements highlight the potential of machine learning to uncover hidden patterns, make precise predictions, and guide decision-making in the healthcare realm.

1.9.2 Anticipated Transformations in Biological Research

The future of biological research is poised for transformative changes due to the continued advancement of machine learning techniques. Interpretable machine learning methods will bridge the gap between complex models and actionable insights, thereby enhancing our understanding of biological processes and disease mechanisms. The integration of quantum computing, as it matures, holds the promise of revolutionizing simulations and analyses, which were once computationally infeasible.

Ethical and privacy concerns surrounding patient data will drive the development of more secure and privacy-preserving machine learning methodologies, enabling collaborative research without compromising data integrity. As machine learning models become more adept at handling heterogeneous data and small sample sizes, researchers will be able to extract meaningful insights from limited datasets, accelerating discoveries in rare diseases, and personalized medicine. These transformations will not only reshape the way we approach biological research, but also pave the way for a new era of precision medicine, data-driven diagnostics, and improved patient outcomes. The fusion of machine learning and biological data analysis is a dynamic field with immense potential to revolutionize healthcare and biological research. As advancements continue to unfold and challenges overcome, the synergy between machine learning and biology will lead to breakthroughs that were previously unimaginable, ultimately contributing to a healthier and more informed society.

References

1. OECD, *Enabling the Next Production Revolution: the Future of Manufacturing and Services-Interim Report*, Technical Report, OECD, France, June 2016.
2. EPO, *India and Europe Explore the Impact of Industry 4.0 on the Patent System*, Technical Report, European Patent Office, Munich, Germany, 2016.

3. Gubbi, J., Buyya, R., Marusic, S., Palaniswami, M., Internet of Things (IoT): a vision, architectural elements, and future directions. *Future Gener. Comput. Syst.*, 29, 7, 1645–1660, 2013.
4. EPSRC, *Delivery Plan 2016-2020 Top Ten Messages*, Technical Report, United Kindgom, 2016.
5. Gunther, W.A., Rezazade Mehrizi, M.H., Huysman, M., Feldberg, F., Debating big data: A literature review on realizing value from big data. *J. Strateg. Inf. Syst.*, 26, 3, 191–209, 2017.
6. Abbas, A., Zhang, L., Khan, S.U., A literature review on the state-of-the-art in patent analysis. *World Pat. Inf.*, 37, 3–13, 2014.
7. Sharma, N., Chakraborty, C., Kumar, R., Optimized multimedia data through computationally intelligent algorithms. *Multimed. Syst.*, 29, 5, 2961–2977, 2023.
8. Sharma, N. and Batra, U., An enhanced Huffman-PSO based image optimization algorithm for image steganography. *Genet. Program. Evolvable Mach.*, 22, 189–205, 2021.
9. Baglieri, D. and Cesaroni, F., Capturing the real value of patent analysis for R&D strategies. *Technol. Anal. Strat. Manage.*, 25, 8, 971–986, 2013.
10. Moehrle, M.G., Walter, L., Bergmann, I., Bobe, S., Skrzipale, S., Patinformatics as a business process: A guideline through patent research tasks and tools. *World Pat. Inf.*, 32, 4, 291–299, 2010.
11. Sruthi, G., Ram, C.L., Sai, M.K., Singh, B.P., Majhotra, N., Sharma, N., Cancer prediction using machine learning, in: *2022 2nd International Conference on Innovative Practices in Technology and Management (ICIPTM)*, vol. 2, IEEE, pp. 217–221, February 2022.
12. Sharma, N., Soni, M., Kumar, S., Kumar, R., Deb, N., Shrivastava, A., Supervised machine learning method for ontology-based financial decisions in the stock market. *ACM Trans. Asian Low-Resour. Lang. Inf. Process.*, 22, 5, 1–24, 2023.
13. Trippe, A.J., Patinformatics: Tasks to tools. *World Pat. Inf.*, 25, 3, 211–221, 2003.
14. Dintzner, J.P. and Van Thieleny, J., Image handling at the european patent office: BACON and first page. *World Pat. Inf.*, 13, 3, 152–154, 1991.
15. Srivastav, G., Rashid, M., Singh, R., Gehlot, A., Sharma, N., Breast cancer detection in mammogram images using machine learning methods and clahe algorithm, in: *2022 5th International Conference on Contemporary Computing and Informatics (IC3I)*, IEEE, pp. 1187-1192, December 2022.
16. Mitra, D., Sharma, N., Rashid, M., Singh, R., Classification rules based breast cancer detection using machine learning approach, in: *2022 5th International Conference on Contemporary Computing and Informatics (IC3I)*, IEEE, pp. 1274–1278, December 2022.
17. Dhiman, P., Kukreja, V., Manoharan, P., Kaur, A., Kamruzzaman, M.M., Dhaou, I.B., Iwendi, C., A novel deep learning model for detection of severity level of the disease in citrus fruits. *Electronics*, 11, 3, 495, 2022.

18. Kukreja, V. and Dhiman, P., A deep neural network based disease detection scheme for citrus fruits, in: *2020 International conference on smart electronics and communication (ICOSEC)*, IEEE, pp. 97–101, September 2020.
19. Kumar, A., Sharma, N., Chauhan, R., Khare, A., Anand, A., Sharma, M., A stack ensemble approach for early alzheimer classification using machine learning algorithms, in: *International Conference on Recent Trends in Image Processing and Pattern Recognition*, Springer Nature Switzerland, Cham, pp. 82–96, December 2023.
20. Goyal, J., Sharma, N., Kumar, A., Anand, A., Prabha, C., Classifying diabetes using artificially intelligent techniques: A comparative analysis, in: *2023 IEEE 2nd International Conference on Industrial Electronics: Developments & Applications (ICIDeA)*, IEEE, pp. 353–358, September 2023.

2

Predictive Analytics in Medical Diagnosis

Vivek Upadhyaya

Department of Electrical & Electronics Engineering, Poornima University, Jaipur, India

Abstract

Medical diagnosis using predictive analytics is a paradigm adjustment in medical care. This chapter analyzes predictive analytics in clinical diagnosis and its effects on clients, medical care workers, and the healthcare system. Predictive analytics predicts and analyzes disease threats using information, statistical formulas, and artificial intelligence. The phase begins by describing the data sources, preprocessing, and predictive modeling methods used in healthcare predictive analytics. We demonstrate the importance of predictive analytics in ailment detection, danger evaluation, and customized treatment suggestions that make use of engaging application instances. In addition to image analysis, it provides medical practitioners with precise insights through picture interpretation, making it a vital analysis device.

Nevertheless, predictive analytics in clinical diagnostics has challenges. The chapter discusses about personal data privacy, model interpretability, principles, and laws. This emphasizes the need to balance a client's legal rights and security. Real-world case studies illustrate exactly how predictive analytics enhances client care, resource circulation, and expenses in medical care firms. Artificial intelligence, electronic wellness documents, telemedicine, and quantum computers may kead to progress in healthcare. Medication might be identified earlier, dealt with more separately, and resourced more efficiently using predictive analytics. This chapter introduces predictive analytics' major impacts on medical care, with a focus on other related issues.

***Keywords*:** Predictive analysis, medical diagnosis, disease progression, early detection, data analysis, risk assessment

Email: vivekupadhyaya@ieee.org

Neha Sharma, Korhan Cengiz and Prasenjit Chatterjee (eds.) Intelligent Data Analytics for Bioinformatics and Biomedical Systems, (27–66) © 2024 Scrivener Publishing LLC

2.1 Introduction to Predictive Analytics in Healthcare

Predictive analytics in the healthcare industry is a cutting-edge field that utilizes sophisticated evaluations and information to forecast health and wellness outcomes and enhance medical therapy for patients [1, 2]. By assessing large datasets that consist of person details, case history, and therapy records, predictive analytics can assist physicians in making informed choices concerning private care, early treatment, and source allowance. This effective tool not only improves patient end results but also raises functional effectiveness in healthcare centers, brings about cost savings, and boosts the total top quality of treatment. This technology makes it possible to identify potential health and wellness dangers, forecast condition development, and individualized treatments for specific individuals, leading to even more individualized and efficient health care. In the healthcare domain, predictive analytics plays a critical role in determining patterns and trends that may not be conveniently noticeable with traditional techniques. This encourages healthcare professionals to adopt a positive strategy for healthcare management, helping with the application of preventive measures and improving diagnostic precision. The application of predictive analytics in the healthcare sector is driving considerable renovations in functional processes and service arrangements resulting in enhanced personal results and general improvements in healthcare systems.

2.1.1 Definition of Predictive Analytics

Predictive analytics, also referred to as using information evaluation, statistical formulas, and artificial intelligence strategies in the clinical field, intends to identify patterns, trends, and prospective end results connected to the health and wellness and clinical problems of people [3]. This procedure includes evaluating historical patient information, including digital wellness records, laboratory results, and treatment documents, to predict future health events, susceptibility to illness, responses to treatments, and patient outcomes. The primary goal of predictive analytics in the medical field is to help healthcare specialists choose based upon proof, making it possible for prompt intervention, personalizing treatment techniques, and improving individual treatment, while optimizing source allowance and improving the performance of the healthcare system.

2.1.2 The Significance of Predictive Analytics in Medical Diagnosis

Making use of predictive analytics in medical diagnosis is very useful because it can dramatically boost healthcare by increasing the accuracy and speed of finding conditions [4]. By assessing huge datasets that include individual information, such as signs, medical history, genetic qualities, and various other appropriate aspects, predictive analytics can identify complicated patterns and links that may be past human monitoring. This helps with the quick recognition of diseases and ailments, leading to proactive therapies, and ultimately, better individual results. In the context of cancer diagnosis, predictive analytics can play a vital role in the absence of delay-finding growth, with the identification of special biomarkers or imaging patterns. This application of predictive analytics has the potential to significantly boost the possibility of achieving positive treatment results.

Furthermore, the exercise of predictive analytics holds a significant capacity in the realm of healthcare expense reduction and source appropriation, as it enables the avoidance of unnecessary medical checkups and interventions. The consideration of specific personal qualities and the prediction of the most efficient medicines contribute to the formulation of customized treatment programs. This method not only ensures that clients receive care that is much more customized and effective but also reduces the economic strain on healthcare systems. The total relevance of predictive analytics in the field of medical diagnosis remains in its capacity to improve individual end results, reduce mortality prices, enhance person contentment, and promote the sustainability of healthcare systems by optimizing analytical precision and therapy methods.

2.2 Overview of the Chapter's Structure

The phase's format was purposely designed to offer an in-depth expedition of predictive analytics in the medical field. This thorough assessment covers a range of subjects, including data resources, evaluation techniques, real-world applications, ethical considerations, challenges, and emerging patterns. The initial sections (2–4) lay the groundwork by discussing data collection, preprocessing, and predictive modeling approaches. The precision and usefulness of predictive versions, especially when working with complex healthcare datasets, rely heavily on top quality information, cleansing, and attribute engineering. The succeeding sections delve deeper into numerous predictive analytics techniques, such as regression evaluation, classification versions, machine learning algorithms, and time-series evaluation, demonstrating their convenience in clinical contexts. Section 2.4 concentrates largely on functional applications where predictive analytics plays an essential role in boosting clinical diagnostics and medical care distribution, consisting of early disease discovery, threat evaluation, personalized therapy referrals, clinical picture analysis, and disease development monitoring. These applications demonstrate the concrete impact of predictive analytics on individual outcomes and the effectiveness of health care systems.

Complying with this phase discovers the value of version interpretability and explainability in the healthcare field, along with the moral and lawful considerations that feature using predictive analytics in a heavily regulated industry that prioritizes privacy. The chapter then explores various challenges and constraints inherent in predictive analytics, including data-related concerns, overfitting, and prejudice mitigation. The chapter later changes its focus to real-world instances of effective application and future fads, featuring a study that demonstrates the positive end results of using predictive analytics in medical care and academic conversations on cutting-edge topics, such as expert systems, deep learning, electronic health and wellness records, telemedicine, and the potential influence of quantum computers. This chapter provides an extensive examination of predictive analytics in the context of clinical diagnosis, and provides a beneficial understanding of its present state and future prospects.

2.3 Data Sources and Data Preprocessing

Information sources and data preprocessing are crucial components of predictive analytics for clinical diagnoses. In the context of healthcare, information originates from various sources, such as electronic health records (EHRs), wearable devices, hereditary data, and medical imaging [5]. Digital health and wellness records provide a bonanza of client information, incorporating case histories, laboratory results, medicines, and scientific notes. Wearable devices offer real-time information on a client's physical criteria, activity levels, and other patterns, while hereditary data provide beneficial insights into a person's genetic predispositions. Clinical imaging information, consisting of X-rays, MRIs, and CT scans, provides visual information that can help in the diagnosis of different conditions. The key obstacle is integrating these diverse data sources, ensuring high quality data, and maintaining personal privacy and protection in conformity with health care guidelines such as HIPAA.

Data pre-processing in medical care involves numerous vital actions, starting with high-quality information and cleaning. This process is important for determining and remedying mistakes, missing values, and disparities within information. Function options and engineering come next, where relevant variables are selected and new functions are produced to enhance version precision. Managing missing information is an additional important facet that requires methods such as imputation or, sometimes, the exclusion of insufficient documents. As predictive analytics versions are as good as the data they are built on, robust data preprocessing is essential to attain accurate and reputable predictions in clinical diagnosis, helping with very early condition detection, threat assessment, and individualized therapy suggestions.

2.3.1 Types of Data Sources (Electronic Health Records, Wearable Devices, Genetic Data, etc.)

In the field of predictive analytics for medical diagnosis, a diverse range of data sources is employed to derive meaningful insights and achieve precise prognostication [6]. In this discipline, several primary categories of data sources are frequently utilized.

- **Electronic Health Records (EHRs):** Electronic Health Records (EHRs) encompass an extensive compilation of a person's case history, including medical diagnoses, therapies, prescriptions, laboratory searches, and medical professional notes. The inclusion of both organized and unstructured data items provides an extensive and useful resource for the application of predictive analytics to assess an individual's wellness problem, keep track of the development of diseases, and identify possible elements that might present threats.
- **Wearable Devices:** Wearable gizmos, such as smartwatches and physical fitness trackers, provide constant surveillance of a series of health-related indicators, including heart price, rest patterns, physical activity, and additional criteria. The exercise of real-time data enables the application of predictive modeling methods to examine general health, identify irregularities, and forecast potential health incidents, such as heart ailments or other concerns.
- **Genetic Data:** Genetic information acquired by methodologies such as DNA sequencing provides valuable insights into

an individual's genetic composition and probable hereditary predispositions towards specific diseases. Predictive analytics has the potential to utilize genetic data to evaluate the likelihood of hereditary disorders or forecast the potential response of a patient to particular therapies.

- **Medical Imaging Data:** Radiographic images, including X-rays, magnetic resonance imaging (MRI), computed tomography (CT) scans, and ultrasound images, offer visual representations of the anatomical structures within a patient's body. The application of predictive analytics to medical imaging data has the potential to facilitate the early diagnosis of diseases, categorization of medical conditions, and ongoing monitoring of disease advancement.
- **Biometric Data:** Biometric data sources encompass many forms of biometric measures, such as fingerprints and retinal scans, which serve the purpose of patient identification and contribute to the improvement of security and precision in healthcare records.
- **Clinical Trial Data:** The utilization of data derived from clinical trials and research studies holds considerable importance in the application of predictive analytics for medical diagnosis. These records facilitate evaluation of the efficacy of novel treatments, pharmaceuticals, and medical interventions.
- **Patient-Reported Data:** The collection of patients' self-reported data, obtained via surveys, questionnaires, or mobile applications, can yield significant insights into symptoms, lifestyle patterns, and adherence to treatment protocols. These data have the potential to provide insights into patient preferences, treatment responses, and the progression of diseases.

In the domain of medical diagnosis, the incorporation of various data sources in conjunction with sophisticated predictive analytics methods empowers healthcare practitioners to make well-informed judgements, enhance the quality of patient treatment, and optimize health outcomes. Through the utilization of data from many sources, predictive analytics plays a significant role in the early diagnosis of diseases, evaluation of risks, provision of personalized treatment recommendations, and facilitation of effective disease monitoring.

2.4 Data Quality and Cleaning

The requirements of information quality and cleaning are of utmost relevance within the domain name of predictive analytics for clinical diagnosis [7, 8]. The efficacy and dependability of prediction versions are directly influenced by the dependability and accuracy of medical care information. Several elements have the potential to add sound and inconsistencies to the healthcare datasets. These problems include mistakes in the process of data input, instances of missing out on worths, duplications within the dataset, and adjustments to the style of the data. Consequently, it is essential to employ extensive treatments for reviewing and refining high-quality of information to maintain the integrity of the data used for predictive analytics.

The process of guaranteeing top information quality begins with a detailed evaluation of the information, where abnormalities and incongruities that have the potential to misshape the outcomes are determined. Innovative data-cleansing approaches incorporate the correction of unreliable entrances, standardization of information layouts, and elimination of redundant records. In the realm of electronic health records (EHRs), the presence of free-text clinical notes presents even more intricacies because of their disorganized nature and variability in language used. Natural language processing (NLP) and message mining methodologies were utilized to remove significant information from clinical notes. This facilitates the assimilation of valuable yet disorganized information into prediction versions.

In addition, it is imperative for data cleaning procedures to successfully manage the obstacle of missing information, which is a prevalent issue in medical care datasets. Several methods such as imputation are utilized to reduce the influence of missing information on predictive designs. Imputation involves estimating the values of missing data points by leveraging the available details. The establishment of suitable high-quality data and cleaning protocols is crucial for the creation of dependable and specific predictive analytics models for clinical diagnoses. The exercise of top-notch data helps boost the accuracy of forecasts, thereby facilitating very early condition recognition, threat evaluation, and personal treatment recommendations. Consequently, this contributes to improved outcomes.

2.4.1 Feature Selection and Engineering

The addition of function choice and design is essential within the realm of predictive analytics for medical diagnosis [9]. The resolution of the most relevant qualities or features and the creation of added attributes that record substantial details are necessary in enhancing the accuracy and effectiveness of forecast designs. In the realm of health care data, the exercise of these approaches is of utmost value to comprehend detailed and frequently multi-dimensional datasets.

Attribute choice is an essential action in data analysis, which entails the identification of the most significant variables or qualities from a more comprehensive pool of prospective attributes. Within the domain name of clinical diagnosis, the objective of attribute selection is to identify and select information qualities with the highest possible level of value in connection with the forecast of health outcomes. The effectiveness and toughness of predictive models can be boosted by reducing the dimensionality of information and prioritizing one of the most important functions, thus mitigating the risk of overfitting. Function option techniques can be classified into three primary groups: filters, wrappers, and embedding strategies. Each group has its own special staminas and limitations. In the context of early disease discovery, such as in cancer cells, the exercise of attribute option techniques can assist in the identification of important biomarkers or clinical attributes that display a high relationship with the provided condition.

Feature design is a process that involves the development of unique attributes or changes in existing ones to accurately record the underlying patterns inherent in the information. Within the realm of medical care, the aforementioned procedure holds substantial relevance, considering that it assists in the acquisition of useful information that might not be easily noticeable from the unrefined data. For example, in the context of forecasting the chance of heart disease in a person, the procedure of feature engineering might encompass the creation of a composite function that integrates information concerning blood pressure, cholesterol levels, and age, thus creating a cardiac risk score. Feature engineering enables the combination of domain-specific knowledge and promoting the establishment of detailed associations between variables. Functional engineering plays a crucial role in the field of medical imaging as it encompasses the removal of structure, form, and strength functions from pictures to assist in the diagnosis procedure.

The application of efficient function selection and design strategies in the field of predictive analytics for medical diagnosis has the potential to boost the precision, interpretability, and functionality of design. These strategies use useful aid to health care specialists by offering an understanding of the prompt recognition of conditions, assessment of risks, and customized suggestions for treatment, consequently enhancing person end results and optimizing the healthcare procedure.

2.4.2 Dealing with Missing Data

The administration of missing data is an important part of predictive analytics in the field of clinical diagnostics given that healthcare datasets frequently exhibit partial information [10]. This incompleteness has the potential to reduce the precision and reliability of the predictive models. Correctly addressing the absence of data is important to ensure that forecasts and diagnoses are founded on the most detailed and precise information that is currently accessible. Multiple methods have been utilized in this certain context:

- **Imputation:** The process of imputation requires changing missing values with estimated or predictive worths stemming from the existing information. Several imputation techniques exist, including mean imputation, mean imputation, and regression imputation. Imputation methods play a critical role in clinical diagnosis, as they add to the preservation of dataset completeness and mitigate the potential loss of essential details. One potential strategy to resolve the concern of missing out on laboratory outcomes or individual demographics is the utilization of imputation methods, in which patterns identified in comparable patients are utilized to estimate the missing out on data.
- **Deletion:** The non-inclusion of missing information can be done without activating substantial hinderance to the accuracy and efficiency of projection variations. The technique utilized in this study is called removal, which requires the removal of records with incomplete details. Nonetheless, it is necessary to work out care while using this technique, considering that excitable removal of information can create a lowered dataset size and may present prejudices right into the obtained outcomes. In the context of dealing with digital health and wellness records or other healthcare datasets, the comprehensive assessment of records to be eliminated presumes vital relevance, specifically when confronted with little detail.
- **Indicator Variables:** Developing indication variables can be beneficial in certain situations, as they explicitly suggest the

presence or absence of information elements. This enables the prediction models to compensate for missing information, potentially boosting their efficiency. Indication variables are particularly beneficial when there is a lack of information contains valuable understanding.

The strategy to address the lack of information in scientific diagnosis relies on the details of the top qualities of the dataset and the objectives of the analysis. Successfully management of missing data is critical for boosting the precision of the designs used in early disease discovery, risk analysis, customized treatment referrals, and various other elements of clinical diagnosis. This guarantees that predictions are made using a comprehensive collection of appropriate variables, ultimately boosting client care and the results.

2.5 Predictive Analytics Techniques

The application of predictive analytics strategies in clinical diagnosis incorporates a variety of approaches [11–13]. These methodologies include regression evaluation, category models (such as logistic regression, decision trees, and random forests), artificial intelligence algorithms (such as support vector machines and semantic networks), and time-collection evaluation. These methods utilize previous client information, medical records, and various other analytical criteria to produce educated prognostications pertaining to illness vulnerability, patient diagnosis, and therapy effectiveness. By carrying out these approaches, healthcare experts can augment the timely recognition of illness, assess the chance of clinical ailments, supply individualized therapy approaches, and look after the innovation of ailments, inevitably resulting in more accurate diagnoses and improved patient treatment.

2.5.1 Regression Analysis

Regression analysis is a highly reliable technique used in predictive analytics for clinical diagnostics [14]. By recognizing connections between different patient qualities and the probability of details of clinical problems, medical care practitioners are equipped to make informed decisions based on information. Currently, regression models such as logistic regression for binary outcomes and straight regression for constant results may be employed. For example, logistic regression can be utilized to predict the event or non-occurrence of medical conditions, such as diabetes or heart problems, using variables such as as age, sex, cholesterol levels, and other appropriate attributes. In contrast, straight regression can be used to approximate the size of a specific sensation, such as forecasting a person's high blood pressure, by considering variables such as weight, age, and various other important features.

The relevance of information quality and feature selection cannot be overemphasized in the context of medical diagnoses. The purchase of a total dataset with pertinent variables, execution of strategies to sanitize certain information via the handling of missing values and outliers, and mindful choice of one of the most helpful features are vital stages in the study procedure. The involvement of doctors in this procedure is important, as their expertise in the field can provide a useful understanding for selecting appropriate attributes and including medically significant variables.

The relevance of comprehending regression coefficients is emphasized in the medical field, as it allows healthcare specialists to understand the elements that form diagnoses and the extent of their influence. This understanding is critical for making effective therapeutic choices. However, making use of regression evaluation in medical diagnosis is not without difficulties, including moral issues, privacy issues, and version validation in real-world professional settings. Overcoming these obstacles calls for a durable partnership between information researchers and medical care professionals to ensure safe and reliable implementation of predictive analytics in health care.

2.5.2 Classification Models (e.g., Logistic Regression, Decision Trees, Random Forests)

In the domain of predictive analytics for clinical diagnosis, a wide variety of category designs, including logistic regression, decision trees, and arbitrary forests, are used to make enlightened and evidence-based choices pertaining to patient well-being. These models are highly useful tools for healthcare employees, as they enable the forecasting and categorization of medical problems by utilizing person information. Classification designs, such as logistic regression, choice trees, and random woodlands, have substantial ramifications in clinical settings. Logistic regression is particularly useful for assessing binary results, such as visibility or lack of an illness. Choice trees provide interpretability, whereas random forests are durable in managing intricate information. By leveraging these versions, clinical diagnoses can be made more precisely and effectively, ultimately resulting in boosted individual care and boost (Table 2.1).

Category versions are of utmost relevance in the field of medicine, as they are necessary for forecasting and medical diagnosis of various clinical

Table 2.1 Classification models for predictive medical diagnosis.

Classification model	Application	Advantages	Considerations
Logistic Regression [15]	Binary classification (e.g., presence/absence of a disease)	Interpretable, easy to understand, feature importance	Assumes linear relationship, may not capture complex patterns
Decision Trees [16]	Binary or multi-class classification, hierarchical decision-making	Interpretability, handling mixed data types, visualization	Prone to overfitting, may require pruning
Random Forests [17]	Binary or multi-class classification, robust ensemble method	Robustness, feature importance, mitigates overfitting	Less interpretable than individual trees
Support Vector Machines (SVM) [18]	Binary classification, finding clear boundaries	Works well in high-dimensional spaces, handles non-linearity	Hyperparameter tuning, data scaling, imbalanced datasets
Neural Networks (Deep Learning) [19]	Medical image classification, sequence data analysis	Handles unstructured data, state-of-the-art performance	Data requirements, model complexity, computational resources
Naïve Bayes [20]	Binary or multi-class classification, simple probabilistic model	Simplicity, efficiency, effective with text data	Naive feature independence assumption

conditions. Each design possesses a distinct toughness and elements that need to be considered. The choice of a model is contingent upon several variables, including the nature of the clinical diagnosis issue, functions of the information, and demand for interpretability of the design. The involvement of healthcare experts and information experts is necessary to efficiently choose and implement one of the most appropriate versions within a particular healthcare setting.

2.5.3 Machine Learning Algorithms (e.g., Support Vector Machines, Neural Networks)

Artificial intelligence formulas have dramatically enhanced the precision of medical diagnoses, providing medical care professionals with effective tools for making even more educated decisions. Support Vector Machines (SVM) are a popular option for binary category jobs because they are knowledgeable when comparing different clinical conditions by discovering clear boundaries. SVMs operate in high-dimensional spaces, can deal with nonlinearity via bit functions, and are durable against overfitting. However, they require a careful choice of bit functions and hyperparameter adjustment and can be conscious information outliers.

Deep-understanding versions, such as Convolutional Neural Networks (CNNs), have become progressively preferred in medical diagnosis, supplying top-notch efficiency in various tasks. These versions excel at taking care of unstructured information, making them suitable for medical photo categories and sequence information analysis. CNNs can draw out complex features from medical images, enabling the identification of refined patterns that might go unnoticed by human observers. Nonetheless, their application needs substantial computational resources and information, and their intricacy can make them much less interpretable, which is a problem in the clinical field.

Random forest, an ensemble method, is widely used for binary or multiclass categories in clinical diagnosis. Their strength hinges on their toughness and capability to evaluate function significance, mitigating overfitting issues commonly related to specific choice trees. The set nature of Random Forests ensures boosted forecast accuracy. However, the trade-off for this precision is that they are less interpretable than the specific trees. In addition, care must be taken when handling imbalanced datasets, as the formula may present prejudice in the predictions.

Logistic regression is a timeless method that remains pertinent in medical diagnosis for binary categories, particularly when the relationships between the features and end results are straightforward. Its simplicity and interpretability make it a favored selection for jobs such as predicting the existence or lack of a disease based on individual information. Nevertheless, logistic regression presumes a linear connection between features and may not capture facility and nonlinear patterns efficiently, restricting its applicability in scenarios with intricate data dynamics.

Decision trees offer an instinctive way to deal with binary or multiclass classification jobs, and they are ideal when decisions adhere to an ordered structure. They are interpretable and can manage blended information types, making them a prominent option in situations in which recognizing the choice procedure is of vital significance. Nevertheless, choice trees are prone to overfitting and may require pruning to maximize their predictive efficiency.

2.5.4 Time Series Analysis

Time series analysis is a highly advantageous method within the world of predictive analytics for medical diagnosis, especially when challenged with information that undertakes temporal changes [21, 22]. The exercise of this modern technology has the potential to offer useful points of view on patterns in person health and wellness, the advancement of illness, and the capability to predict clinical events (Table 2.2).

Time series analysis is of great importance in enhancing patient care, as it enables healthcare practitioners to effectively monitor chronic ailments, forecast the occurrence of diseases, and evaluate the efficacy of treatments across a span of time. In the realm of medical diagnostics, it serves to enhance decision-making processes, enable the timely identification of potential concerns, and ultimately improve patient outcomes.

2.6 Use Cases in Medical Diagnosis

The area of clinical diagnosis has undergone substantial modifications due to the implementation of advanced modern technologies and analytics based on information. The use of predictive analytics and artificial intelligence has considerably boosted the capacity of healthcare professionals to examine client conditions properly and quickly. Numerous applications, such as early disease discovery, picture analysis, and individual threat classification, demonstrate how cutting-edge devices can improve and support the experience of doctors. Therefore, individual end results are improved and medical care systems are more efficient.

Table 2.2 Time series analysis components and description.

Component	Description
Data Collection	Gather time-stamped medical data, such as patient records, vital signs, lab results, and more, ensuring data consistency and accuracy.
Data Preprocessing	Clean the data, handle missing values, remove outliers, and ensure regular time intervals for the time series data.
Feature Extraction	Derive relevant features from the time series data, such as aggregating data over specific time intervals, extracting seasonality patterns, or calculating trends.
Exploratory Data Analysis (EDA)	Visualize and explore the time series data to understand trends, seasonal patterns, and anomalies indicative of medical conditions.
Time Series Modeling	Utilize time series models, such as ARIMA (Autoregressive Integrated Moving Average), ETS (Exponential Smoothing), or Prophet, to make forecasts or capture trends and seasonality.
Machine Learning Models	Incorporate time series data as features into traditional machine learning models, like decision trees, random forests, or gradient boosting, for predictive tasks.
Anomaly Detection	Employ time series analysis to identify anomalies or outliers in the data that might indicate unusual patient conditions or medical events.
Model Validation	Split the data into training and testing sets or use cross-validation to assess model performance, using metrics like MAE or RMSE.
Clinical Validation	Collaborate with medical professionals to validate model predictions, ensuring clinical relevance and safety.
Deployment	If validated, integrate the model into a healthcare system for real-time monitoring or early diagnosis of medical conditions.
Ethical Considerations	Ensure data used adheres to privacy regulations and develop and deploy predictive models with patient privacy and data security in mind.

2.6.1 Early Detection of Diseases (e.g., Cancer, Diabetes)

The prompt identification of diseases, consisting of ailments such as cancer and diabetes mellitus, is an essential facet of contemporary medical diagnostics and has significant implications for both individuals and healthcare systems [23]. The timely discovery of cancer cells is often associated with better therapeutic outcomes and increased chances of survival. Evaluating programs, such as mammography for the discovery of breast cancer cells and colonoscopy for the recognition of intestinal cancer cells, play a crucial role in the early discovery of cancer cells. In addition, this area is being transformed by developments in Artificial Intelligence (AI) and machine learning. Deep learning versions, such as convolutional neural networks (CNNs), have been effectively utilized in the field of clinical imaging. These designs can analyze radiological images, including X-rays and mammograms. By leveraging this modern technology, radiologists can identify subtle indications of malignancies at an earlier stage, thus boosting the possibility of more efficient treatment alternatives. In addition, within the context of diabetic issues, predictive analytics utilizes a series of data resources, such as blood glucose levels, hereditary factors, and way-of-life details, to determine those that are at a heightened threat. Artificial intelligence algorithms can be used to forecast the onset of diabetes mellitus. This enables medical care practitioners to deliver customized preventive approaches that can cover lifestyle adjustments to medication. These strategies hold the possibility of restraining the improvement of health problems or possibly avoiding events. The utilization of these use instances not only has the potential to maintain human lives but also to reduce the monetary stress on healthcare systems by mitigating the need for extensive and expensive therapies linked to the progression of illness to innovative stages.

2.6.2 Risk Assessment and Stratification

In the field of medical diagnosis and healthcare management, threat assessment and stratification are of utmost relevance. They aid in providing customized treatment and effectively allocate sources [24, 25]. These treatments entail examining the chance of a private or group creating particular clinical problems or experiencing unfavorable health and wellness outcomes. The crucial elements of threat evaluation and stratification are as follows:

- Individual Risk Assessment
- Population Risk Assessment

- Predictive Modeling
- Stratification
- Preventive Interventions
- Chronic Disease Management
- Cost-Effective Resource Allocation

In conclusion, risk assessment and stratification play essential roles in modern medical care. Supporters assist the arrangement of individualized medical care, ideal allocation of resources, and successful execution of approaches for ailment avoidance and administration. With the utilization of data-driven methodologies and predictive modeling strategies, medical care professionals and policymakers possess the ability to boost the stipulation of services to both people and the populace, thus bringing about the amelioration of health and wellness end results and the reduction of healthcare expenses.

2.6.3 Personalized Treatment Recommendations

Personal therapy recommendations are an essential element of contemporary health care; they are frequently described as accuracy medicine or customized medicine [26]. Personalizing medical therapies and interventions to the distinctive characteristics of individual people, including yet not restricted to their genetic make-up, clinical background, way of living, and particular health demands, is the essence of these suggestions. Adhering to are vital elements of individualized therapy recommendations (Table 2.3).

The application of personal therapy recommendations represents a change from a standardized method to patient-centric and data-driven healthcare. Doctors can enhance patient outcomes, reduce unfavorable effects, and optimize treatment efficacy by tailoring interventions to match the distinct characteristics of private patients. In challenging and complicated conditions, such as cancer and uncommon diseases, where traditional treatments might have restricted effectiveness, this approach is especially encouraging.

2.6.4 Image Analysis and Medical Imaging

Image analysis and medical imaging are essential components in the process of clinical diagnosis because they provide crucial aesthetic data that are essential for the evaluation, diagnosis, and surveillance of diverse medical

Table 2.3 Personalized treatment components and description.

Component	Description
Genomic and Genetic Information	Analyzing an individual's genomic and genetic data to identify mutations, variations, and susceptibilities that impact treatment decisions.
Biomarker Analysis	Evaluation of biomarkers, such as proteins or genetic markers, to understand a patient's health status and treatment response.
Targeted Therapies	The use of treatments that focus on specific molecular or genetic abnormalities associated with a patient's condition, delivering more effective and less harmful interventions.
Treatment Pathways	Development of individualized treatment pathways that outline the specific steps and interventions tailored to a patient's condition, stage, and genetic profile.
Pharmacogenomics	Examination of how a patient's genetic makeup affects their response to medications, guiding healthcare providers in selecting the most appropriate drugs and dosages.
Clinical Decision Support Systems	Computer-based tools providing healthcare professionals with evidence-based guidance for making personalized treatment decisions.
Patient Preferences and Values	Incorporating patient preferences, values, and quality of life considerations into the treatment plan through shared decision-making with healthcare providers.
Ongoing Monitoring and Adjustments	Continuous monitoring and modification of treatment recommendations based on patient responses, disease progression, and evolving medical information.
Precision Medicine Trials	Enrolment of patients in precision medicine clinical trials to test novel treatments designed to target specific genetic or molecular factors in their condition.
Ethical and Privacy Considerations	Addressing ethical and privacy concerns related to the use of personal genetic and health data for treatment recommendations, ensuring data security and patient consent.

Table 2.4 Different imaging modalities with use cases and description.

Imaging modality	Use case	Description
X-ray	Chest X-rays	Diagnosing lung diseases, heart conditions, and rib fractures.
CT Scan	Head and Body Scans	Visualizing internal structures for identifying tumors, injuries, and vascular issues.
MRI	Brain and Soft Tissue Imaging	Examining soft tissues, neurological disorders, and musculoskeletal conditions.
Ultrasound	Obstetrics and Abdominal Imaging	Monitoring fetal development and assessing abdominal organs.
Mammography	Breast Cancer Screening	Detecting breast cancer in its early stages.
Endoscopy and Colonoscopy	Gastrointestinal Visualization	Diagnosing ulcers, colorectal cancer, and gastrointestinal disorders.
Pathology and Histopathology	Tissue Examination	Identifying diseases through microscopic analysis of tissue samples.
Dermatology Imaging	Skin Condition Diagnosis	Diagnosing skin conditions, including melanoma and psoriasis.
Ophthalmology Imaging	Eye Disease Assessment	Detecting eye diseases such as glaucoma and macular degeneration.
Digital Pathology	Digital Slide Analysis	Using digital scans and image analysis to enhance pathology diagnosis.
Machine Learning and AI	Automated Image Analysis	Using AI to detect abnormalities and assist radiologists in interpretation.
Image-Guided Interventions	Surgical and Minimally Invasive Procedures	Real-time imaging for precision during surgical interventions.
Radiomics	Tumor Characterization	Extracting quantitative features from images to assess tumors and predict treatment response.
3D Imaging and Virtual Reality	Enhanced Visualization	Visualizing complex anatomical structures for surgical planning and education.

problems [27]. Key medical diagnosis applications for image analysis and medical imaging include the following (Table 2.4).

Medical imaging and image analysis are crucial for disease diagnosis because they improve patient care and provide useful insights. Healthcare providers can easily and quickly diagnose a wide range of medical diseases and specializations with their help.

2.6.5 Disease Progression Tracking

Monitoring the progression of a condition is an important part of providing care and making medical diagnoses, particularly for chronic and dynamic problems [28–30]. This procedure involves constantly observing and examining an individual's health to establish how the condition advances. There are three crucial elements for monitoring illness development:

Early Detection and Intervention: The utilization of illness progression monitoring enables doctors to identify early indications of illness exacerbation or complications. In the case of chronic diseases such as diabetes mellitus, early detection of degraded blood glucose control can prevent extreme complications, which is of great importance. Keeping track of the improvement of deadly developments using imaging or biomarker analysis can educate on modifications to restorative techniques and boost the likelihood of effective treatment. By maintaining normal surveillance, physicians have the capacity to quickly implement changes to clients' way of living or therapies, which ultimately contributes to enhanced personal results.

Treatment Efficacy Assessment: Checking the development of a disease makes it possible to analyze the effectiveness of clinical interventions and therapies. This is particulalrly advantageous in the case of rheumatoid joint inflammation, a problem for which the treatment objectives are to minimize inflammation and hold-up joint deterioration. Medical professionals can examine the effectiveness of the chosen treatment with routine security of illness indications and client symptoms. With the occurrence of adverse effects or inefficacy, changes may be made, such as drug substitutions or alterations to the treatment routine. The aforementioned iterative procedure of analysis and modification boosts the precision and effectiveness of personal care.

Data-Driven Decision-Making: Condition development tracking is significantly dependent on a variety of data sources such as patient-reported end results, imaging, medical records, and lab outcomes. The utilization of information analytics and electronic health records (EHRs) has enabled doctors to make choices based on this wealth of information. By evaluating longitudinal client information, artificial intelligence algorithms can forecast the progression of illness, thereby assisting doctors in predicting upcoming wellness events. Additionally, the dissemination of personal information to multidisciplinary care groups can foster cooperation and boost the criterion of care given in its entirety. In essence, disease development monitoring enables physicians to improve client care by assisting in educated decision-making and therapy technique optimization, specifically for those afflicted with chronic and progressive ailments.

In summary, condition development tracking is an ever-evolving data-centric treatment that has a substantial influence on the provision of clinical diagnosis and client care. It helps with the assessment of treatment efficiency, early detection of condition exacerbation, and progression of data-driven decision-making in the medical care market. Medical care experts can enhance the quality of life of people with chronic and modern conditions, optimize client treatment, and boost treatment results through continuous monitoring and adaptation to disease development.

2.6.6 Model Interpretability and Explainability

Within the domain of predictive analytics for clinical diagnosis, where the ability to make timely and exact decisions can have critical effects, the interpretability and explicability of the versions are important [31, 32]. These components are essential in ensuring that the intricate predictive models employed in healthcare are not non-transparent mysteries, but rather clear instruments that healthcare practitioners can rely on and comprehend. The capacity to interpret models enables clinicians to understand the procedure through which these models produce prognostic or analytical choices, consequently ensuring that algorithmic understanding is consistent with their medical expertise. Along with promoting conformity and acceptance, such openness enables the prompt recognition of errors, the decrease of bias, and adherence to moral and governing concepts; hence, it inevitably enhances the requirement of care offered to clients and ensures the safety and security of medical judgements.

2.6.7 The Importance of Model Interpretability in Healthcare

The value of design interpretability in the healthcare industry is of utmost and it has a direct influence on patient well-being, professional judgement, and the reliability of predictive analytics. Predominantly, interpretability is an essential prerequisite for developing confidence and understanding among medical professionals regarding the outcomes produced by predictive models [33]. The effects are incredibly high in the medical care sector; consequently, clinicians need to have full confidence in the recommendations of algorithms for fruit and vegetables. Utilizing an interpretable design allows healthcare providers to gain an understanding of the decision-making process by elucidating the rationale behind a certain diagnosis or treatment suggestion. This understanding is crucial for promoting confidence and assisting the application of AI-powered analysis instruments. Healthcare professionals are more inclined to welcome and integrate these tools into their medical techniques, thus helping with informed medical choices when they have the capacity to interpret design outcomes.

In addition, the capacity to translate models is essential for spotting and fixing mistakes. In the healthcare sector, where guaranteeing patient safety and security is of utmost importance, any kind of mistake or prejudice present in the information or design forecasts can lead to life-threatening outcomes. Utilization of an interpretable version boosts the ability of medical professionals to acknowledge and detect problems. They possess the capacity to determine the essential resources of a problem, such as imprecise information, a misconfigured version, or an unrepresentative training dataset, without delaying the implementation of therapeutic activities. By doing so, incorrect medical choices are less likely to occur, which ultimately results in life savings and a diminished threat of medical negligence.

2.6.8 Techniques for Making Predictive Models More Interpretable

To boost the interpretability of the predictive versions, attribute selection and design must precede [34]. Select functionalities that are not exclusively pertinent, but likewise easy to use and in accordance with the location of worry. This may be achieved via the development of easy-to-use qualities such as information aggregation or the application of domain-specific proficiency. In addition, interpretability is enhanced by favoring simplified design styles, such as choice trees or linear regression, over even more intricate styles. An extra way to boost this is by implementing regularization methods, such as L1 or L2 regularization, which serve to advertise attribute choice and enhance design.

An additional effective technique is to employ visualization devices, such as attribute importance charts and partial dependence plots, to equip explicit insights concerning the impact of certain attributes on the forecasts generated by the model. In addition, the inclusion of domain name specialists during the model-building stage can strengthen the self-confidence that the model's efficiency represents functional predictions. The openness, measurability, and integrity of predictive versions can be increased by using visualization devices, cooperation with professionals, and documents of the modeling process.

2.6.9 Regulatory Considerations (e.g., GDPR, HIPAA)

Predictive analytics plays an essential role in transforming clinical diagnoses by leveraging sophisticated data-driven techniques to improve medical care outcomes [35]. However, its application within the healthcare domain name demands robust understanding and adherence to rigorous governing frameworks, such as the General Data Protection Regulation (GDPR) and the Health Insurance Portability and Accountability Act (HIPAA). These laws are created to protect individual privacy, ensuring the safe, secure, and moral handling of sensitive clinical data. Therefore, the effective and accountable deployment of predictive analytics in clinical diagnosis calls for a unified combination of sophisticated innovation with detailed compliance techniques to ensure personal confidentiality and data security, while supplying boosted analysis accuracy and individual care (Table 2.5).

Table 2.5 Regulatory aspects for predictive analytics in medical diagnosis.

Regulatory aspect	**GDPR (general data protection regulation)**	**HIPAA (health insurance portability and accountability act)**
Scope	Applies to the processing of personal data within the European Union (EU).	Applies to the handling of protected health information (PHI) in the United States.
Data Privacy Principles	Emphasizes principles of lawfulness, fairness, transparency, purpose limitation, data minimization, accuracy, storage limitation, integrity, and confidentiality.	Focuses on privacy and security of health data, including access controls, data encryption, and audit trails.
Patient Consent	Requires explicit and informed consent for data processing, with specific opt-in mechanisms.	Allows for data sharing without patient consent in certain situations, but with strict limitations.

(Continued)

Table 2.5 Regulatory aspects for predictive analytics in medical diagnosis. (*Continued*)

Regulatory aspect	GDPR (general data protection regulation)	HIPAA (health insurance portability and accountability act)
Data Anonymization	Encourages the use of anonymized or pseudonymized data for research and analytics.	Recognizes de-identified health data as non-PHI and allows its use for research and analysis.
Data Security	Mandates robust data protection measures, including encryption and data breach reporting.	Requires healthcare organizations to implement security safeguards and report data breaches.
Data Subject Rights	Grants data subjects' rights to access, rectify, erase, and restrict the processing of their data.	Gives patients' rights to access their health records and request amendments.
Data Transfer	Requires special mechanisms (e.g., Standard Contractual Clauses) for transferring data outside the EU.	Allows PHI transfer within the U.S. for healthcare operations, payment, and treatment without consent.
Penalties	Non-compliance may result in fines of up to 20 million euros or 4% of the company's global annual revenue.	Non-compliance can lead to civil and criminal penalties, including fines and imprisonment.
Regulatory Authority	Enforced by national data protection authorities within EU member states.	Enforced by the U.S. Department of Health and Human Services (HHS) and the Office for Civil Rights (OCR).

Important regulatory issues include protecting patient privacy and ensuring the appropriate use of predictive analytics for medical diagnosis.

2.6.10 Ethical and Legal Considerations

The execution of predictive analytics in clinical diagnosis has significant potential for enhancing individual care; nonetheless, it involves a multifaceted terrain of moral and lawful deliberations that require precise navigating [36, 37]. Concern is given to honest factors to consider, starting with the foundational principle of individual authorization. Permissions that are both volunteer and notified are critical when using clients' medical data for predictive analytics. Individuals must possess full expertise concerning the designated exercise of their information and be provided the freedom to choose whether to take part in analysis processes powered by data. In addition, it is a legal responsibility and ethical requirement to guard the confidentiality and stability of information. Avoiding unsanctioned accessibility, breaches, or exploitation of patient information is essential to protect the self-confidence and credibility of medical care systems.

Lawfully, adherence to regulations cannot be compromised. The GDPR in the European Union and HIPAA in the USA developed specific standards relating to the collection, storage, and disclosure of individual information. Disobedience to these guidelines might result in considerable legal ramifications, such as financial charges and penalties. To ensure legal compliance, it is important that healthcare providers and innovation companies engaged in predictive analytics, information researchers, and companies carry out strong data protection procedures, obtain safe informed approval from clients, and stick to developed information dealing with standards.

On top of that, responsibility is an important lawful element to consider. Appointing responsibility in the case of unfavorable results can become a formidable task when diagnostic and therapy decisions are influenced by predictive analytics. The application of these innovations by doctors might potentially subject them to obligation, while information researchers can face legal consequences for creating models that produce incorrect diagnoses or therapy suggestions. It is crucial to establish unambiguous boundaries of accountability and duty to reduce lawful obligations and guard the legal rights of clients. In an ever-evolving domain name such as this, it is essential to continue to upgraded policies and proactively confront legal and honest problems to ensure that predictive analytics boosts individual care while supporting personal privacy and legal demands.

2.7 Challenges and Limitations

The implementation of predictive analytics in the field of medical diagnosis has yielded significant developments in the medical care sector through the utilization of machine learning algorithms and information to enhance the accuracy and effectiveness of disease detection and client treatment. Nonetheless, this cutting-edge modern technology is not without its challenges and restraints, which necessitate careful examination. To optimize the advantages of predictive analytics while promoting patient security and data ethics, it is essential to comprehend and challenge the compliance with obstacles: data top quality and personal privacy problems, model interpretability, and regulative compliance. Given these situations, it is important to carry out a complete evaluation of these obstacles and

Table 2.6 Challenges and limitations for predictive analytics in medical diagnosis.

Challenge/ limitation	Description
Data Quality	Inaccurate or incomplete patient data can lead to unreliable predictions. Data cleaning and validation are essential.
Data Privacy	Safeguarding patient data and complying with regulations like HIPAA and GDPR can be complex and costly.
Bias and Fairness	Biased training data or algorithms can lead to unfair or discriminatory outcomes, especially affecting underrepresented groups.
Interpretability	Complex predictive models may lack transparency, making it difficult to understand their decisions.
Model Overfitting	Overly complex models can lead to overfitting, causing poor generalization and unreliable predictions.
Limited Sample Size	Some medical conditions are rare, leading to challenges in building predictive models due to limited data.
Regulatory Compliance	Adhering to evolving healthcare and data privacy regulations requires ongoing efforts and resources.
Clinical Adoption	Resistance from medical professionals to adopt predictive analytics can hinder its integration into clinical workflows.
Human Expertise	Predictive models may lack the nuanced clinical expertise of healthcare professionals, potentially missing critical context.
Cost and Resource Constraints	The implementation and maintenance of predictive analytics systems can be expensive and resource-intensive.
Ethical Concerns	Decisions made based on predictive models can raise ethical dilemmas, such as the potential to override clinical judgment.

constraints to successfully pass through the elaborate terrain of predictive analytics, as it concerns clinical diagnosis.

The following is a tabular compilation of the obstacles and constraints inherent in the use of predictive analytics for medical diagnoses (Table 2.6).

It is imperative to confront these obstacles and constraints to guarantee the effective incorporation of predictive analytics into medical diagnosis and guarantee its precision, dependability, and ethical application within healthcare environments.

2.7.1 Data-Related Challenges (Data Volume, Quality, Interoperability)

The utilization of information plays a critical role in the field of clinical diagnostics, especially in the application of predictive analytics, as it allows the generation of accurate and significant understandings [38]. Nevertheless, dependence on data presents a collection of significant challenges. Primarily, the large amount of clinical data is a considerable challenge for healthcare systems and calculation infrastructure, necessitating considerable storage space and processing capabilities. Successfully managing a substantial quantity of information while concurrently ensuring its safety and security, poses a recurring problem, particularly in the context of the exponential growth of medical care information.

Moreover, high-quality data and interoperability are considerable challenges. The value of the top quality of clinical information cannot be overstated when making accurate projections. Nevertheless, it frequently encounters challenges such as mistakes, missing out on worths, and incongruities, which have the potential to lead to incorrect findings. Furthermore, it is common for clinical information to be stored in diverse types and systems within medical care organizations, which offers a challenging and continuous initiative to attain smooth information assimilation and interoperability. The aforementioned issues call for comprehensive efforts in information curation and the establishment of standardized information layouts to preserve the dependability and efficacy of predictive analytics in clinical diagnostics as a means of enhancing personal care.

2.7.2 Overfitting and Model Generalization

The value of avoiding overfitting and ensuring model generalization cannot be overstated in the field of medical diagnostic predictive analytics [39]. Overfitting occurs when a forecast design becomes overly intricate and winds up suitable noise in the training information instead of identifying meaningful patterns. Although overfit models may execute well during training, they are unable to properly apply their understanding to unidentified situations, making them unstable for medical diagnosis. This poses a significant danger as these designs might produce inaccurate medical diagnoses and treatment suggestions, ultimately jeopardizing individuals' health and wellness. To avoid overfitting and remove reputable medical understandings, it is needed to use strategies such as regularization, cross-validation, and design intricacy reduction. Furthermore, accomplishing durable version generalization is essential, as versions educated on particular individual populations or healthcare institutions may not work in different environments or in other patient teams. To ensure the generalizability of models, it is necessary to use depictive and diverse training data, consider client demographics, and represent variants in professional methods and high quality data. Close cooperation between doctors and information scientists is required to establish accurate and adaptable designs related to various medical care scenarios. By accomplishing excellent generalization across different circumstances, predictive analytics versions can dramatically boost client treatment and improve the results.

2.7.3 Addressing Bias and Fairness in Predictive Models

To eliminate social predispositions and obtain reasonable results for all, forecast designs must determine and reduce prejudice and promote justice [40]. Prejudice based on sex, race, age, and socioeconomic standing can result in unfair or prejudiced actions. To overcome these issues, equity-promoting methods should be used in predictive modeling to get over these issues.

Prior to anything else, data pre-processing is important. This approach recognizes and reduces the predisposition to training information. This might consist of resampling underrepresented populations or creating new information to reduce discrepancies. Data augmentation and cleaning can reduce sounds and mistakes, which can enhance biases.

Furthermore, model justness is important for version development. Fairness-aware formulas, which reduce the disproportionate effect on specific market teams, can benefit you. Design analysis should include fairness standards consisting of disproportionate influence, a level-playing field, and calibration. This technique aids developers in discovering and fixing predispositions in model forecasts.

A multidisciplinary approach is required to constantly examine forecast design predisposition and justness. Justness concerns may be integrated into information prep work, design structure, and real-world applications to create forecast versions with high precision, justice, and equity. These efforts have made predictive analytics much more dependable and ethical in medical care diagnoses, economic financing, and the criminal justice system.

2.7.4 Successful Implementation and Case Studies

The successful integration of predictive analytics in medical diagnosis holds the promise of transforming the healthcare industry through advancements in early disease identification, treatment suggestions, and, ultimately, patient outcomes. The following are a few noteworthy case studies that illustrate the efficacy of predictive analytics in this particular field:

- **Breast Cancer Diagnosis with Deep Learning:** In a famous example study, scientists employed deep learning versions to carry out an analysis of mammograms with the goal of discovering breast cancer cells at its early stages [41]. The convolutional semantic network (CNN)-based model was trained using a comprehensive dataset comprising mammography photos. The system showed a substantial level of precision in the recognition of breast cancer cells, which is beyond the diagnostic capacities of human radiologists. This implementation exemplifies the capacity of predictive analytics to enhance and improve the precision of diagnosis in a critical clinical domain.
- **Early Sepsis Detection:** Predictive analytics have been used by healthcare facilities to determine sepsis in individuals at an early stage [42]. With the examination of a convergence of essential physical indications, laboratory searching for, and added client details, prognostic versions can determine the possible circumstances of blood poisoning prior to their development into critical stages. The use of this aggressive method has resulted in expedited interventions and enhanced rates of patient survival.
- **Diabetic Retinopathy Screening:** Predictive analytics have been used to screen for diabetic retinopathy by examining retinal photos [43]. Using machine learning models, the exact indications of diabetic retinopathy can be identified, permitting prompt treatment to decrease the threat of vision loss. Modern technology has been used in telemedicine,

making diabetic eyes evaluating a lot more easily accessible to people in geographically remote locations.

- **Stroke Risk Assessment:** Medical facilities and healthcare organizations utilize predictive designs to assess the chance of stroke events in individuals [44]. These versions include diverse individual data, such as age, medical history, and lifestyle characteristics, to forecast the chance of a stroke event. This information can assist medical care experts in personalizing preventive measures and restorative treatments.
- **Predicting Disease Outcomes:** Predictive analytics is being employed by scientists and healthcare professionals to predict the evolution of diseases and forecast outcomes for clients. For example, predictive versions can forecast the treatment action and healthcare facility readmission likelihood of people suffering from chronic health problems, such as heart failure or diabetes mellitus.
- **Genomic Medicine:** The application of predictive analytics to genomic information to identify hereditary pens connected with various illnesses is experiencing a growing fad [45]. This information is used by researchers to individualize treatment programs, wherein the choice of optimal medications for cancer individuals is educated by their hereditary profiles.

The aforementioned case studies demonstrate predictive analytics for medical diagnoses. These examples demonstrate how this technology may improve diagnostic precision, intervention time, and patient care. Integrating predictive analytics into healthcare systems is expected to improve patients' well-being and results.

2.7.5 Real-World Examples of Healthcare Institutions Successfully Using Predictive Analytics

Many medical care organizations have successfully utilized predictive analytics to enhance individual outcomes, streamline operations, and minimize costs. For example, [46] offers numerous real-world instances of institutions that have successfully executed this

- **Cleveland Clinic:** The Cleveland Clinic, a renowned clinical establishment, uses predictive analytics to predict and forecast person intakes. Predictive designs are employed to regulate staffing levels effectively, thereby guaranteeing the appropriate allowance of registered nurses, physicians, and other employees to sufficiently resolve client requirements. This not only improves the quality of individual treatments yet also reduces functional costs.

- **Mayo Clinic:** The Mayo Facility uses predictive analytics to identify patients who experience an increased risk of blood poisoning, a clinical illness that poses a considerable threat to an individual's life. Through the examination of electronic health records (EHR) and the continuous tracking of important indications, it is possible to prepare for the event of sepsis and implement prompt interventions, thereby leading to the conservation of human life.
- **Kaiser Permanente:** Kaiser Permanente, a leading care of treatment organization in the US, leverages predictive analytics to recognize individuals that may be much less likely to abide by vaccination routines. By releasing personalized pointers and instructional resources, they have successfully enhanced inoculation rates among these people, resulting in improved wellness.
- **Geisinger Health System:** The Geisinger Wellness System's use of predictive analytics focuses on determining people who are likely to establish chronic problems, such as diabetes mellitus and heart disease. By leveraging data-driven threat analyses, the health and wellness system can supply customized care plans and aggressive treatments to aid in the prevention or effective management of these ailments.
- **Intermountain Healthcare:** Integrating predictive analytics, Intermountain Medical care proactively expects prospective equipment problems inside their clinical facilities. By making predictions regarding the timing of maintenance required for equipment and gadgets, organizations might properly reduce device downtime and ensure the continuous supply of individual treatment.
- **Mount Sinai Health System:** At Mount Sinai, scientists have performed predictive analytics in genome studies to understand hereditary information and identify individuals who might be predisposed to certain illnesses or conditions based on their hereditary profiles. This makes it possible for

healthcare providers to provide personalized and efficient healthcare and therapy methods.

- **Children's Hospital of Philadelphia (CHOP):** The application of predictive analytics by CHOP makes it possible to forecast individual admission patterns in the emergency department. By making precise predictions regarding the arrival of patients, doctors can enhance their source allowance approaches and ensure prompt distribution of therapy to pediatric clients.

The aforementioned instances in real life illustrate the comprehensive applicability of predictive analytics within the medical care market. These applications incorporate enhancements in operational performance, individualized individual care, timely identification of conditions. These organizations utilize information and innovative analytics to optimize their operations and enhance individual outcomes.

2.8 Future Trends and Innovations

The potential effect of predictive analytics in medical diagnostics is the prediction of considerable advancements that will essentially redefine the healthcare landscape. Among the most noteworthy fads over the last few years is the development made in the field of artificial intelligence (AI) and machine learning methods. Artificial intelligence (AI) systems, especially deep-discovering versions, are predictive of boosting their efficiency in evaluating detailed medical data and incorporating radiological photos and genes. This innovation will lead to the advancement of analytical tools with a high level of precision, facilitating the early identification of conditions and the customization of treatment approaches. The increased explainability and interpretability of AI versions will likely lead health care specialists to increasingly rely on them for helping in medical decision-making, thereby improving the overall quality of personal care.

More significant advancements include the unification of predictive analytics with real-time tracking and wearable tools. The increasing frequency of wearable gadgets and constant tracking systems will certainly cause a substantial quantity of individual information to come in real time. The exercise of predictive analytics is expected to have a considerable impact on the interpretation of these data, making it possible to promptly recognize health and wellness concerns and implement preventive measures to mitigate potential consequences. The integration of remote client monitoring, combined with predictive analytics, will promote aggressive medical care interventions and transition towards telehealth and home-based treatment. Moreover, there will certainly be an ongoing focus on promoting individual privacy, fairness, and openness in the production and implementation of predictive versions in healthcare, thus highlighting the moral use of predictive analytics.

2.8.1 The Role of Artificial Intelligence and Deep Learning

The transformational nature of artificial intelligence (AI) and deep discovery in the realm of predictive analytics for medical diagnostics cannot be rejected. Artificial intelligence (AI), particularly deep discovery, has the potential to substantially change the precision, efficiency, and speed of medical diagnosis, inevitably leading to enhanced patient-end results. The following is an evaluation of its substantial duty:

Advanced Pattern Recognition: Deep discovery models succeed in identifying complicated patterns and connections within large and complex datasets. This efficiency holds substantial value in clinical diagnosis, especially in image-based areas, such as radiology and pathology. Convolutional neural networks (CNNs) have revealed remarkable precision in assessing clinical pictures, enabling the discovery of refined abnormalities that might run away from human vision. Timely and precise disease discovery has significant value.

Personalized Medicine: The artificial intelligence capabilities of expert system models significantly lessen the period necessary for analysis treatments and the procedure of making informed judgments. In emergency situations, prompt and precise recognition of a problem is of utmost importance. For example, expert system algorithms can swiftly check a client's medical records and professional information to assess the probability of establishing a particular condition. This enables healthcare professionals to react quickly and intervene as required.

Speed and Efficiency: The expeditious computational capacities of expert system models considerably diminish the duration essential for analysis treatments and the process of making notified judgements. In emergency situations, the timely and precise identification of a condition is of utmost relevance. For example, artificial intelligence formulas can swiftly examine a patient's medical records and clinical information to determine their likelihood of creating a particular disorder. This allows healthcare experts to respond quickly and intervene, as necessary.

Continuous Learning: Deep learning designs have the capacity to discover and constantly improve. Because they are subjected to new information and real-world outcomes, they can improve their predictions, resulting in improved precision over time. This versatility is particularly beneficial in health care, where predictive models can remain up-to-date and in sync with the latest medical advancements, owing to the frequent schedule of brand-new research and information.

2.8.2 Integration with Electronic Health Records and Telemedicine

The assimilation of predictive analytics into electronic health records (EHRs) and telemedicine has been a significant milestone in the medical care sector, enabling much better patient treatment, structured information accessibility, and remote healthcare delivery. EHRs consist of a substantial amount of personal data, including case history, lab outcomes, and treatment information. By applying predictive versions to this information, health care professionals can recognize risky individuals, forecast illness results, and enhance treatment approaches. For example, predictive analytics can notify doctors about people likely to be readmitted, allowing timely interventions and personalized post-discharge treatment.

Additionally, the combination of predictive analytics and EHRs boosts the accuracy and efficiency of medical diagnosis. By leveraging historical patient data, these designs can assist in the early discovery of diseases and supply medical professionals with data-driven insights for notified decision-making. For instance, predictive formulas can recognize people in jeopardy of establishing persistent diseases while additionally assisting radiologists in finding clinical imaging abnormalities, inevitably resulting in earlier interventions and enhanced patient outcomes.

2.8.3 The Potential Impact of Quantum Computing on Medical Diagnosis

Quantum computers show a significant capacity for transformative innovations in medical diagnosis, using the opportunity of substantial ramifications for the area of medical care. Quantum computers have the potential to significantly influence medical diagnoses in numerous crucial domain names.

- **Optimization of Diagnostic Algorithms:** Quantum computing's ability to manage large amounts of information and carry out complicated estimations at exceptional speeds permits the growth of advanced diagnostic formulas. These algorithms can efficiently assess diverse individual data, including genomic, medical, and imaging details, to provide rapid and accurate medical diagnoses. By leveraging quantum computers to resolve integral optimization challenges in medical diagnosis, illness patterns can be determined more quickly, resulting in earlier discovery and better patient outcomes.
- **Drug Discovery and Personalized Medicine:** Quantum computer can accelerate the medicine discovery process by imitating complicated molecular communications that are past the capacity of timeless computers. This allows researchers to recognize possible medication candidates more effectively and to predict their effectiveness for specific clients based on their genetic makeup. Therefore, quantum computing has the potentials to significantly advance customization medication by enabling the customizing of therapies for every client's unique biological features.
- **Complex Data Processing:** Modern clinical diagnosis creates complicated, high-dimensional data that a quantum computer can handle. When assessing the threat of illness via evaluation of genetic details, quantum computer systems can execute computations that are both quick and precise. They can accelerate the analysis of complicated images in the context of medical imaging, which might increase the accuracy of medical diagnoses.
- **Enhanced Security and Privacy:** In medical care, the security and decryption of delicate personal data, which are crucial for preserving confidentiality, can be reinforced with quantum-resistant encryption algorithms. In addition, quantum computer systems have unique leads for the safe and secure exchange of information, which may enable more detailed and protected diagnosis processes based on data while preserving client discretion.

Practical and scalable quantum computing for medical care is still in its infancy, regardless of the fascinating prospective influence of quantum computers on medical diagnosis. It is important to address barriers pertaining to mistake modifications, hardware security, and the availability of quantum sources. Nevertheless, with the recurring innovations in quantum computers, the profound effects they may have on medical diagnosis remain to captivate interest and warrant further examination and development.

2.9 Conclusion

In summary, the execution of predictive analytics in medical diagnosis signifies an essential adjustment in the healthcare field, presenting unrivalled potential customers to enhance individual end results, optimize medical care treatments, and boost overall medical decision-making. With the exercise of innovative analytical methods and the integration of data from different resources, healthcare providers have the capacity to transition from a responsive to a proactive stance. This standard change provides clinicians with the capability to discover diseases in their inceptive phases, dressmaker therapy approaches to specific patients, and oversee person care with higher effectiveness.

Additionally, the incorporation of predictive analytics into the area of clinical diagnosis has the capacity to fundamentally transform the healthcare domain through the resolution of numerous barriers. Using early illness discovery, danger evaluation, and personalized therapy suggestions, healthcare providers can ease the pressure on healthcare systems, optimize the circulation of resources, and ultimately elevate the lifestyle of individuals. In addition, the unification of clinical imaging and photoanalysis into predictive analytics facilitates the accomplishment of more precise and timely diagnoses, thus boosting the effectiveness and accuracy of medical treatments.

Despite the continuous makeover of clinical diagnosis caused by predictive analytics, it continues to be crucial to browse the moral and lawful complexities that concern individual discretion, information defense, and adherence to regulatory requirements. Guaranteeing the prudent application of predictive analytics is critical for maintaining public confidence and optimizing its advantages while reducing potential dangers. In conclusion, the application of predictive analytics in clinical diagnosis is a powerful tool that, when utilized reasonably and ethically, has the potential to significantly boost the stipulation of health care, ushering in a paradigm shift towards proactive and patient-focused practices.

References

1. Hegde, S.K. and Mundada, M.R., Machine Learning-Based Approach for Predictive Analytics in Healthcare, in: *Deep Learning Applications for Cyber-Physical Systems*, pp. 182–206, IGI Global, Hershey, Pennsylvania, 2022.
2. Hassan, M.M., Billah, M.A.M., Rahman, M.M., Zaman, S., Shakil, M.M.H., Angon, J.H., Early predictive analytics in healthcare for diabetes prediction using machine learning approach, in: *2021 12th International Conference on Computing Communication and Networking Technologies (ICCCNT)*, IEEE, pp. 01–05, 2021.
3. Aishvarya, G. and Janarthanan, K., Predictive Medical Image Analytics for Covid-19 Diagnosis, in: *2022 International Conference on Computer Communication and Informatics (ICCCI)*, IEEE, pp. 1–4, 2022.
4. Yahyazadeh, S.R., Izadi, S.S., Inanloo, S.H., Clinical Significance of Intravesical Prostatic Protrusion Index in Patients with Clinical Diagnosis of Benign Prostatic Hyperplasia. *Nephro-Urol. Mon.*, 14, 2, 1–6, 2022.
5. Metsker, O., Magoev, K., Yakovlev, A., Yanishevskiy, S., Kopanitsa, G., Kovalchuk, S., Krzhizhanovskaya, V.V., Identification of risk factors for patients with diabetes: diabetic polyneuropathy case study. *BMC Med. Inf. Decis. Making*, 20, 1, 1–15, 2020.
6. Taquet, M., Geddes, J.R., Husain, M., Luciano, S., Harrison, P.J., 6-month neurological and psychiatric outcomes in 236 379 survivors of COVID-19: a retrospective cohort study using electronic health records. *Lancet Psychiatry*, 8, 5, 416–427, 2021.
7. Jiang, D., Wang, Z., Li, K., Zhang, J., Zhang, S., Predictive Modeling and Control Analysis of Fuel Ratio in Blast Furnace Ironmaking Process Based on Machine Learning. *JOM*, 75, 9, 3975–3984, 2023.
8. Etaati, L. and Etaati, L., Data Wrangling for Predictive Analysis, in: *Machine Learning with Microsoft Technologies: Selecting the Right Architecture and Tools for Your Project*, pp. 75–92, 2019.
9. Xing, R. and Meng, J., Machine Learning for Ischaemic Heart Disease Diagnostic Analysis, in: *2022 IEEE 4th Eurasia Conference on Biomedical Engineering, Healthcare and Sustainability (ECBIOS)*, IEEE, pp. 207–211, 2022.
10. Gorter, R., Fox, J.P., Eekhout, I., Heymans, M.W., Twisk, J.W.R., Missing item responses in latent growth analysis: Item response theory versus classical test theory. *Stat. Methods Med. Res.*, 29, 4, 996–1014, 2020.
11. Omana, J. and Moorthi, M., Predictive analysis and prognostic approach of diabetes prediction with machine learning techniques. *Wirel. Pers. Commun.*, 127, 1–14, 2021.
12. Godara, S. and Singh, R., Evaluation of predictive machine learning techniques as expert systems in medical diagnosis. *Indian J. Sci. Technol.*, 9, 10, 1–14, 2016.

13. Agrawal, R., Predictive analysis of breast cancer using machine learning techniques. *Ing. Solidar.*, 15, 3, 1–23, 2019.
14. Ai, M.T., Sumiati, S., Rosalina, V., Predictive model for heart disease diagnosis based on multinomial logistic regression. *Inf. Technol. Control*, 50, 2, 308–318, 2021.
15. van den Goorbergh, R., van Smeden, M., Timmerman, D., Van Calster, B., The harm of class imbalance corrections for risk prediction models: illustration and simulation using logistic regression. *J. Am. Med. Inf. Assoc.*, 29, 9, 1525–1534, 2022.
16. Huyut, M.T. and Üstündağ, H., Prediction of diagnosis and prognosis of COVID-19 disease by blood gas parameters using decision trees machine learning model: a retrospective observational study. *Med. Gas Res.*, 12, 2, 60, 2022.
17. Benbelkacem, S. and Atmani, B., Random forests for diabetes diagnosis, in: *2019 International Conference on Computer and Information Sciences (ICCIS)*, IEEE, pp. 1–4, 2019.
18. Drosou, K., Georgiou, S., Koukouvinos, C., Stylianou, S., Support vector machines classification on class imbalanced data: a case study with real medical data. *J. Data Sci.*, 12, 4, 727–753, 2014.
19. Djavanshir, G.R., Chen, X., Yang, W., A Review of artificial intelligence's neural networks (deep learning) applications in medical diagnosis and prediction. *IT Prof.*, 23, 3, 58–62, 2021.
20. Fauziyyah, N.A., Abdullah, S., Nurrohmah, S., Reviewing the consistency of the Naïve Bayes Classifier's performance in medical diagnosis and prognosis problems. *AIP Conf. Proc.*, 2242, 1, 030019-1–030019-6, AIP Publishing, 2020.
21. Hong, D., Lv, D., Wu, J., Li, X., Zhao, Q., Lu, X., Li, L., The Influence of Diagnosis Intervention Packet Policy Intervention on Medication Structure and Drug Cost of Elderly Hypertensive Inpatients in China: A Multicenter Interrupted Time-Series Analysis. *Risk Manage. Healthcare Policy*, 16, 2023, 1781–1790, 2023.
22. Fukaguchi, K., Goto, T., Yamamoto, T., Yamagami, H., Experimental Implementation of NSER Mobile App for Efficient Real-Time Sharing of Prehospital Patient Information With Emergency Departments: Interrupted Time-Series Analysis. *JMIR Form. Res.*, 6, 7, e37301, 2022.
23. Khaled, A.Y., Aziz, S.A., Bejo, S.K., Nawi, N.M., Seman, I.A., Onwude, D.I., Early detection of diseases in plant tissue using spectroscopy–applications and limitations. *Appl. Spectrosc. Rev.*, 53, 1, 36–64, 2018.
24. Simpson, L.A., Macdonald, K., Searle, E.F., Shearer, J.A., Dimitrov, D., Foley, D., Morales, E., Shenoy, E.S., Rapid Response for Notification of Monkeypox Exposure, Exposure Risk Assessment and Stratification, and Symptom Monitoring. *Infect. Control Hosp. Epidemiol.*, 43, 8, 2022–06, 2022, medRxiv.
25. Simpson, L.A., Macdonald, K., Searle, E.F., Shearer, J.A., Dimitrov, D., Foley, D., Morales, E., Shenoy, E.S., Development and deployment of tools for rapid

response notification of Monkeypox exposure, exposure risk assessment and stratification, and symptom monitoring. *Infect. Control. Hosp. Epidemiol.*, 43, 8, 963–967, 2022.

26. Pierce, M. and Emsley, R., Estimating and evaluating personalized treatment recommendations from randomized trials with ptr. *Stata J.*, 21, 2, 348–359, 2021.
27. Abdou, M.A., Literature review: Efficient deep neural networks techniques for medical image analysis. *Neural Comput. Appl.*, 34, 8, 5791–5812, 2022.
28. Fonseka, R.D., Natarajan, P., Maharaj, M.M., Mobbs, R.J., Tracking the disease progression of lumbar spinal stenosis using objective gait metrics: a case report. *J. Spine Surg.*, 8, 1, 163, 2022.
29. Abeyasinghe, P.M., Long, J.D., Razi, A., Pustina, D., Paulsen, J.S., Tabrizi, S.J., Poudel, G.R., Georgiou-Karistianis, N., Tracking Huntington's disease progression using motor, functional, cognitive, and imaging markers. *Mov. Disord.*, 36, 10, 2282–2292, 2021.
30. Nilashi, M., Ahmadi, H., Sheikhtaheri, A., Naemi, R., Alotaibi, R., Alarood, A.A., Munshi, A., Rashid, T.A., Zhao, J., Remote tracking of Parkinson's disease progression using ensembles of deep belief network and self-organizing map. *Expert Syst. Appl.*, 159, 1135625, 2020.
31. Si, B., Biecek, P., Burzykowski, T., *Explanatory Model Analysis: Explore, Explain, and Examine Predictive Models*, vol. 324, pp. 486–486, Chapman and Hall/CRC, Boca Raton, FL, 2021, 2022, $99.95, Reference book, ISBN-13: 978-0-3671-3559-1.
32. Ekuma, G., Hier, D.B., Obafemi-Ajayi, T., An Explainable Deep Learning Model for Prediction of Severity of Alzheimer's Disease, in: *2023 IEEE Conference on Computational Intelligence in Bioinformatics and Computational Biology (CIBCB)*, IEEE, pp. 1–8, 2023.
33. ElShawi, R., Sherif, Y., Al-Mallah, M., Sakr, S., Interpretability in healthcare: A comparative study of local machine learning interpretability techniques. *Comput. Intell.*, 37, 4, 1633–1650, 2021.
34. Thiagarajan, J. J., Sattigeri P., Rajan D. and B. Venkatesh, B., Calibrating Healthcare AI: Towards Reliable and Interpretable Deep Predictive Models. No. LLNL-CONF-809718. Lawrence Livermore National Lab.(LLNL), Livermore, CA, United States, 2020.
35. Abràmoff, M.D., Tarver, M.E., Loyo-Berrios, N., Trujillo, S., Char, D., Obermeyer, Z., Eydelman, M.B., Foundational Principles of Ophthalmic Imaging and Algorithmic Interpretation Working Group of the Collaborative Community for Ophthalmic Imaging Foundation, Washington, DC, Maisel, W.H., Considerations for addressing bias in artificial intelligence for health equity. *NPJ Digit. Med.*, 6, 1, 170, 2023.
36. Voigt, P. and Von dem Bussche, A., The eu general data protection regulation (gdpr), in: *A Practical Guide*, 1st Ed., vol. 10, no. 3152676, pp. 10–5555, Springer International Publishing, Cham, 2017.

37. Edemekong, P.F., Annamaraju, P., Haydel, M.J., Health insurance portability and accountability act. In: *StatPearls [Internet]*, Treasure Island (FL), StatPearls Publishing, 2024.
38. Pike, J., Leidner, A.J., Chesson, H., Stoecker, C., Grosse, S.D., Data-related challenges in cost-effectiveness analyses of vaccines. *Appl. Health Econ. Health Policy*, 20, 4, 457–465, 2022.
39. Basatini, F.M. and Chinipardaz, R., Softmax model as generalization upon logistic discrimination suffers from overfitting. *J. Data Sci.*, 12, 4, 563–574, 2014.
40. Branchaud-Charron, F., Atighehchian, P., Rodríguez, P., Abuhamad, G., Lacoste, A., Can active learning preemptively mitigate fairness issues?, 2021, arXiv preprint arXiv:2104.06879.
41. Houssein, E.H., Emam, M.M., Ali, A.A., An optimized deep learning architecture for breast cancer diagnosis based on improved marine predators algorithm. *Neural Comput. Appl.*, 34, 20, 18015–18033, 2022.
42. Kijpaisalratana, N., Sanglertsinlapachai, D., Techaratsami, S., Musikatavorn, K., Saoraya, J., Machine learning algorithms for early sepsis detection in the emergency department: A retrospective study. *Int. J. Med. Inf.*, 160, 1046895, 2022.
43. Grzybowski, A., Brona, P., Lim, G., Ruamviboonsuk, P., Tan, G.S.W., Abramoff, M., Ting, D.S.W., Artificial intelligence for diabetic retinopathy screening: a review. *Eye*, 34, 3, 451–460, 2020.
44. Chicco, D. and Jurman, G., Arterial disease computational prediction and health record feature ranking among patients diagnosed with inflammatory bowel disease. *IEEE Access*, 9, 78648–786575, 2021.
45. Kumuthini, J., Zick, B., Balasopoulou, A., Chalikiopoulou, C., Dandara, C., El-Kamah, G., Findley, L. *et al.*, The clinical utility of polygenic risk scores in genomic medicine practices: a systematic review. *Hum. Genet.*, 141, 11, 1697–1704, 2022.
46. Mandreoli, F., Ferrari, D., Guidetti, V., Motta, F., Missier, P., Real-world data mining meets clinical practice: Research challenges and perspective. *Front. Big Data*, 99, 1–07, 2022.

3

Skin Disease Detection and Classification

M. Aamir Gulzar[1], Salman Iqbal[1], Akhtar Jamil[1]*, Alaa Ali Hameed[2] and Faezeh Soleimani[3]

[1]*Department of Computer Science, National University of Computer and Emerging Sciences, Islamabad, Pakistan*
[2]*Department of Computer Engineering, Istinye University, Istanbul, Turkey*
[3]*Department of Mathematical Sciences, Ball State University, Muncie, IN, USA*

Abstract
Dermatology and dermoscopy pose unique challenges due to their inherent complexity and the high level of expertise required for accurate diagnosis. To address these challenges, this study proposes an automated image-based approach that leverages deep and machine learning to diagnose skin disorders. By harnessing state-of-the-art computational technology, our objective is to overcome the limitations of conventional diagnostic methods. Initially, we explored more straightforward strategies that integrate traditional machine learning models with image processing techniques. This involved employing methods such as Histogram of Oriented Gradients (HOG) and Fast Fourier Transform (FFT) for feature extraction, in conjunction with image enhancement techniques. These extracted features were then utilized to train various traditional machine learning models for the classification of skin disorders. Subsequently, we delved into deep learning and trained models, such as ResNet18, ResNet50, Efficient-Net, and Inception-Net. Compared with human techniques, these deep learning models exhibit superior accuracy and efficiency, signifying the potential for a more reliable and effective diagnostic system. The utilization of cutting-edge technologies revolutionizes dermatological practice by offering a more precise diagnosis and streamlining the diagnostic process.

Keywords: Skin disease classification, feature extraction, image processing, machine learning, deep learning

**Corresponding author*: akhtar.jamil@nu.edu.pk

Neha Sharma, Korhan Cengiz and Prasenjit Chatterjee (eds.) Intelligent Data Analytics for Bioinformatics and Biomedical Systems, (67–92) © 2024 Scrivener Publishing LLC

3.1 Introduction

Skin disease is a prevalent global health concern, and although its prevalence is high, its diagnosis remains a complex task requiring substantial experience. Approximately 24% of the population seek consultation with their general practitioner (GP) for skin conditions within a year. The inconsistency in dermatology education at the undergraduate level underscores the need for trainees to reevaluate their current skills and knowledge in this specific field. Presently, primary care successfully manages approximately 90% of skin diseases, emphasizing the importance of early intervention. Skin diseases significantly affect both the patient's quality of life and skin. The incidence of skin diseases continues to increase, making early diagnosis crucial. GPs play pivotal roles in the early detection of skin diseases [16]. Various efforts have been made worldwide to integrate traditional medicines into dermatological care. Skin diseases often result from environmental factors and other underlying causes. Unfortunately, tools necessary for early disease detection are not readily accessible to all individuals. In this paper, we introduce a method for identifying various types of skin diseases. The user submits an image of the skin condition, which the system then processes using Convolutional Neural Networks (CNNs) for feature extraction [9]. The diagnosis is conducted using machine learning algorithms and softmax image classifiers, making it suitable for a wide range of individuals worldwide [7, 17]. If no disease is detected, the system will yield a negative result. Several classification methods based on convolutional neural networks have been proposed for dermoscopy tests [10, 12], and we will delve further into these in the related work section.

The remainder of this study is organized as follows: In Section 3.2, we delve into existing approaches for skin disease detection. Section 3.3 introduces the dataset and provides examples of various classes of skin diseases. Section 3.4 discusses the machine learning algorithms employed in our research, including decision trees, K-nearest neighbors (KNN), artificial neural networks (ANNs), and ResNet50. We detail their architectural design and training methods and assess their effectiveness in image-classification tasks. We elucidate the operational principles of these algorithms, outline their advantages, and explain their applicability to skin disease classification tasks. Section 3.5 presents the experimental results, where we evaluate different models' performance using the HAM10000 dataset. We compared accuracy, precision, recall, and F1-score across various models, including those trained without feature extraction, Histogram of Oriented Gradients (HOG) feature extraction, and Fast Fourier Transform (FFT) feature extraction. In Section 3.6, we discuss the implications of our findings and underscore the effectiveness of image enhancement, feature extraction, and deep learning techniques in skin disease detection and classification. Section 3.7 outlines potential future directions, including the utilization of larger and more diverse datasets, the integration of these techniques with other technologies, and the exploration of their performance in different populations. Finally, we conclude by summarizing the key findings and emphasizing the pivotal role of advanced techniques in the field of skin disease detection and classification.

3.2 Related Work

Several methods have been developed to automate the identification and classification of skin diseases. These methods primarily rely on imaging technology because recognizing this type of skin disease does not require radiographic imaging technology. They can be implemented using various image processing techniques, including image conversion, equalization, enhancement, and edge detection [13]. One notable method in this category is the cross-correlation feature extraction classification model [3]. This model utilizes both spatial and frequency features for feature selection and ensures visual continuity. The cross-correlation model demonstrated robustness against background fluctuations, rendering it more accurate than alternative approaches. However, this requires the establishment of experimental settings and the acquisition of results in the frequency domain.

Skin diseases can also be categorized based on image color and features using image processing methods. These approaches typically yield higher accuracy than those relying solely on image texture [15]. The most commonly employed techniques for detecting and diagnosing radiographic abnormalities are Artificial Neural Networks (ANN) [8] and Convolutional Neural Networks (CNN) [10–12]. In advanced artificial intelligence applications such as machine learning and deep learning, skin images serve as inputs for disease recognition and classification [4, 6]. The utilization of the CNN method for skin disease diagnosis has shown promising results. However, it is worth noting that the CNN model lacks scaling and rotation invariance [14]. This limitation arises because CNN models are trained on fixed-size input images, preventing them from effectively generalizing to images of varying sizes or rotations. This presents a particular challenge when dealing with images captured by mobile devices or digital cameras because such images often exhibit variations in size and rotation. In a study by the authors [14], a deep learning model designed for skin disease classification was introduced. This model is built upon the MobileNet V2 architecture, which is known for its lightweight and efficient nature, making it suitable for deployment on mobile devices. In addition, the model is enhanced with an LSTM layer, which aids in enhancing the model accuracy by capturing long-term dependencies in the data. The authors evaluated their model using the extensive HAM10000 dataset, which comprises a substantial collection of skin images. The model successfully categorized the lesion into one of seven categories, achieving an accuracy rate of 85%, which is comparable to that of other state-of-the-art deep learning models designed for skin disease classification. In another study by the authors [1], they proposed a deep learning method for reliable early stage diagnosis of melanoma, distinguishing between malignant, superficial spreading, and nodular melanoma types. This differentiation enables early diagnosis of the condition, facilitating prompt isolation and the necessary therapy to prevent further infection transmission. The authors conducted a comparative analysis of their method with state-of-the-art techniques, including K-nearest Neighbors, Support Vector Machines, and Decision Trees. They demonstrated that their method surpassed the state-of-the-art approaches in terms of diagnostic accuracy. Another proposed technique for skin disease classification and detection involves the use of image processing and machine learning techniques [2]. Initially, image preprocessing was employed to enhance the image quality, followed by image segmentation to identify the region of interest. Subsequently, features were extracted from the images, which were then utilized to train a machine learning model to classify the images into distinct skin disease categories. The authors evaluated their model using a dataset of skin images and achieved an impressive accuracy rate of 98.8%. However, it is important to note that this dataset comprises only six classes of skin disease. This method begins by filtering skin photographs to eliminate unwanted noise, followed by image enhancement to improve overall image quality. Advanced techniques such as convolutional neural networks (CNNs) are used for feature extraction, and image classification is performed using the softmax classifier algorithm, ultimately generating a diagnostic report as the output [5]. The authors evaluated their approach on a dataset containing images of six prevalent skin diseases and achieved an accuracy of 94.6%.

3.3 Data

The HAM10000 dataset is a comprehensive collection of dermatoscopic images that depict pigmented skin lesions. This dataset comprises a total

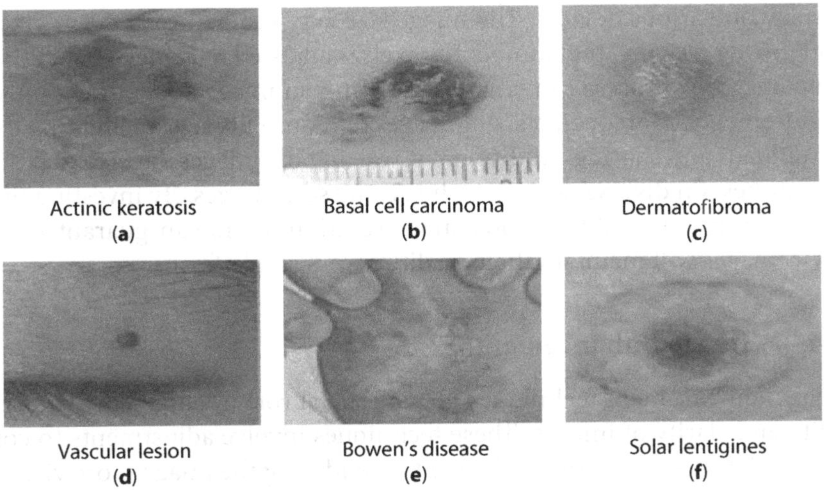

Figure 3.1 Dataset images.

of 10,015 images, each falling into one of 12 distinct skin lesion classes, including actinic keratosis (ak), basal cell carcinoma (bcc), dermatofibroma, hemangioma, intraepithelial carcinoma, lentigo, melanoma, nevus, pyogenic granuloma, squamous cell carcinoma (scc), seborrheic keratosis (sebk), and wart. This is a large and diverse dataset that enables the development of more accurate and robust models. It is worth noting that the dataset exhibited class imbalance, with certain classes being overrepresented. This imbalance can pose challenges when training models to classify classes with equal precision. In our study, we opted to work with seven selected classes, utilizing approximately 4,000 instances from the dataset. These instances were then divided in an 80:20 ratio for training and testing purposes. Some types of disease images in the dataset are shown in Figure 3.1.

3.4 Methodology

3.4.1 Data Pre-Processing

The image provided as an input may not necessarily have the required dimensions for the algorithm. Therefore, it underwent a resizing process to attain a standardized size before being fed into the machine learning model. Image resizing plays a significant role in the digital imaging process, enabling users to tailor the size and resolution of the image for an optimal display on various devices. The image size is typically measured in pixels, and during resizing, the number of pixels is adjusted to achieve the desired outcome. This process can enlarge or shrink an image depending on user requirements. Moreover, resizing serves to reduce file size, facilitating easier uploads and sharing. Additionally, resizing the images ensures that they appear best on diverse devices with varying screen sizes. By investing time in adjusting image dimensions and resolution, users can guarantee that their images will maintain their quality across all platforms.

3.4.2 Image Enhancement

Image-enhancement techniques play a crucial role in enhancing the visibility and clarity of images. These techniques involve adjustments to contrast, brightness, and color, all aimed at rendering the image more visually appealing. By employing these methods, finer details within an image can be accentuated and clarified, thereby serving a multitude of purposes. For instance, in the realm of medical imaging, image enhancement techniques have proven invaluable in assisting doctors in diagnosing diseases more accurately. Similarly, in security applications, these techniques are instrumental in facilitating the easier identification of objects. Before feeding the data into our models, we applied a set of image-enhancement techniques. Some of the image enhancement techniques that we employed are outlined below:

Sharpening

Unsharp masking is a technique employed to enhance the sharpness of an image by accentuating the contrast between neighboring pixels. This process entails subtracting a blurred and desaturated version of the original image and emphasizing edges and other intricate details. This technique is particularly advantageous in the realm of digital image editing, offering a more precise and targeted approach for sharpening. Moreover, unsharp masking is a relatively straightforward procedure that can be accomplished by adjusting a few key parameters such as the blur radius and degree of sharpening. These minor parameter adjustments can yield subtle effects and provide a spectrum of sharpening options. In our dataset image processing, we applied an unsharp masking technique for sharpening.

Blurring

The median blurring technique is a potent image-processing method employed to diminish noise visibility or introduce a controlled level of blur into an image. This technique involves substituting each pixel in an image with the median value derived from its neighboring pixels. Its primary use revolves around diminishing the image contrast, thereby facilitating the identification of features and patterns. Additionally, it serves the purpose of noise reduction by imparting a smoother and more natural appearance to the image. The median blurring technique offers an effective means of blurring an image, while minimally affecting its overall composition. Often, the results obtained using this technique are more aesthetically pleasing than those obtained using other methods, such as Gaussian blurring. In our image-processing workflow, we initially ved our images to grayscale and subsequently applied Gaussian blurring.

Smoothing
Gaussian blurring is a popular method used for smoothing digital images. This technique operates on the principle of convolution, which involves replacing each pixel in an image with a weighted average of its neighboring pixels. This operation results in a blurred image where the sharp edges and intricate details of the original image are softened. Gaussian blurring is a well-established method that is widely employed in numerous image-processing applications. It offers a straightforward approach for enhancing the overall visual quality of an image while mitigating the presence of noise. Moreover, Gaussian blurring is useful for reducing the computational complexity of more advanced image-processing techniques.

Thresholding
Thresholding is an image processing technique employed to transform a grayscale image into a binary image. Among the various methods for thresholding images, binary thresholding is the most commonly used. This entails assigning a threshold value to each pixel in the image. Pixels with values above the threshold receive a value of 1, whereas those with values below the threshold are assigned a value of 0. This technique is valuable for image segmentation, which allows the isolation of objects within an image, and for the extraction of various features, including edges and intricate details.

3.4.3 Feature Extraction

We employed various algorithms for feature extraction from our dataset, some of which are outlined below:

Histogram of Oriented Gradients (HOG)
The Histogram of Oriented Gradients (HOG) feature extractor is an effective tool for object detection and image recognition. It extracts a set of

features from an image, including gradients, edges, and color information, and subsequently constructs a histogram based on these features. Through analysis of this histogram, the HOG feature extractor can identify the presence of objects within an image, rendering it an indispensable tool for tasks such as object detection and image recognition.

BRIEF

A BRIEF Feature Extractor is a type of machine learning algorithm employed to extract features from data. Its primary purpose is to discern patterns within the data, thereby diminishing the volume of data that require processing. This algorithm functions by isolating crucial characteristics from the data, such as size, shape, and texture. Once these features are extracted, they can be used to construct models capable of identifying patterns within a dataset. This, in turn, streamlines data processing, making data analysis and interpretation manageable. We attempted to implement the BRIEF feature extractor to extract the features from our dataset. However, it yielded null results and failed to extract features from our data. Consequently, we opted not to include these results in the *Results* section.

Fast Fourier Transform (FFT)

Fast Fourier Transform (FFT) is an algorithm used for feature extraction that transforms a signal from the time domain into the frequency domain. This algorithm is widely used in signal-processing applications due to its computational efficiency and capacity for precise feature extraction. This is accomplished by employing a frequency-domain technique to break down a signal into its constituent sine and cosine components. This transformation into the frequency domain enables the identification of crucial features such as noise levels, frequency bands, and other patterns. FFT is a powerful tool for feature extraction and is frequently applied in audio- and image-processing applications. We implemented FFT to extract features from our dataset and subsequently fed these features into machine learning models. However, in our case, there were no improvements in the results.

3.4.4 Machine Learning Algorithm Used

We employed various machine learning models during the training of our classifier to enhance the classification performance. Given our dataset with 12 distinct classes, each appropriately labeled, our approach incorporates both traditional supervised machine learning algorithms and deep-learning models. Below, you will find detailed descriptions and explanations of the models that we utilized:

Logistic Regression

Logistic regression is a pivotal machine learning algorithm that is versatile enough to tackle various tasks, including binary classification, probability estimation, and medical diagnosis. It operates as a supervised learning algorithm, that establishes a model that captures the connection between one or more independent variables and a categorical dependent variable. At its core, this algorithm relies on a logistic function, a sigmoid function that yields probability values ranging from 0 to 1. The model's training objective was to predict the probability of the dependent variable belonging to a particular class. Employing a logistic regression model enabled us to make predictions regarding the likelihood of a specific outcome based on the provided input. Logistic regression has widespread utility across multiple domains, including finance, medicine, marketing, and numerous others. It serves as a vital tool for forecasting the probability of an event occurring and constitutes a pivotal component of predictive analytics.

$$y = \frac{\exp(\beta_0 + \beta_1 \text{F1} + \beta_2 \text{F2} + \cdots + \beta_{12} \text{F3})}{1 + \exp(\beta_0 + \beta_1 \text{F1} + \beta_2 \text{F2} + \cdots + \beta_{12} \text{F3})} \tag{3.1}$$

for the value of y is $y > 0.5 == 1$ and $y < 0.5 == 0$.

Optimal tune able parameters found for Logistic Regression using GridSearchCV are Best Penalty: l2 and Best C: 1.0.

Support Vector Machines (SVM)

Support Vector Machines (SVMs) represent a popular supervised learning algorithm suitable for both classification and regression tasks. The primary objective of the SVM algorithm is to identify a hyperplane within a high-dimensional space that effectively separates the distinct classes. Among the data points, those closest to this hyperplane are referred to as support vectors and have the most substantial influence on their placement. SVMs achieve this separation by maximizing the margin, i.e., the distance between the hyperplane and the support vectors. This margin optimization helps mitigate overfitting, while enhancing the model's generalization capability. An inherent advantage of SVMs is their capacity to handle high-dimensional and nonlinear data, rendering them a versatile tool for a wide array of applications. Furthermore, the optimization problem addressed by SVMs yields a global solution. This property results in the model's reduced sensitivity to initial conditions and local minima, setting SVMs apart from the other algorithms. In summary, SVMs constitute an effective and widely adopted machine learning tool that consistently shows robust performance across a variety of tasks.

First, let us consider a training set comprising n points $\{\mathbf{x}_i, y_i\} i = 1,\ldots,n$, where $y_i \in \{-1,1\}$ signifies the class label of point x_i. For ease of representation, we designate the two classes as $y_i = 1$ and $y_i = -1$. Our goal is to discover a classifier, effectively a hyperplane, capable of mapping the x_i points into a higher-dimensional space, facilitating the division of points belonging to two different classes. In addition, we aim to maximize the margin of this hyperplane, ensuring the greatest separation distance between the hyperplane and the nearest points from both classes. In linear cases, the hyperplane can be written as:

$$\mathbf{x}_i\mathbf{w} + b = 0 \tag{3.2}$$

Our objective is to discover two parallel hyperplanes capable of effectively separating data while maximizing the distance between them. This distance can be described as follows:

$$\mathbf{x}_i\mathbf{w} + b = +1 \tag{3.3}$$

$$\mathbf{x}_i\mathbf{w} + b = -1 \tag{3.4}$$

It is not challenging to demonstrate that the distance between these two hyperplanes is $\frac{2}{||w||}$:

$$d_+ + d_- = \frac{|1-b|}{||w||} + \frac{|-1-b|}{||w||} = \frac{2}{||w||} \tag{3.5}$$

which means we want to minimize $||w||$ since it is always positive. Besides, we want for every $i \in (1,n)$, x_i and y_i follows the constraints:

$$\mathbf{x}_i\mathbf{w} + b \geq +1, \qquad y_i = +1 \tag{3.6}$$

$$\mathbf{x}_i\mathbf{w} + b \leq -1, \qquad y_i = -1 \tag{3.7}$$

$$y_i(\mathbf{x}_i\mathbf{w}+b)-1\geq 0, \quad \forall i \tag{3.8}$$

Optimal tune able parameters found for SVM using GridSearchCV are 'C': 10, 'gamma': 1 and 'kernel': 'rbf.'

Decision Tree

Decision trees are widely acclaimed and frequently employed machine learning algorithms suitable for both classification and regression tasks. This algorithm operates by constructing a tree-like model of decisions based on input data. At each internal node of the tree, the algorithm splits the data based on a feature value and guides the data points down to the branches of the tree. The terminal nodes of the tree, referred to as leaf nodes, contain either the predicted class label or the predicted value for the regression tasks. One of the advantages of decision trees is their ease of interpretation and comprehensibility, rendering them a top choice for tasks in which interpretability holds significance. Furthermore, decision trees are sufficiently versatile to handle both categorical and numerical data and exhibit resistance to noise. This robustness positions decision trees as reliable algorithms suited for a broad spectrum of applications. In summary, decision trees constitute a valuable and efficient machine learning tool capable of addressing a variety of problems.

To construct a decision tree, we must calculate two types of entropy using frequency tables, as outlined below:

a) Entropy using the frequency table of one attribute:

$$E(S)=\sum_{c=1}^{M}-P_i\log_2(p_i) \tag{3.9}$$

b) Entropy using the frequency table of two attributes.

$$E(X,T)=\sum_{c=1}^{M}-P(C)\log_2\left(E(c)\right) \tag{3.10}$$

Information gain hinges on the reduction in entropy that occurs following the partitioning of a dataset based on an attribute. The process of constructing a decision tree involves identifying an attribute that yields the greatest information gain, thereby creating the most homogenous branches.

$$Gain(T,X) = Entropy(S) - Entropy(T,X) \tag{3.11}$$

We selected the attribute with the highest information gain as the decision node, partitioned the dataset into its respective branches, and then iterated through the same process for each branch.

K-Nearest Neighbor (KNN)

The K-nearest neighbor (KNN) algorithm is a simple yet highly effective approach for both classification and regression tasks. The algorithm operates by storing all available data and subsequently making predictions for a new data point's class label or value based on the class labels or values of the stored data points. Specifically, the algorithm identifies the 'k' number of data points that are closest to the new data point and then predicts the class label or value by considering the majority among these neighbors. One of the principal advantages of the KNN algorithm is its simplicity of implementation and minimal training time requirement, rendering it a rapid and efficient algorithm that is suitable for a wide range of applications. Additionally, KNN exhibits flexibility, accommodating both categorical and numerical data, as well as addressing multiclass problems. In summary, the KNN algorithm represents a valuable and effective machine-learning tool applicable to a diverse array of problem-solving scenarios.

To implement the KNN algorithm, the initial step involved calculating the distances between the input data point and other points in our training dataset. Let us assume that x denotes a point with coordinates $(x_1, x_2, \ldots, x_p)$ and y is a point with coordinates $(y_1, y_2, \ldots, y_p)$. Then, the distance between these two points is:

$$d(x,y) = \sqrt{\sum_{i=1}^{p} (x_i - y_i)^2} \tag{3.12}$$

For a given positive integer k, the k-nearest neighbors algorithm examines the k observations closest to a test observation x_0 and estimates the conditional probability that it belongs to class 'j' using the following formula:

$$Pr(Y = j|X = x_0) = \frac{1}{k}\sum_{i\in\mathcal{N}_0} I(y_i = j) \tag{3.13}$$

Optimal tune able parameters found for KNN using GridSearchCV are 'metric': 'Manhattan,' 'neighbors': 11 and 'weights': 'distance.'

Artificial Neural Networks (ANNs)

Artificial Neural Networks (ANNs) represent a category of machine learning algorithms inspired by the structure and function of the human brain. ANNs consist of interconnected nodes, referred to as artificial neurons, that process and transmit information. These nodes are organized into layers, with the input layer receiving the input data, and the output layer generating the predicted output. One or more hidden layers are situated between the input and output layers, housing the majority of artificial neurons. The artificial neurons within the hidden layers process the input data and relay the processed information to the output layer. ANNs undergo training using various techniques, such as backpropagation, which adjusts the weights of connections between artificial neurons to minimize the error between the predicted and true outputs. One of the pivotal advantages of ANNs is their capacity to model intricate relationships and patterns in data, rendering them a potent tool across a wide spectrum of applications. Furthermore, ANNs exhibit flexibility, handle both categorical and numerical data, and tackle multi-class problems. In summary, ANNs serve as valuable and efficient machine learning tools for addressing a myriad of problems.

First calculate Y using random weights

$$Y = w_0 + w_1\text{F}1 + w_2\text{F}2 + \cdots + w_n\text{Fn} \tag{3.14}$$

Then calculate the error.

$$Err = (y - \bar{y})^2 \tag{3.15}$$

Then back-propagate the error to update the weights.

$$\frac{dE}{dw_{ij}} = \frac{dE}{dy_j}\frac{dy_j}{dw_{ij}} = \frac{dE}{dy_j}\frac{dy_j}{d(\sum_{k=1}^{n} w_{kj}x_k)}\frac{d(\sum_{k=1}^{n} w_{kj}x_k)}{dw_{ij}}$$
$$= \frac{dE}{dy_j}\frac{dy_j}{d(\sum_{k=1}^{n} w_{kj}x_k)}x_i = \frac{dE}{dy_j}y_j\left(1-y_j\right)x_i \tag{3.16}$$

Then update the weights

$$w_i = w_i + \alpha * \frac{\partial E}{\partial w_i} \tag{3.17}$$

Resenet50

The ResNet50 algorithm is a deep neural network architecture specifically designed for object recognition and image classification tasks. It is as one of the most successful deep learning models in the realm of computer vision and has been widely adopted for various image classification tasks. The ResNet50 model was built based on the ResNet architecture initially developed by Microsoft Research in 2015. This algorithm functions by employing a series of convolutional layers to extract essential features from input images, and subsequently utilizes a series of fully connected layers for image classification, as shown in Figure 3.2. Notably, the ResNet50 model

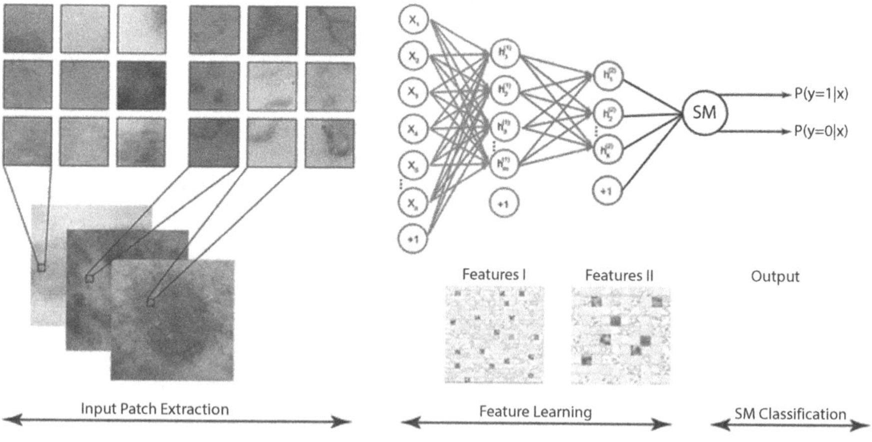

Figure 3.2 Classification using softmax.

demonstrated remarkable success in image recognition tasks, achieving state-of-the-art results, particularly on datasets such as ImageNet. The ResNet50 algorithm has emerged as a pivotal tool in computer vision applications, and has been extensively used in diverse fields, including autonomous vehicles, medical imaging, and natural language processing. In our application, we leverage the ResNet50 algorithm. ResNet-50 is a pre-trained deep convolutional neural network with 50 layers. This network underwent training on a dataset exceeding 1 million images from the ImageNet dataset, enabling it to classify over 1,000 classes. It operates on input images with a size of 224 × 224 pixels. ResNet50 employs transfer learning to extract features from the input images and further refines its learning based on these features.

3.5 Results

This section presents experimental results. First, we provide a description of the experimental setup, followed by an overview of the data preprocessing steps. Subsequently, we delve into the discussion of the evaluation metrics employed in our experiments and finally, present the classification results.

3.5.1 Experimental Setup

We conducted experiments using the HAM10000 dataset, which comprises 4,000 dermatoscopic images belonging to seven distinct skin lesion classes. These images were randomly divided into three sets: a training (70%), validation (15%), and test (15%).

Programming Language and Libraries:
This research work utilized Python as the primary programming language due to its versatility and extensive library ecosystem, making it an ideal choice for tasks involving image processing and deep learning. An overview of the key libraries employed is as follows:

- **NumPy:** This fundamental library provides essential support for numerical operations, enabling efficient handling of multidimensional arrays and matrices. It plays a pivotal role in data pre-processing and manipulation.
- **Python Imaging Library (PIL):** PIL was employed for various image processing tasks, including reading and

comprehending images. This library offers a comprehensive set of tools to open, manipulate, and save images in various formats.

- **OpenCV:** Leveraging the capabilities of OpenCV, a powerful computer vision library, we performed advanced image analysis. OpenCV facilitates tasks such as image enhancement (sharpening and smoothing), feature extraction, and other critical image-processing techniques essential for dermoscopy analysis.
- **Scikit-learn and sklearn.metrics:** For tasks related to data management and machine learning, we relied on scikit-learn. This library provides an extensive range of tools for tasks, such as data splitting, preprocessing, and model evaluation. The sklearn.metrics module offers a variety of metrics for assessing model performance.
- **Matplotlib and Seaborn:** To create clear and informative visual representations of our results, we used visualization libraries. Matplotlib offers a wide array of plotting functions, whereas Seaborn provides a high-level interface for generating visually appealing statistical graphics.
- **PyTorch:** PyTorch serves as the core framework for constructing and training deep learning models. Specifically, models such as ResNet 18 and 50 were implemented using PyTorch's flexible and efficient deep-learning capabilities.

Hardware Configuration:

The study was conducted on a local machine with specific hardware configurations:

- **GPU:** The machine is equipped with a Radeon GPU, providing substantial computational power. GPU acceleration significantly expedited the training of deep learning models, which is a crucial factor for handling large datasets and complex neural network architectures.
- **RAM:** The system boasts 16 GB of RAM, ensuring abundant memory for efficient data processing and model training.
- **Storage:** A 512 GB SSD was utilized, offering fast read/write speeds. This is crucial for swift data access, particularly when dealing with large image datasets.

3.5.2 Data Preprocessing, Feature Extraction, and Model Selection

This section discusses the intricacies of data preprocessing, which is a pivotal foundation for an accurate skin condition diagnosis. It commences with the meticulous application of image-enhancement techniques aimed at enhancing the quality and information content of the dataset. Subsequently, the process involved data extraction. Subsequently, we employ sophisticated image processing methods to extract features, with particular emphasis on techniques such as the Histogram of Oriented Gradients (HOG), which is renowned for its effectiveness in capturing texture and shape information. These extracted attributes served as the bedrock for subsequent machine learning analyses. An essential step involves the application of multiple fundamental machine learning algorithms to the extracted features. This initial effort allowed us to assess the effectiveness of traditional approaches in addressing the complexity of dermatological diagnoses. To fine-tune our models, we leveraged GridSearchCV, a potent hyperparameter optimization technique, to exhaustively search for parameter combinations and determine the optimal configuration for our machine learning algorithms. The optimal values of the parameters for different machine learning models are presented in Table 3.1. This not only enhances the predictive capabilities of the models, but also refines them. In our experiments, we employed the following machine learning models:

- Support vector machines (SVMs)
- Logistic Regression (LR)
- Random forests
- K-Neighbors Classifier (KNN)
- Artificial Neural Network (ANN)

In cases where the results fail to meet our stringent standards, we shift our focus towards prioritizing deep-learning models. This transition represents a move into a domain of analysis that is more intricate and nuanced. We conducted a comparative investigation by testing two to three distinct deep-learning architectures, each customized for the extraction of latent features from dermoscopic images. This multifaceted approach enabled us to uncover the subtleties and complexities that may be pivotal for achieving diagnostic precision. The chosen deep learning models were trained using PyTorch. Depending on the experimental results, we chose either Adam or RMSprop as the optimizer, with categorical cross-entropy chosen

Table 3.1 Optimal parameter selection.

Model	Parameter	Reference range	Optimal value
SVM	C	0.1–100	10
	Kernel	'linear,' 'poly,' 'rbf'	rbf
	Gamma	0.0001–1	1
Logistic Regression	Penality	l1,l2	l2
	C	0–10	1
RandomForestClassifier	Max depth	80,90,100,110	90
	Max Features	2,3	3
	No. of estimators	100,200,300,1,000	300
K-NeighborsClassifier	No. of Neighbors	3,5,11,19	11
	Weights	'Uniform,' 'Distance'	Distance
	Metric	'Euclidean,' 'Manhattan'	Manhattan
ANN	Solver	'lbfgs,' 'sgd,' 'adam'	lbfgs
	Alpha	0.01–0.0000001	1e–5

as the loss function. Below, we outline the deep learning models utilized in our experiments:

- Inception Net
- ResNet-18
- ResNet-50
- Efficient-Net

By meticulously traversing this exhaustive path of data preprocessing, feature extraction, and model selection, we can equip ourselves with a diverse array of techniques. This ensured that our diagnostic system was well prepared to handle the intricate nuances of dermatological images. This approach, characterized by its adaptability and rigor, lays the foundation for the robust results and reliable insights presented in subsequent sections. The experimental design provides a strong foundation for research on dermoscopy and dermatology. The combination of powerful programming languages, specialized libraries, and high-performance hardware facilitates efficient image processing and analysis. The utilization of deep learning models, such as Inception-Net, ResNet-50, and Efficient-Net, has yielded promising results in automating skin condition diagnoses, with the potential to revolutionize dermatological practice. A comprehensive approach and meticulous experimental design enhanced the dependability and credibility of the research findings.

3.5.3 Evaluation Metrics

We employed the 'ClassificationReport' function from the 'sklearn.metrics' module to conduct a comprehensive analysis of the models' performance. This function provides a detailed breakdown of key metrics, including accuracy, precision, recall, and F1-score, for each class within our dataset. Analyzing these metrics individually allowed us to gain insights into the models' ability to accurately identify various skin conditions. Furthermore, to gain a comprehensive perspective on model performance, we calculated both macro and weighted averages. The macro average assigns equal weight to each class, providing an objective measure of the overall model efficacy across various skin diseases. In contrast, the weighted average considers class imbalance by assigning more weight to classes with more instances. This ensured that our evaluation process was robust and representative of real-world scenarios. Our primary objective was to achieve high accuracy and precision in our diagnostic system, thereby ensuring reliable and dependable outcomes. Through a systematic evaluation of both basic machine learning and deep learning models, we were able to discern their respective strengths and weaknesses. This thorough evaluation process facilitated selection of the most suitable models for our dermatological diagnostic system. All the aforementioned models were trained and tested using the same dataset to enable a fair comparison of their performance. To assess their performance, we calculated their accuracy, precision, recall, and F1-score as performance metrics. *Accuracy* represents the ratio of correctly identified data samples to the total number of samples. This is calculated as follows:

$$Accuracy = \frac{TP + TN}{TP + FP + TN + FN} \tag{3.18}$$

where TP is True Positive, TN is True Negative, FP is False Positive, and FN is False Negative. *Precision* measures the number of correctly identified data samples divided by the sum of correctly identified positive samples and falsely identified positive samples. Ideally, in a good classifier, precision should be high. This is calculated as follows:

$$Precision = \frac{TP}{TP + FP} \tag{3.19}$$

Recall is the ratio of correctly identified positive samples to the sum of correctly identified positive samples and falsely identified negative samples. Recall is calculated as follows:

$$Recall = \frac{TP}{TP + FN} \tag{3.20}$$

F1-Score considers both the precision and recall. F1-Score is calculated as

$$F1 = 2 * \frac{Precision * Recall}{Precision + Recall} \tag{3.21}$$

We compared these scores of the chosen machine learning models, as shown in Table 3.2.

3.5.4 Classification and Outcomes

In this section, we present a comprehensive evaluation of skin disease classification using a diverse range of machine learning and deep learning models. Each phase was meticulously designed to ensure optimal performance, with hyperparameter fine-tuning enabling the models to reach their full potential. We employed cutting-edge feature extraction techniques, including Histogram of Oriented Gradients (HOG) and Fast Fourier Transform (FFT), to enhance discriminative capabilities. Additionally, we implemented image enhancement techniques such as filtering and sharpening to improve the quality of both our dataset and the inputs to our models. Initially, our investigation focused on the effectiveness of FFT and HOG feature extraction in combination with various machine-learning models. This comparative analysis revealed the superior performance of the HOG in capturing crucial patterns indicative of various skin conditions. Guided by this realization, we continued our experiments with a focus on the HOG-based characteristics. The results of both FFT and HOG feature extraction techniques are listed in Tables 3.2 and 3.3.

Incorporating image enhancement techniques yielded a significant improvement in classification accuracy, underscoring the substantial impact of pre-processing steps on model performance, as shown in Table 3.4. This progress prompted us to venture into deep learning.

Table 3.2 Results with FFT feature extraction technique.

Model	Accuracy	Precision	Recall	F1-score
SVM	0.29	0.24	0.28	0.25
Logistic Regression	0.21	0.19	0.23	0.23
Random Forest	0.20	0.16	0.21	0.19
KNN	0.23	0.20	0.24	0.22
ANN	0.23	0.7	0.23	0.10

Table 3.3 Results with HOG feature extraction technique.

Model	Accuracy	Precision	Recall	F1-score
SVM	0.42	0.45	0.42	0.40
Logistic Regression	0.42	0.44	0.42	0.42
Random Forest	0.32	0.31	0.42	0.26
KNN	0.32	0.30	0.32	0.30
ANN	0.27	0.16	0.33	0.19

Table 3.4 Results with HOG feature extraction technique and image enhancement.

Model	Accuracy	Precision	Recall	F1-score
SVM	0.69	0.61	0.69	0.62
Logistic Regression	0.68	0.59	0.68	0.61
Random Forest	0.66	0.49	0.66	0.54
KNN	0.68	0.58	0.68	0.60
ANN	0.62	0.52	0.62	0.55

After introducing Inception Net, ResNet-18, ResNet-50, and Efficient-Net into our toolkit, we embarked on a journey of unprecedented complexity. These architectures showed an exceptional ability to autonomously learn intricate hierarchies of features, solidifying their positions as formidable instruments for dermatoscopic image analysis. Among them, Efficient-Net emerged as the top performer, demonstrating unparalleled proficiency, as shown in Table 3.5.

As this section draws to a close, it is essential to note that our chosen path, commencing with feature extraction, dataset augmentation, and culminating in deep learning, was a deliberate progression toward refining our diagnostic system. The forthcoming tables of results and visualizations, including confusion matrices in Figure 3.3, training/testing errors, and more, illustrate the transformative potential of this methodology. This section serves as a testament to the effectiveness of careful experimentation, showcasing the journey that has brought us to the cusp of a revolutionary diagnostic approach to dermatology.

To succinctly present the outcomes of our experiments, we included tables displaying the performance of each model. These tables summarize the key metrics, enabling straightforward comparisons, and highlighting the strengths of each approach. In addition, we generated confusion matrices to provide a comprehensive breakdown of the model predictions for each class. This visual aid aids in identifying specific areas of strength and potential areas for improvement. In conclusion, the culmination of our exhaustive evaluation process, which encompasses both conventional machine learning techniques and cutting-edge deep learning models, has yielded a refined and dependable dermatological diagnostic system poised to revolutionize clinical practice. Our classification framework is robust and reliable, owing to the meticulous consideration of the training epochs, error analysis, and confusion metrics.

Table 3.5 Results of deep-learning models.

Model	**Accuracy**	**Precision**	**Recall**	**F1-score**
Inception-Net	0.60	0.62	0.60	0.60
ResNet-18	0.65	0.70	0.65	0.66
ResNet-50	0.70	0.70	0.70	0.68
Efficient-Net	0.85	0.87	0.85	0.85

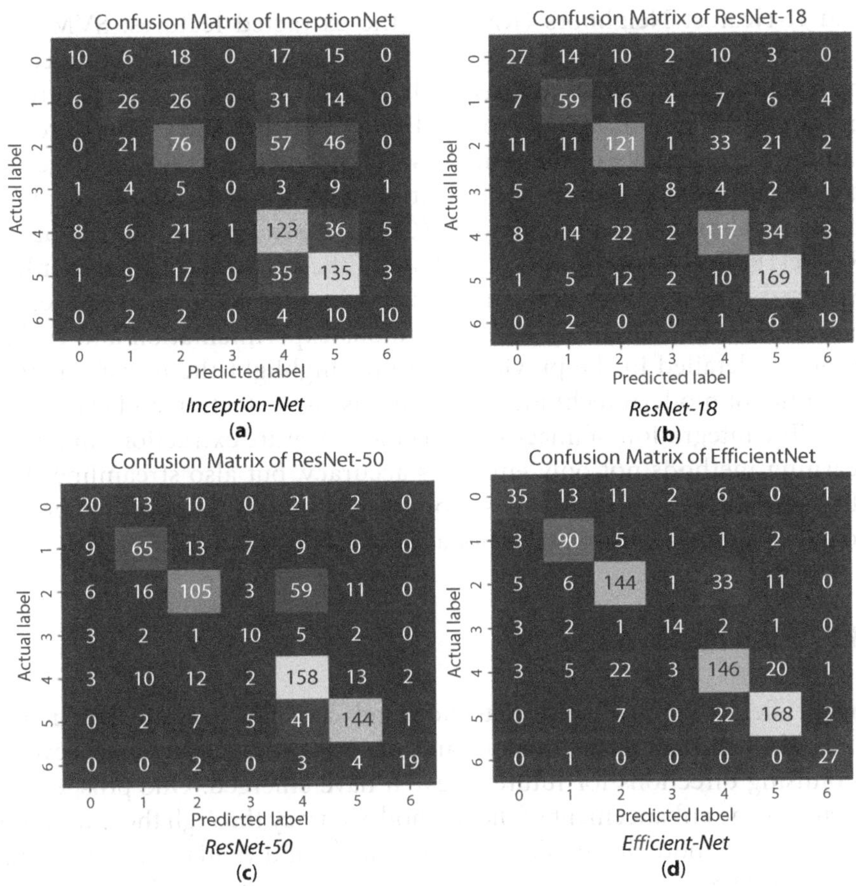

Figure 3.3 Confusion metrics.

3.6 Conclusion

In this study, we aimed to enhance the skin disease detection and classification capabilities in dermoscopy and dermatology. We meticulously refined our dataset using image-enhancement techniques, recognizing the importance of high-quality data for accurate disease classification. We explored a range of feature extraction methods, including Fast Fourier Transform (FFT) and Histogram of Oriented Gradients (HOG). Comparative analysis revealed HOG's superiority in capturing vital patterns within dermatoscopic images, laying the foundation for subsequent experiments. We initially applied conventional machine learning models such as SVM, Random Forest, Logistic Regression, and K-Nearest Neighbors (KNN) to the extracted features. SVM and Logistic Regression have emerged as frontrunners, demonstrating commendable accuracy in skin disease classification. The iterative nature of our approach emphasizes the pivotal role of feature extraction in refining the performance of these models. Acknowledging the challenges of manual feature extraction, we transitioned to deep learning by deploying Convolutional Neural Network (CNN)-based models. We evaluated ResNet18, ResNet50, Inception-Net, and Efficient-Net. Efficient-Net has emerged as a standout performer, surpassing its counterparts in terms of accuracy and efficiency. Our meticulous experimentation and evaluation, as detailed in the previous sections, highlight the transformative potential of modern techniques for skin disease detection and classification. The integration of image enhancement, feature extraction, and deep learning methods not only enhances accuracy, but also streamlines the diagnostic process and provides promising invaluable support to dermatologists and healthcare professionals.

3.7 Future Work

In the field of skin disease detection and classification utilizing image enhancement, feature extraction, and deep learning techniques, several promising directions for future research have emerged. One prospective avenue is the enhancement of the method accuracy through the utilization of larger and more diverse datasets for training and validation. Expanding the scope of data can potentially lead to more precise results. Another fruitful area of investigation could involve exploring the integration of these techniques with other technologies such as wearable devices or telemedicine platforms. This integration has the potential to enhance the accessibility and convenience of skin disease detection and treatment, thereby improving patient care. Furthermore, it would be valuable to delve into the application of these techniques in different populations, such as children or older adults. Understanding how these methods are performed in diverse groups can shed light on their efficacy and potential challenges or limitations. In conclusion, the field of skin disease detection and classification has great potential for future research. We believe that these techniques will continue to play a pivotal role in advancing the field and improving the diagnosis and treatment of skin conditions.

References

1. Allugunti, V.R., A machine learning model for skin disease classification using convolution neural network. *Int. J. Comput. Program. Database Manage.*, 3, 1, 141–147, 2022.
2. Bordoloi, D., Singh, V., Kaliyaperumal, K., Ritonga, M., Jawarneh, M., Kassanuk, T., Quinonez-Choquecota, J., Classification and detection of skin disease based on machine learning and image processing evolutionary models. *Comput. Assist. Methods Eng. Sci.*, 30, 2, 247–256, 2023.
3. Chatterjee, S., Dey, D., Munshi, S., Gorai, S., Extraction of features from cross-correlation in space and frequency domains for classification of skin lesions. *Biomed. Signal Process. Control*, 53, 101581, 2019.
4. Dabowsa, N.I., Amaitik, N.M., Maatuk, A.M., Aljawarneh, S.A., A hybrid intelligent system for skin disease diagnosis, in: *2017 International Conference on Engineering and Technology (ICET)*, IEEE, pp. 1–6, 2017.
5. Inthiyaz, S., Altahan, B.R., Ahammad, S.H., Rajesh, V., Kalangi, R.R., Smirani, L.K., Hossain, M.A., Rashed., A.N.Z., Skin disease detection using deep learning. *Adv. Eng. Softw.*, 175, 103361, 2023.
6. Li, L.F., Wang, X., Hu, W.J., Xiong, N.N., Du, Y.X., Li, B.S., Deep learning in skin disease image recognition: A review. *IEEE Access*, 8, 208264–208280, 2020.
7. Liu, Y., Jain, A., Eng, C., Way, D.H., Lee, K., Bui, P., Kanada, K., de Oliveira Marinho, G., Gallegos, J., Gabriele, S. *et al.*, A deep learning system for differential diagnosis of skin diseases. *Nat. Med.*, 26, 6, 900–908, 2020.
8. Mehdy, M.M., Ng, P.Y., Shair, E.F., Saleh, N.M., Gomes, C., Artificial neural networks in image processing for early detection of breast cancer. *Comput. Math. Methods Med.*, 2017, 2610628, 2017.
9. Polat, K. and Koc, K.O., Detection of skin diseases from dermoscopy image using the combination of convolutional neural network and one-versus-all. *J. Artif. Intell. Syst.*, 2, 1, 80–97, 2020.
10. Rathod, J., Waghmode, V., Sodha, A., Bhavathankar, P., Diagnosis of skin diseases using convolutional neural networks, in: *2018 Second International Conference on Electronics, Communication and Aerospace Technology (ICECA)*, IEEE, pp. 1048–1051, 2018.
11. Hasan, M., Barman, S.D., Islam, S., Reza, A.W., Skin cancer detection using convolutional neural network, in: *Proceedings of the 2019 5th International Conference on Computing and Artificial Intelligence*, pp. 254–258, April 2019.
12. Shanthi, T., Sabeenian, R.S., Anand, R., Automatic diagnosis of skin diseases using convolution neural network. *Microprocess. Microsyst.*, 76, 103074, 2020.
13. Srinivasu, P.N., Rao, T.S., Balas, V.E., A systematic approach for identification of tumor regions in the human brain through haris algorithm, in: *Deep Learning Techniques for Biomedical and Health Informatics*, pp. 97–118, Academic Press, 2020.

14. Srinivasu, P.N., SivaSai, J.G., Ijaz, M.F., Bhoi, A.K., Kim, W., Kang, J.J., Classification of skin disease using deep learning neural networks with mobilenet v2 and lstm. *Sensors*, 21, 8, 2852, 2021.
15. Wei, L.S., Gan, Q., Ji, T., Skin disease recognition method based on image color and texture features. *Comput. Math. Methods Med.*, 2018, 8145713, 2018.
16. Zhang, X., Wang, S., Liu, J., Tao, C., Towards improving diagnosis of skin diseases by combining deep neural network and human knowledge. *BMC Med. Inf. Decis. Making*, 18, 2, 69–76, 2018.
17. Zhou, H., Xie, F., Jiang, Z., Liu, J., Wang, S., Zhu, C., Multi-classification of skin diseases for dermoscopy images using deep learning, in: *2017 IEEE International Conference on Imaging Systems and Techniques (IST)*, IEEE, pp. 1–5, 2017.

4

Computer-Aided Polyp Detection Using Customized Convolutional Neural Network Architecture

Palak Handa[1]*, Nidhi Goel[2], S. Indu[1] and Deepak Gunjan[3]

[1]Department of E & C Engineering, DTU, New Delhi, India
[2]Department of E & C Engineering, IGDTUW, New Delhi, India
[3]Department of Gastroenterology and HNU, AIIMS, New Delhi, India

Abstract

The manual detection of polyp frames is a laborious task, even for specialized gastroenterologists. The automatic detection of polyps using deep learning algorithms may be helpful in reducing the time required by gastroenterologists. This work proposes an automated system to detect polyps using a customized Convolutional Neural Network (CNN) architecture. It was developed with the help of extensive hyperparameter tuning of parameters, namely optimizers, filter size, color space, image dimension, and kernel initializers. A systematic ablation study, test set evaluation, and feature mapping were conducted to evaluate the efficacy of the proposed architecture. The proposed architecture achieved accuracy, specificity, precision, F1-score, F2-score, and recall levels of 92.76%, 94.50%, 94.47%, 94.50%, 90.82%, and 87.44%, respectively, utilizing 1,629,473 trainable parameters. The evaluation of the test set revealed a maximum of 206 accurately identified polyp frames out of 215, accompanied by an enhanced Jaccard index of 83.18% and a specificity level of 94.50%. The proposed pipeline was compared with state-of-the-art deep learning architectures in this field. It achieved optimum results with higher precision while detecting polyps, with a reduced execution time and number of trainable parameters.

***Keywords*:** Polyp detection, artificial intelligence, endoscopy

**Corresponding author*: palakhanda_2k21phdec05@dtu.ac.in

Neha Sharma, Korhan Cengiz and Prasenjit Chatterjee (eds.) Intelligent Data Analytics for Bioinformatics and Biomedical Systems, (93–108) © 2024 Scrivener Publishing LLC

4.1 Introduction

The incidence of gastrointestinal disorders worldwide is approximately 35%, with 10% of cases involving colorectal abnormalities [1]. Colorectal lesions, commonly known as polyps, are crucial diagnostic indicators of colorectal disease (CRC). These small protrusions on the bowel lining have the potential to develop into cancer over time if not addressed. In as many as 90% of instances, it has been discovered that prompt identification and removal of adenomatous polyps can help avoid colorectal cancer [1].

One of the most effective methods to diagnose the presence of polyps in the gastrointestinal tract is to perform a colonoscopy procedure, wherein an endoscope is inserted within the GI tract through the mouth or anus opening.

The camera recorded a video of the lining of the colon. This generated video is analyzed after the procedure in a frame-by-frame manner by a skilled gastroenterologist to produce a differential diagnosis [1]. Manual detection of polyps in these videos is prone to physician errors and high false-positive rates [2]. Human error can be reduced with the help of Artificial Intelligence (AI). Many state-of-the-art (SOTA) pipelines have been developed for polyp identification [1].

Previous methods employed manually designed feature engineering, traditional image processing, machine learning, various forms of deep learning (end-to-end, hybrid, and feature extractor-based approaches), and transfer learning to address these tasks [1–6]. One example of such networks is Convolutional Neural Networks (CNNs), which excel at pattern recognition due to their grid-like structures. They can automatically extract profound features, including texture, shape, color, intensity, and statistical parameters [1, 7, 8]. However, they still fall short of explaining their model as to why certain blocks and schemes can produce poor or good results. This demands a thorough experimental analysis of the parameters used in their models; the reproduction of the results is also an important factor. Keeping these points in view, this study focused on overcoming the problem related to generalization in polyp detection while designing a customized CNN. This study presents a generalized detection of polyps (Figure 4.1) consisting of three steps: (i) data preparation, (ii) search and hyper-parameter tuning experiments to develop a customized CNN, and (iii) analysis with the help of training, testing evaluation, feature mapping, and ablation study of the customized CNN architecture. The major contributions of this study are as follows:

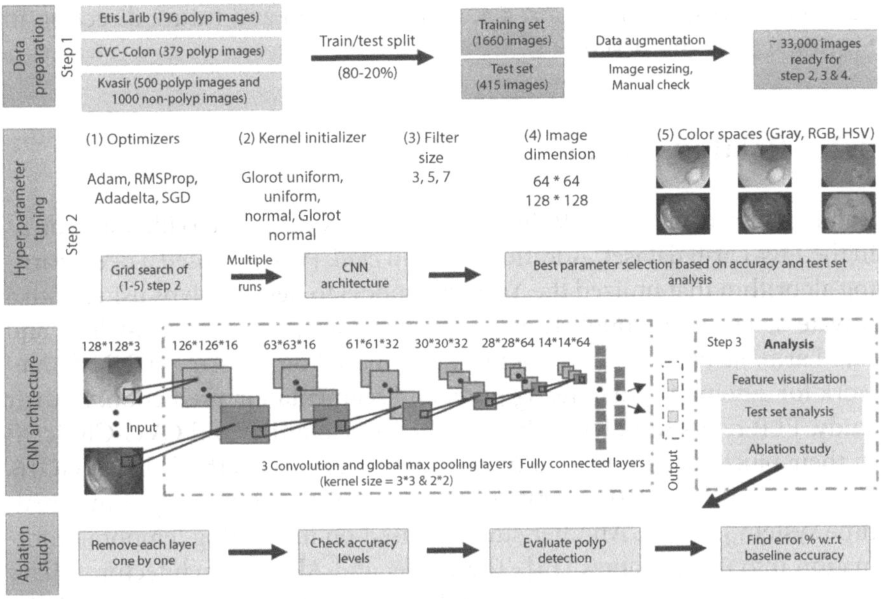

Figure 4.1 Experiment protocol for computer-aided polyp detection.

- The proposed work focuses on the development of an end-to-end customized architecture for computer-aided detection of polyp frames. Hyperparameters, test set evaluation, feature mapping, and ablation studies were conducted to demonstrate the generalization and reproducibility of the work.
- The proposed work includes hyperparameter tuning and variation in optimizers, namely Adam, RMSProp, Adadelta, and SGD; kernel initializers, namely glorot uniform, uniform, normal, and glorot normal; filter size of 3, 5, and 7; image dimension of 64 × 64 and 128 × 128; and color space of gray, RGB, and HSV.
- The effectiveness of the proposed architecture was confirmed by creating 33,000 polyp and nonpolyp frames from three publicly accessible colonoscopic databases. The reported results included an enhanced Jaccard index of 83.18%, along with specificity and validation loss values of 94.50% and 0.187, respectively.

The following sections are discussed in the remaining book chapter. Related works are discussed in Section 4.2. The materials and methods in

Section 4.3, results in Section 4.4, and conclusion and future direction in Section 4.5 are discussed.

4.2 Related Works

Rahim, Hassan, and Shin [9] introduced a CNN designed to identify polyps in the Etis-Larib dataset. Additionally, Cao *et al.* [10] proposed a deep learning algorithm that utilized the YOLOv3 model to detect polyps using both a private database and publicly accessible databases, namely, CVC-Clinic and Etis-Larib. Jia *et al.* [11] proposed PLPnet based on a faster R-CNN framework for automatic polyp recognition and segmentation prediction. In their study, PLP refers to polyps. They used CVC-ColonDB and CVC-ClinicDB in their pipeline. Another study used deep learning methods like VGG16, VGG19, and ResNet50 separately to localize and identify polyps in a real-time system [12, 13]. Another study focused on integrating temporal information into polyp frames [14]. The U-Net and AlexNet architecture s have also been used for automatic polyp detection [15, 16]. The reproducibility of the obtained results has been a concern in this field [8]. Further improvements can be made in this field. The present study paves the way for advancements in this field by proposing an end-to-end automatic pipeline, with the importance of hyperparameter tuning, test set analysis, and ablation studies to show the reproducibility of the pipeline.

4.3 Materials and Methods

4.3.1 Description of the Used Datasets and Their Preparation

In this study, three datasets namely—ETIS-Larib, CVC-Colon, and Kvasir (v1)—were employed. The training and test split ratios were consistently set to 80%–20%. Specifically, 196 images were obtained from the ETIS-Larib database. A total of 379 images were obtained from the CVC-Colon database. A total of 500 images were obtained from the "polyp" category in the Kvasir database were utilized for the polyp class. Regarding the non-polyp class, around a thousand frames were chosen from the Kvasir dataset.

4.3.2 Data Augmentation

Following data preparation, the image data underwent a crucial step in the implementation of deep learning for smaller datasets, namely, data augmentation [1]. The specified model employs data augmentation techniques, including re-scaling of the images, shear range of the images, zoom range (in and out), and horizontal flipping of the images. After performing augmentation on the stated model, 33,000 new images were formed, which was almost 20 times the available dataset. All the augmentation methods were applied on-the-fly in such a manner that they introduced as much variability in the images so that the model could be trained with varied polyp and non-polyp frames. After data augmentation, a manual check was performed to ensure that each frame looked different and the same image was not present in the training and testing datasets to avoid data leakage.

4.3.3 Customized CNN

The proposed custom CNN architecture comprises four main parts: an input layer that acts as an input to the set of images for training, three convolutional layers and three max-pooling layers for feature extraction, and two fully connected layers for identification purposes. All images were resized to a specific dimension (n) of 128 × 128, with (nc) representing the number of channels. This resizing ensured consistency across the three datasets and required fewer computational resources. Each convolutional layer consisted of a filter and associated size f (a set of weights), which was applied to the input data to create a feature map. Multiple feature maps were obtained using different filters for, e.g., a total of 32 filters (nf) for one layer with default stride, s, i.e., 1, and padding, p produced an output volume of dimension 126 × 126 × 32.

The tensor obtained from the convolutional layer was passed between the layers by connecting channels that included biases, weights, and activation functions. The outcome of the activation function determines whether the neuron is activated and each activated function carries information to the next layer. In CNN architecture, the "Relu" activation function has been widely employed, enhancing nonlinearity in the image [17]. The "Relu" @ctivation function is recognized for expediting the convergence of stochastic gradient by minimizing the cost function with fewer activations [18]. The volume remained unchanged, resulting in an output volume with dimensions 126 × 126 × 32.

The max-pooling layer selects the maximum element from the region of the feature map covered by the filter. The importance of this layer is to reduce the size of the image and prevent overfitting. During this operation, a 2 × 2 filter and a stride of 2 produced a resultant volume of 63 × 63 × 32. The fully connected layers were regular neural network layers. This helped in computing the prediction scores of the test set images. The processing of the images by the neural network continued up to the second-last layer. One neuron activated in the output layer corresponds to an input image. Random weights were defined to generalize the network further.

Based on the experimental protocol, the hyperparameters available in the CNN architecture underwent a grid search to achieve the best parameters for polyp detection. A constant seed was set for all the experiments, wherein a seed was a Python integer that helped to generate the same tensor for a given shape and type. This setup helped the pipeline to produce reproducible results.

4.4 Results and Discussion

The proposed custom CNN architecture comprises of four parts, as stated above. Augmentation parameters were carefully considered in an on-the-fly mode to augment the data and introduce variability into the colonoscopy datasets.

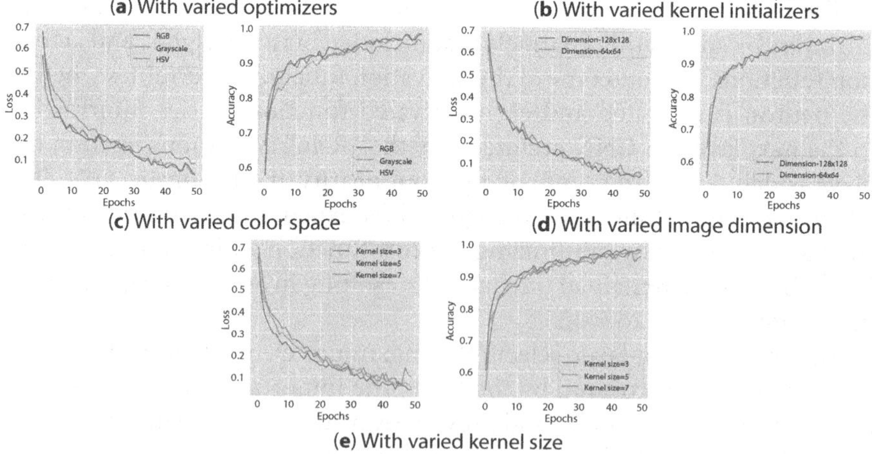

Figure 4.2 Accuracy and loss graph w.r.t 50 epochs when hyperparameters are varied.

A custom CNN architecture was developed to perform the binary classification. Hyperparameter tuning was performed for various parameters of the CNN. All experiments presented in Figure 4.2 were evaluated for accuracy and the number of polyps detected from the test set (215 images). The experiments were repeated and tested for approximately 50 epochs. The optimal hyperparameters obtained from the grid search for the optimizer, kernel initializer, RGB, image dimension, and kernel size were Adam, Glorot uniform, RGB, 128 × 128 matrix, and 3 × 3 matrix.

4.4.1 CNN Optimizers

In deep learning models, optimizers play a crucial role in handling system complexity by adjusting the weight parameters to minimize the loss function [18]. Numerous optimizers are at disposal, and each employs distinct algorithms to converge to a global minimum with respect to the loss function, yielding diverse outcomes. To identify the most effective optimizer for polyp detection, the proposed architecture was trained with various optimizers, including Adam, RMSProp, SGD, and Adadelta, utilizing grid searching as part of the process.

The Adam optimizer, operating based on the stochastic gradient descent method, demonstrated superior performance, achieving a validation accuracy of 91.66% and successfully identifying 206 polyp images among 215 images in the test folder. Adam is considered the most robust optimizer as it does not need much tuning of the hyper- parameters and has little memory requirement [19]. The RMSProp optimizer yielded results close to those of Adam with a validation accuracy of 88.62% and correctly predicted 192 images of polyps.

The SGD optimizer achieved an accuracy of 82.95% and correctly predicted 120 polyps. The SGD algorithm is preferred for shallow networks and requires longer convergence time [20]. The Adadelta optimizer was the least optimal for our tasks, achieving a validation accuracy of 62.74% while predicting only 103 polyps. This is because the Adadelta algorithm uses an exponentially decaying average of the learning rates to increase the convergence of the loss function [21].

4.4.2 Kernel Initializers

The neural network starts training with some default values of weights and keeps updating the weights with each iteration to achieve global minima. A kernel initializer is used in the CNN layers to initialize these weights with predefined values. In the Keras library, different types of kernel initializers are available: random normal, zero class, one class, glorot uniform, and normal [22].

Each initializer generates a tensor (an array of components in a vector space) based on a unique distribution. For e.g., an identity initializer generates an identity matrix as tensor. We checked four initializers: glorot uniform, glorot normal, random normal, and uniform class.

The best kernel initializer came out to be glorot uniform, which is also the default weight initializer in the Keras library settings [22]. It produced a validation accuracy of 90.93% and detected 182 of 215 polyps. The least results were found for glorot normal, where the model was only able to predict 81 of 215 polyps.

4.4.3 Color Space

There is a wide range of color spaces such as Red, Green, Blue (RGB), Rec. 2100, Cyan, Magenta, Yellow, and Key (CMYK), Hue, Saturation, Value (HSV) etc., that can be used for training of images in a deep learning model. Each color space has its own importance and significance for human perception [23]. The different color spaces used in this work are RGB, grayscale, and HSV.

The RGB color space is the most commonly used color space for training deep-learning models [23, 24]. In this method, colors are obtained by a linear combination of red, green, and blue. This is the simplest available color space. The grayscale color space works on the principle of intensity and focuses on the brightness of a pixel.

The higher the value, the greater the intensity. The pixel level values are between 0 and 255, leading to different white and black shapes. The Hue Saturation Value (HSV) color space is recognized as a psychological color space, where hue signifies the dominant color, saturation indicates the purity or degree of gray in the color, and value represents the brightness or intensity of the color. This color space is achieved through a nonlinear transformation of the RGB model.

To analyze the best possible results, the architecture was trained on the RGB, grayscale, and HSV color spaces. The validation accuracy of the RGB model reached 90.60%, and the architecture detected 206 of the 215 polyps in the test set. In the grayscale color space model, the accuracy was 84.84%, and 103 polyps were detected. The HSV model performed poorly, achieving an accuracy of 51.27%. However, when observed with the naked eye, it shows distinct colors for the anomaly present in the frame (Figure 4.1).

We observed that the customized CNN architecture extracted different features from the HSV frames, such as sharp edges and boundaries.

However, the color space has not been able to detect polyps uniquely and produced produces low accuracy. HSV contains a separate image intensity parameter apart from color information, which is considered to provide better information. In the chosen dataset, colonoscopy frames were collected with a high resolution and bright intensity. The analysis may differ in the scenario where the camera and its light are observed in a darker area inside the colon and may change the value of the hue due to indirect lighting.

A separate study should be conducted to check light and intensity variations among colonoscopy frames. In the present work, it can be seen that the RGB color space has been the most successful because of the linear combinations of the color space in colonoscopic polyp and non-polyp frames. An improved validation accuracy and loss was achieved for the RGB color space during grid search in comparison to the above-stated color spaces; hence, it was chosen for further evaluation.

4.4.4 Image Dimension

The dimensions of the images in the dataset play a very important role in the training of the model [18]. If the image dimension is too small or too large, the model might fail to detect polyps correctly and with a higher accuracy [18]. Analysis of the proposed architecture revealed that when the image dimension was 64 × 64, the model validation accuracy was 89.74%, and 201 out of 215 polyps were detected. However, when the dimensions were changed to 128 × 128, the validation accuracy increased to 95.54%, and detected 202 out of 215.

The increase in this accuracy level is dependent on various factors such as kernel size, color space, and optimizers. The polyps present in the colonoscopy image frames were small in dimension and best detected with a kernel size of 3 and an image dimension of 128 × 128. The model with dimension 128 × 128 outperformed the former model by approximately a 6% increase in the validation accuracy in comparison with the 64 × 64 image dimension result. Hence, 128 × 128 was considered for further analysis.

4.4.5 Kernel Size

Kernel size refers to the dimension of the filter used in the convolution layers of the CNN architecture. It slides over every pixel block individually to produce an output. It defines the receptive field of a network and varies from application to application [18]. Smaller kernel sizes are preferred

Table 4.1 Achieved results.

Parameter	Accuracy values achieved during training stage	Loss values achieved during training stage	Accuracy values achieved during validation stage	Loss values achieved during validation stage	No. of polyps classified (out of 215)
(a) Optimizers					
Adam	93.01%	0.163	91.66%	0.251	206
SGD	81.56%	0.393	82.95%	0.377	120
RMSProp	91.58%	0.204	88.62%	0.328	192
Adadelta	65.80%	0.661	62.74%	0.673	103
(b) Kernel initializers					
Glorot uniform	92.77%	0.167	90.93%	0.253	182
Uniform	91.02%	0.211	88.54%	0.314	141
Normal	91.82%	0.187	90.74%	0.276	156
Glorot normal	65.17%	0.664	64.72%	0.672	81
(c) Color space					
RGB	92.25%	0.177	90.60%	0.269	206
Grayscale	91.08%	0.202	84.84%	0.515	103
HSV	91.30%	0.194	51.27%	6.055	98
(d) Image dimension					
128 × 128	92.30%	0.172	95.54%	0.291	202
64 × 64	92.62%	0.171	89.74%	0.22	201
(e) Kernel size					
3	92.75%	0.169	89.7%	0.279	183
5	91.51%	0.194	89.45%	0.286	144
7	91.06%	0.205	89.34%	0.309	84

because they are relatively faster in training the model and require less computational cost while achieving receptive fields similar to those of larger kernel sizes [18]. Generally, kernel sizes with even dimensions are not used because even-sized filters cannot divide the pixels around the output pixel symmetrically.

From the comparison in Table 4.1, it was observed that a 3 × 3 kernel size produced the best results with a validation accuracy of 89.7% and detected 183 polyps correctly, whereas 5 × 5 and 7 × 7 kernel sizes were able to correctly detect 144 and 84 polyps out of 215 polyp images, respectively. This is because the larger the kernel size, the less it slides over the respective pixel blocks and fetches minute image details. The 5 × 5 and 7 × 7 kernel sizes scanned the entire receptive field and found superficial features (edges/boundaries, etc.) in comparison to the 3 × 3 kernel size, which traversed more and computed deeper minute features of polyp pixels in the image. The obtained results show that medical images that contain rich and minute details should consider the use of smaller kernel sizes to achieve better receptive fields while extracting more complex and deeper features from the images.

4.4.6 Sample Maps of the CNN Features

Feature maps serve as representations of the output generated by applying a single filter to the preceding layer in the CNN pipeline. These maps were constructed using various units within the CNN architecture that shared the same weights and biases. In Figure 4.3, the feature visualization of a polyp test image, which shows its various feature maps. The feature maps of the initial and final convolutional layers and dense layers are shown in the figure. They are responsible for the feature extraction and class mapping, respectively. As shown in Figure 4.3, the CNN filters extracted features, such as image boundaries, tissue texture, and surface linings.

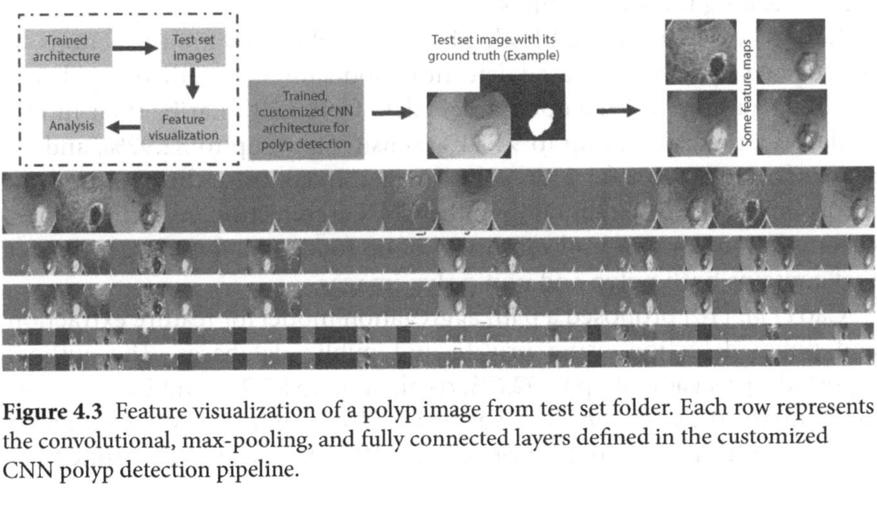

Figure 4.3 Feature visualization of a polyp image from test set folder. Each row represents the convolutional, max-pooling, and fully connected layers defined in the customized CNN polyp detection pipeline.

4.4.7 Ablation Study

An ablation study is a method employed to assess the performance of a pipeline by systematically excluding or omitting specific blocks, portions, or components [25]. The term "ablation" originates from the surgical removal of an organ or tissue. This study is particularly valuable in deciphering the inner workings of deep learning methods, often perceived as "black boxes." Each layer was individually commented on to conduct the ablation study, and the model was run to evaluate the accuracy and losses without that layer. This process aids in understanding the significance of each convolutional layer with its distinct filters and customized settings. An average decrease of 1%–5% was observed in the testing accuracy compared to the baseline accuracy of 90.84% when any layer was removed. Extending the number of epochs beyond 50 could achieve a training accuracy of up to 100%. However, the maximum number of polyps detected was 206 out of 215. Consequently, the ablation study incorporated the early stopping criteria to observe the greatest variations in accuracy and loss levels when any layer was omitted.

4.4.8 Comparison of the Proposed Architecture with Existing Deep-Learning Algorithms in This Field

The proposed architecture was compared with existing SOTA pipelines that utilize deep-learning methods for polyp detection. The comparison was performed using various objective parameters, namely, the number of trainable parameters, number of images used as input, their ablation study, feature mapping, F1-score, precision, and recall score obtained after training and testing the architectures.

Rahim *et al.* [9] utilized both Mish and ReLu activation functions to develop a deep learning-based detection model for automatic polyp detection. The authors utilized open-access data from ETIS-Larib. Their model achieved a precision of up to 94.44%, sensitivity of up to 82.92%, and F1 score of up to 88.30% for 2156 polyp images. In contrast, the present work incorporated the ReLu function in the CNN architecture, resulting in precision of up to 94.47% and sensitivity of up to 87.44% for a larger dataset that contains both polyp and non-polyp images.

Cao *et al.* [10] proposed a path aggregation model for feature extraction and polyp detection using private and public databases. The authors reported a precision of up to 92.6%, recall of up to 87.9%, and F1 score values of up to 90.2% for the ETIS-Larib and CVC-Clinic datasets. Compared to the model proposed by Cao *et al.* [10], the proposed architecture demonstrated superior evaluation metrics for a larger dataset, achieving a precision of up to 94.47% and an F1 score of up to 90.82%. A similar recall of up to 87.44% value was achieved. Li *et al.* [16] developed a deep learning algorithm using AlexNet architecture for automatic polyp detection. This is a type of transfer-learning model. The authors only performed training and testing using the open-access datasets. After augmenting their images, the authors reported an overall accuracy of up to 86%, a sensitivity of up to 73%, and specificity values of up to 96%. In contrast to the algorithm proposed by Li *et al.* [16], the proposed architecture achieved an improved overall accuracy of up to 87.99% and a specificity of up to 87.44%.

In addition to the widely used parameters such as accuracy, precision, and recall, the present work also validated the proposed architecture on various objective parameters. The results were obtained from a local machine with 16GB RAM, AMD Ryzen 7 2700 eight-core processor, NVIDIA GeForce GTX 1050Ti, and 4 GB RAM graphics card. It was noticed that the loss was reduced to 0.187 upon appropriate hyperparameter tuning with optimum precision, recall, specificity, F1-score, F2 score, Jaccard index, and testing accuracy of up to 94.47%, 87.44%, 94.50%, 90.82%, 88.76%, 83.18%, and 90.84%, respectively, upon multiple runs.

4.5 Conclusion and Future Scope

Automated identification of polyp frames holds significant value for gastroenterologists. This study concentrated on creating an end-to-end customized CNN architecture for the automated detection of both polyp and non-polyp frames. Ensuring the generalizability of the proposed architecture involves a comprehensive analysis of various hyperparameters within the deep-learning model. Special attention was paid to evaluating the test set performance under different hyperparameter settings. Through meticulous hyperparameter tuning, the specificity, precision, and testing accuracy reached impressive values of 94.50%, 94.47%, and 90.84%, respectively. Fine-tuning of the hyperparameters also resulted in a reduction in the loss to 0.187. A comparative analysis demonstrated that our architecture outperformed existing pipelines in terms of the evaluation metrics. Future investigations should focus on occlusion testing.

Availability Statement

The code is available upon request from the corresponding author. The dataset used was an open-source dataset.

References

1. Sánchez-Peralta, L.F., Bote-Curiel, L., Picón, A., Sánchez-Margallo, F.M., Pagador, J.B., Deep learning to find colorectal polyps in colonoscopy: A systematic literature review. *Artif. Intell. Med.*, 108, 101923, 2020.
2. Mangotra, H., Goel, N. *et al.*, Effect of selection bias on automatic colonoscopy polyp detection. *Biomed. Signal Process. Control*, 85, 104915, 2023.
3. Ali, S., Zhou, F., Daul, C., Braden, B., Bailey, A., Realdon, S., East, J., Wagnieres, G., Loschenov, V., Grisan, E. *et al.*, Endoscopy artifact detection (ead 2019) challenge dataset, 2019, arXiv preprint arXiv:1905.03209.
4. Kaur, S. and Goel, N., A dilated convolutional approach for inflammatory lesion detection using multi-scale input feature fusion (workshop paper), in: *2020 IEEE Sixth International Conference on Multimedia Big Data (BigMM)*, pp. 386–393, 2020.
5. Nogueira-Rodríguez, A., Domínguez-Carbajales, R., López-Fernández, H., Iglesias, Á., Cubiella, J., Fdez-Riverola, F., Reboiro-Jato, M., Glez-Peña, D., Deep neural networks approaches for detecting and classifying colorectal polyps. *Neurocomputing*, 423, 721–734, 2021.
6. Azer, S.A., Challenges facing the detection of colonic polyps: what can deep learning do? *Medicina*, 55, 8, 473, 2019.
7. Sánchez-Montes, C., Bernal, J., García-Rodríguez, A., Córdova, H., Fernández-Esparrach, G., Review of computational methods for the detection and classification of polyps in colonoscopy imaging. *Gastroenterol. Hepatol. (English Edition)*, 43, 4, 222–232, 2020.
8. Houwen, B.B.S.L., Nass, K.J., Vleugels, J.L.A., Fockens, P., Hazewinkel, Y., Dekker, E., Comprehensive review of publicly available colonoscopic imaging databases for artificial intelligence research: availability, accessibility and usability. *Gastrointest. Endosc.*, 97, 2, 184–199, E16, February 2023.
9. Rahim, T., Hassan, S.A., Shin, S.Y., A deep convolutional neural network for the detection of polyps in colonoscopy images. *Biomed. Signal Process. Control*, 68, 102654, 2021.
10. Cao, C., Wang, R., Yu, Y., Zhang, H., Yu, Y., Sun, C., Gastric polyp detection in gastroscopic images using deep neural network. *PLoS One*, 16, 4, e0250632, 2021.
11. Jia, X., Mai, X., Cui, Y., Yuan, Y., Xing, X., Seo, H., Xing, L., Meng, M.Q.-H., Automatic polyp recognition in colonoscopy images using deep learning and two-stage pyramidal feature prediction. *IEEE Trans. Autom. Sci. Eng.*, 17, 3, 1570–1584, 2020.
12. Hasan, M.M., Islam, N., Rahman, M.M., Gastrointestinal polyp detection through a fusion of contourlet transform and neural features. *J. King Saud Univ. - Comput. Inf. Sci.*, 34, 3, 526–533, March 2022.
13. Urban, G., Tripathi, P., Alkayali, T., Mittal, M., Jalali, F., Karnes, W., Baldi, P., Deep learning localizes and identifies polyps in real time with 96% accuracy in screening colonoscopy. *Gastroenterology*, 155, 4, 1069–1078, 2018.

14. Qadir, H.A., Balasingham, I., Solhusvik, J., Bergsland, J., Aabakken, L., Shin, Y., Improving automatic polyp detection using cnn by exploiting temporal dependency in colonoscopy video. *IEEE J. Biomed. Health Inf.*, 24, 1, 180–193, 2019.
15. Tashk, A., Herp, J., Nadimi, E., Fully automatic polyp detection based on a novel u-net architecture and morphological post-process, in: *2019 International Conference on Control, Artificial Intelligence, Robotics & Optimization (ICCAIRO)*, IEEE, pp. 37–41, 2019.
16. Li, T., Glissen Brown, J.R., Tsourides, K., Mahmud, N., Cohen, J.M., Berzin, T.M., Training a computer-aided polyp detec tion system to detect sessile serrated adenomas using public domain colonoscopy videos. *Endosc. Int. Open*, 8, 10, E1448–E1454, 2020.
17. Dureja, A. and Pahwa, P., Analysis of non-linear activation functions for classification tasks using convolutional neural networks. *Recent Pat. Comput. Sci.*, 12, 3, 156–161, 2019.
18. Goodfellow, I., Bengio, Y., Courville, A., *Deep learning*, MIT press, 2016.
19. Kingma, D.P. and Ba, J., Adam: A method for stochastic optimization, 2014, arXiv preprint arXiv:1412.6980.
20. Yazan, E. and Talu, M.F., Comparison of the stochastic gradient descent based optimization techniques, in: *2017 International Artificial Intelligence and Data Processing Symposium (IDAP)*, IEEE, pp. 1–5, 2017.
21. Dogo, E.M., Afolabi, O.J., Nwulu, N.I., Twala, B., Aigbavboa, C.O., A comparative analysis of gradient descent-based optimization algorithms on convolutional neural networks, in: *2018 International Conference on Computational Techniques, Electronics and Mechanical Systems (CTEMS)*, IEEE, pp. 92–99, 2018.
22. Ketkar, N., Introduction to keras, in: *Deep learning with Python*, pp. 97–111, Springer, 2017.
23. Sidorov, O., Novel approach to uniformization of a color space via generic deep learning-based transformation, in: *2018 Colour and Visual Computing Symposium (CVCS)*, IEEE, pp. 1–4, 2018.
24. Agrawal, A. and Mittal, N., Using cnn for facial expression recognition: a study of the effects of kernel size and number of filters on accuracy. *Vis. Comput.*, 36, 2, 405–412, 2020.
25. Du, L., How much deep learning does neural style transfer really need? an ablation study, in: *Proceedings of the IEEE/CVF Winter Conference on Applications of Computer Vision*, pp. 3150–3159, 2020.

5

Computational Intelligence Induced Risk in Modern Healthcare: Classical Review and Current Status

Nitish Ojha[1]* and Shrikant Ojha[2]

[1]Amity University, UP, India
[2]Sharda University, Greater Noida, India

Abstract

The proliferation of IT has turned the healthcare industry up to a different level of automation, and this big leap in healthcare has also invited new challenges. Whether it is a small sensor or a complete room-based operating system, IoT plays a major role in saving lives while involving the new methodologies of medicines. From the remote collection of patient data, storage of electronic health records, facilitating drug delivery, demonstration of research-based drug trials, and synthesis or implementation of pathological results while providing functionality to patients and doctors, AI with IoT is transforming each and every component in this field. While providing great hand-holding capacity, IoT with AI also poses some major challenges and risks for both patients and doctors, such as handling sensitive data, patient consent and implementation of EULA, compliance of security standards in preserving the integrity of data either at transit or at storage, handling the socio-economics-based digital divide in remote areas, discrepancies in multiple vendors' agreements, and its hierarchical implementation to achieve a common goal. This study catalogs all the major studies that have been conducted focusing on AI-based risks in IoT devices used in the field of medicine and healthcare. Challenges and future research directions have also been discussed, which can be helpful for creating better safeguards for minimizing the risk in automation-based devices where AI and IoT are at an intersection.

***Keywords*:** Risk in IoT, risk in healthcare, computational intelligence, risk in diagnosis

**Corresponding author*: nitishkumarojha@gmail.com

Neha Sharma, Korhan Cengiz and Prasenjit Chatterjee (eds.) Intelligent Data Analytics for Bioinformatics and Biomedical Systems, (109–144) © 2024 Scrivener Publishing LLC

5.1 Introduction

The growth of technology has its own pros and cons, and this phenomenon is also quite prevalent in areas that are highly affected by the amalgamation of new technology; the healthcare field is the field that observes the highest level of innovation, and these innovations of technology supported by AI are bringing some inevitable issues at the same time [1]. The concept of connecting devices to the Internet emerged in the late 20th century, and the motivation was to develop a robust computer network where data sharing could be made easy. In the 1980s and the 1990s, the focus was on connecting computers and laying the foundation for the Internet, which happened successfully while giving birth to numerous technologies, i.e., LAN, MAN, and WLAN IEEE 802.11 series. In the early 2000s, with the invention of mobile devices, mobile-to-mobile communication technology emerged, allowing devices to communicate with each other without human intervention [2]. This was a significant leap in the field of data transfer, where the file was shared on the move [3].

Later, security also improved, so mobile telephony gave birth to a new subject, distributed computing. This established connectivity between devices and laid the foundation for IoT. Moreover, as sensor technology has evolved from the electronic sciences, it has become more affordable, and the integration of sensors into everyday objects has increased. These sensors allow devices to collect and transmit data about their surroundings such as temperature, humidity, and movement [4]. This sensor-based technology, which emerged from embedded systems, has created a path for the development of IoT devices. The proliferation of wireless technologies such as Wi-Fi, Bluetooth, and cellular networks has enabled devices to connect to the Internet virtually anywhere [5]. This expansion of connectivity has been important to the growth of the IoT, as it allows devices to transmit data wirelessly. As a result, IoT is well matured and continues to grow, and finally, IoT has become a fully developed device [6].

As the number of IoT devices and applications has improved, standardization and interoperability have become necessary. Organizations working in this field have developed several standards and protocols to ensure optimized and seamless communication and integration between various IoT devices and platforms in different segments of daily life [7]. Examples include the emergence of IoT-specific standards, such as MQTT, CoAP, Zigbee, and Z-Wave.

In the early months of 2010, combining IoT with artificial intelligence (AI) and machine learning (ML) opened new possibilities for better research and outcomes in many fields. AI and ML algorithms can analyze massive amounts of IoT data, termed Big Data, enabling predictive analytics, anomaly detection, and automated decision making [8]. This integration has enabled advancements in areas such as smart homes, financial services, driverless cars, and personalized healthcare, as discussed in this chapter.

If we relate the network of IoT devices to healthcare, it may look like this (see Figure 5.1).

Figure 5.2 shows the setup of the IoT architecture implementation in healthcare organizations.

From the above architecture, it is clear how information flows in the AI-enabled IoT setups in smart hospitals. The security-based risk may arise at any stage, or at any step, be it a user, or any exchange of information or processing of data to achieve the final objective [9].

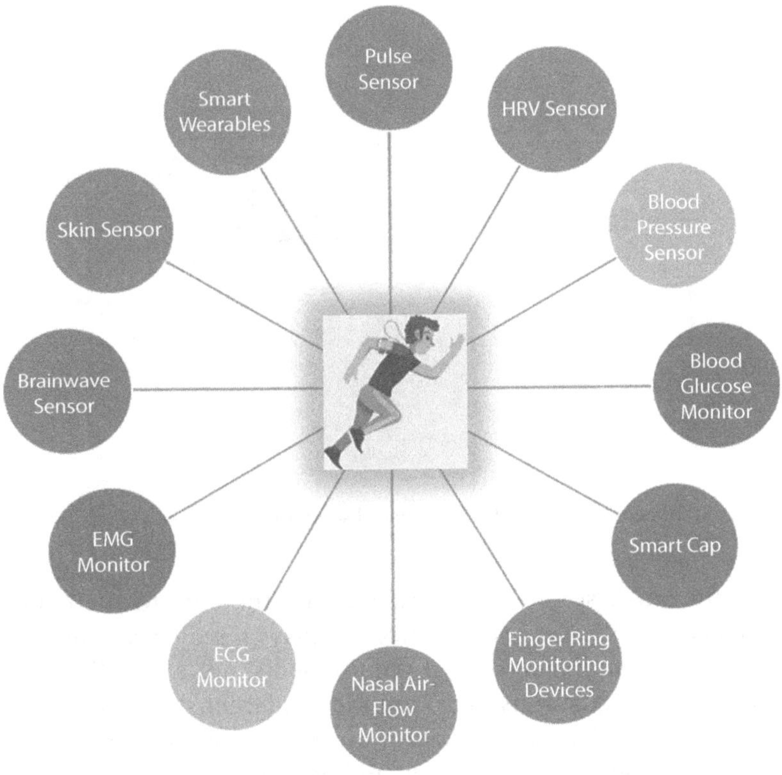
Pulse Sensor
Smart Wearables
HRV Sensor
Skin Sensor
Blood Pressure Sensor
Brainwave Sensor
Blood Glucose Monitor
EMG Monitor
Smart Cap
ECG Monitor
Nasal Air-Flow Monitor
Finger Ring Monitoring Devices

Figure 5.1 Network of IoT devices in healthcare.

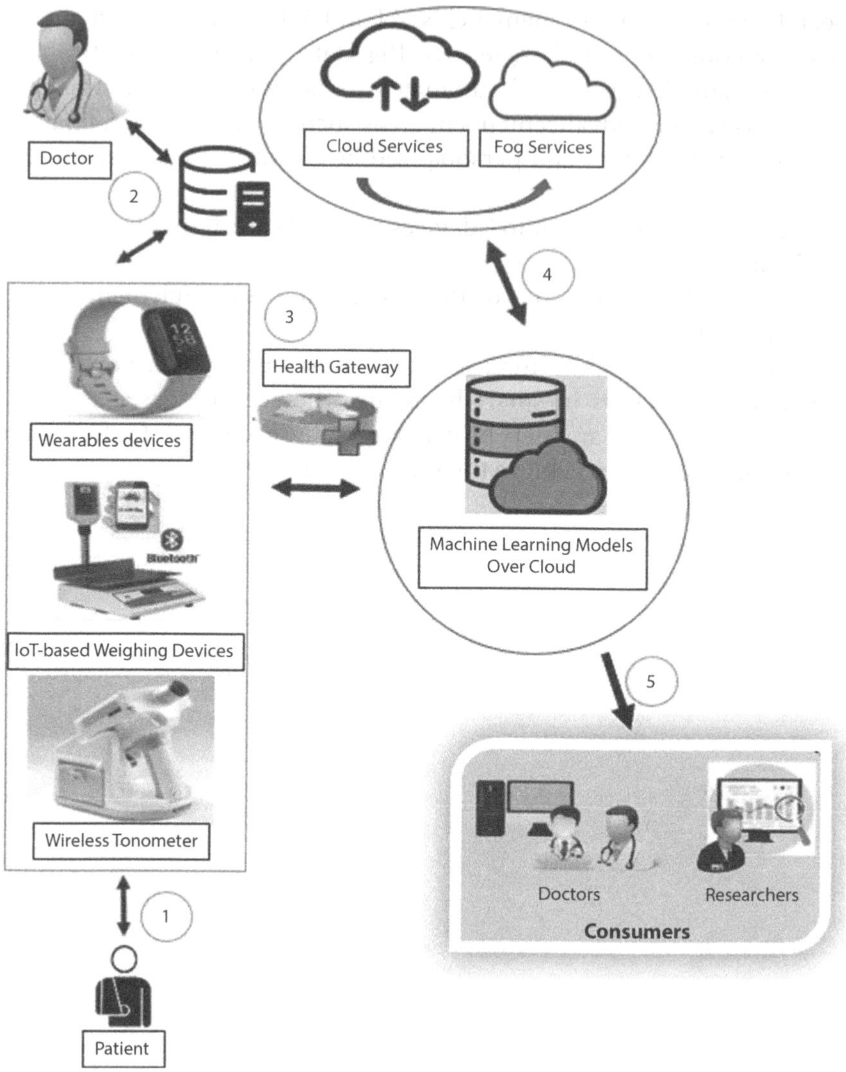

Figure 5.2 Architecture of AI enabled IoT based setup in healthcare.

From the small sensor up to transferring the data to the computer that is located at the longest distance, AI plays a major role but does it follow all the compliance-related requirements, are we really checking those rules and regulations, what are then different standards that have to be followed, and what the failure areas or gray areas that need the formulation of the new requirement and how the new research is able to address those traditional issues, all these issues, factors, and problems

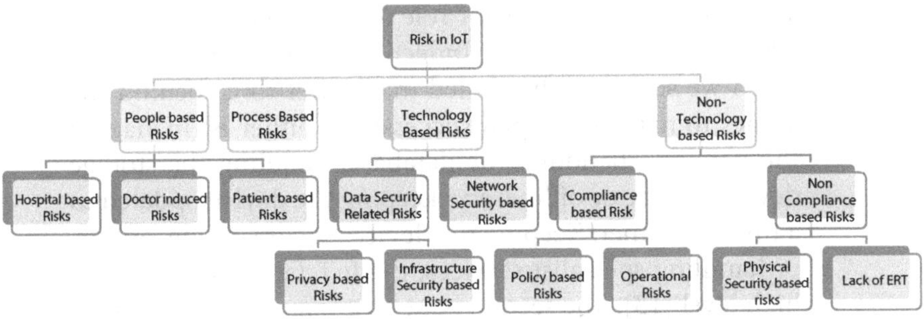

Figure 5.3 Hierarchical classification of risk involved with IoT devices as used in healthcare.

have to be addressed with a healthy approach because ultimately they induce framework-based risk that causes the low performance of the overall system [10] (see Figure 5.3).

5.2 People-Based Risk

Risks inherent to all types of manpower involved with IoT devices are categorized into this classification. Many people do not see any challenges or risks with normal sensors or transducers; however, when that sensor is an IoT-based device, the chances of loss of data and privacy-based issues may arise, as people are not aware of the dark side of the technology, and they have no idea how IoT devices affect them passively. People-based risk can be categorized into three levels

a. **Hospital-Based Risks:** If hospital premises are not secure enough, IoT devices can bring big problems to their users. Many hospitals are fully under surveillance, and the diagnosis is also computer-assisted with the help of AI-based technology, which is important for a better and more secure environment for people who are dealing with IoT devices, and their related data must be trained in a timely manner. There are several reports that determine the lack of skilled people for handling different types of IoT devices and their related components [11]. The market and hospitals are adopting this highly sophisticated technology very fast and by the year 2025, the hospital will be connected at double the rate we have seen in the last decade as AI and chatbots are also playing their major role to boost the current situation in the long term [12]. Indeed, it is a good situation, but when we scale out the skilled manpower force behind the scenes to make it happen successfully, either by managing the network, handling the database, handling the storage devices online or offline, and keeping the device updated in a timely manner. Keeping the devices secure offline, online, or handling specialist services, the IoT faces this issue at a high level [13]. The second issue that many research papers and reviews studies chalk out is the lack of experts to train employees. This problem is not only with IoT but also with devices that have AI-based support [14]. Most AI-based companies invest huge amounts of money in training their employees and training them for upcoming technologies so that further innovations can be made. Another research report reveals that the major gap between the available manpower and the requirement in this field is making production worse as two other major technologies intersect each other, such as big data and Machine Learning. Less skilled employees are the main reason behind the loss in financial outcomes, as vulnerable software and hardware are the outcomes of those employees; if they are less updated with the new technology, the company is going to pay the price of loss; in the long term, the company brand will be shaken, which ultimately phases out that company from its peers in the long run [15].

One of the major IT firms, Price Water House Coopers (PwC) reported an alerting situation about the less skilled employees and the need for skilled employees and the gap. The education level and the subjects at the school level also play an important role as the changing technology needs new subjects and course curricula redesigned because most IoT devices are equipped with AI algorithms to make detection and predictions and for that data analytics subject plays a base in the long term if it would have been part of the course [16]. Data science is an intricate blend of knowledge and expertise. IoT is similar to high-performance computing and real-time analytics in that it generates a large amount of information in the hope of receiving quick feedback, which helps to produce a more complete picture of what is being monitored [17].

Hospital staff involved in patient care in relation to IoT- and AI-enabled devices can be classified into the following categories:

a) **Monitoring Staff:** A nurse or ward boy maintains all records in the traditional hospital environment. In smart hospitals, these tasks are performed by staff trained in surveillance-related activities by keeping an eye on IoT devices. If any nurse is going to miss any patient, then there should be a trigger-based system which is going alerts both the patient and nurse, and in case of any emergency, the higher authorities must be notified in a timely manner [18]. In this chain, if any breakpoint lies, then the performance of smart hospitals will suffer, as well as patient care. A standard model should be used to track and alert the system at any time if a failure occurs. Basically, supply chain management models can be used to make the system robust and trustworthy [19].
b) **Patient Record Keeping Staff:** IoT is increasing annually, especially in the healthcare sector. It influences the way hospitals operate, the way they treat patients, and the way they keep the record by providing many opportunities to improve the safety, security, efficiency, and usability of the data [20]. The better utilization of data makes it available for the long term in case it is needed for the diagnosis of a rare disease; therefore, keeping patient-related records in a digital manner is very important. As more devices are built into IoT and technology becomes smarter and more purposeful, IoT could become an integral part of the medical industry [21].
c) **Administration Staff:** Some staff may be involved in different duties related to record keeping through IoT-based devices such as

- Recording their sleep pattern
- Recording the bowel movement
- Recording the number of steps during walking
- Recording the HRV (Heart Rate Variability)
- Recording of ECHG pattern and its deviation.

In the case of the above reading, any missing recording is entered, which will create a catastrophic result in the end. If any negative result is happening or any fatal outcome is observed because of this mishandling of the data by the administration, it will be a trust issue that will phase out trust in these IoT-based devices. The trust that has been acquired through many years only because of great results and better diagnosis and its loss will again push the patient close to traditional doctor-based diagnosis [22].

d) **Automation Staff:** If for a particular patient, some extra or special care is needed, and at the same time, more sophisticated software is required, then automation staff must be ready to come up with the new idea all the time. During the pandemic time, many hurdles were observed while connecting the patient to doctors, and it became complex if any unknown requirement came, like mapping the oxygen level in a ward where most of the patients had similar kinds of problems. At that time, the automation team may be very useful, provided that the team is sufficiently trained and performs the duty without any errors [23].

e) **Feedback Department Staff:** There should be a dedicated team to record the outlier activities in patients who are being treated in the hospital and undergoing different procedures, in case any rare event is seen that should be recorded and this complete observation is only possible if we have a team. In rare diseases, some completely new unknown variables may be observed, which may a factor behind certain sudden issues in patient falling vitals [24].

f) **Research Staff:** If better efficiency is expected from IoT-based devices, the research team must work tirelessly. For example, faster diagnosis is expected from IoT-based devices; however, accurate results also matter for better treatment, so accuracy and fast detection are contradictory. How this tradeoff is balanced is determined by the research staff. Can we reduce the error occurrence in IoT devices, can we improve the detection rate, can defects be reduced, reducing the defects affects efficiency anyway, and how can the overall cost saving be increased, all of which can be answered if the hospital is equipped with research staff and who is well trained with the current latest technology so that any new or rare disease can be identified easily [25].

5.3 Doctor-Induced Risk

Currently, acute disease detection is efficiently achieved with the help of AI-based IoT devices, such as image processing or data analysis, medical imaging, or interpretation of images into malignant or healthy cells, all of which are possible when assisted by a trained doctor. Successful IoT projects require proper orchestration of the project and professionally trained medical practitioners; if we can train them in-house if needed, it will improve the positive outcome. For example, Kumar and Gandhi, proposed an IoT architecture with machine learning algorithms for the early detection of heart diseases. This includes a three-layer architecture for collecting sensor data from wearable devices, storing data in the cloud, and a regression-based heart disease prediction model. In this study, the biggest challenge is that if a doctor who is on duty is less aware of the IT-based services, then the diagnosis and treatment processes are affected. In addition to this case, there are other similar projects that are fully-fledged designed in AI-based algorithms, and their output, the result, etc., which are generated must match the knowledge of the user [26].

A fully-fledged trained medical practitioner will leverage security control too if any kind of attack is going to happen because of some vulnerability in the infrastructure. Another case of lack of awareness may cause a situation where the doctor is not trained enough to handle the different types of honeypots and accidentally shares the private information of the patient with some hacker over the Internet. To overcome these issues and challenges, regular training and mock drills must be organized in a timely manner in which outcome-based monitoring must be recorded, and demonstration by each user should be monitored to indicate how everyone is going to handle a practical situation [27]. Some internship-based training can be provided to doctors regarding compliance and regulation of the country in which AI-based healthcare devices have been installed. Each country has its own set of ordinances that must be followed: HIPAA and SOX [28].

Risks induced at the practitioner level in AI-based IoT devices can be classified into three categories:

i. **Diagnosis-induced risks:** Are machines going to replace doctors in hospitals in the future? This question may be difficult, but at this stage, the chances of saying 'Yes' is high because of the accuracy of the diagnosis. This is the first attribute asked by any person if he/she is suffering from a biological problem. The best part is that accuracy in disease detection devices is increasing day by day and year by year; however, this is not the case in humans (doctors). There may be several reasons behind the lack of updates, but devices have the major benefit of a global database, which is very useful in case any disease is observed for the first time in a group of people, especially in a developing country where there is a lack of resources and education.

The number of superspecialty hospitals remains very low. The second biggest challenge that was observed is that the detections are accurate; however, they are useful in preventing the spread of the disease. There are other challenging case scenarios in which serious research is required from academic fraternity and with medical experts. For instance, the detection of suicide and its prevention are still very difficult, even when considering the data of wearable devices recovered from the person. In his study, the author points out that we need to take a step back and gain a better understanding of the nature of human cognition, suicide, and machine learning to understand why this is the case and why humans are unable to effectively forecast suicide. Based on several research findings, it is still very inaccurate to detect and forecast human suicide. This explanation is straightforward. Therefore, it should refer to one or more objects. For instance, depression is a succinct justification for suicide [29, 30].

Second, the explanation was deterministic. This means that there is a single explanation that explains all or most of something. For instance, it is simple to see why depression is a major contributing factor to suicide. This straightforward explanatory approach is logical and effective. It helps us survive, reproduce, and get through our days. All of these quoted concepts are difficult to implement and process in IoT-based devices if they are implemented at a larger level [31].

ii. **Treatment-Induced Risk:** A flood of healthcare data, which can be described as the flow of streaming health-related data, is now being used to develop and create new AI applications that aim to enhance the efficacy and efficiency of patient care. Health related big data are accessible via sources such as electronic medical records (EMRs) and wearable health monitoring devices, or they can be stored in the cloud and used for a variety of novel analyses. The rise of AI in the era of big data can help doctors improve patient care, but at the same time, it poses the risk of disease misclassification if we do not have enough data related to a disease [32]. An expert says that AI is going to be future-ready, and its treatment will have a long-term impact on the healthcare industry;

however, the challenges remain strong because AI-based treatment-based decision-making is more accurate at the primary level but not in the majority. AI-based treatment-based classification and decision-making are suitable in areas such as radiology, pathology, and cardiology, where the signals acquired from humans are sufficient and are of very high quality; this high-quality data availability and a large amount of research in this field from a very long time make the decision-making more accurate, so the treatment is more accurate in terms of proper line length. In some other areas, such as oncology and ophthalmology, skin-based disease detection and treatment are still not very promising. One of the major issues in other challenging fields is the availability of standard electronic health record (EHR) or electronic medical record (EMR), and the lack of standardization in this direction has raised concerns regarding many issues [33]. Because of these uneven methodologies of designing health records, the storage pattern is also different at the hospital and country levels. Many conferences and meetings have been held globally at regular intervals; however, these are still improving. The use of a particular technology for a particular problem area is also a major concern, i.e., in the 38th Radiology Intersociety Conference held in the USA, it was decided that image processing techniques are best for cancer detection, and its methodologies were also decided. It can be said that the maturity of methodology can fix the rising challenges in this field which come as an outcome of long-term research [34].

iii. **Prognosis-Induced Risk:** AI can significantly contribute to the simplification of healthcare systems and advancements in medical research. Large datasets are required for Machine Learning (ML) and Deep Learning (DL) models to correctly categorize and forecast illnesses for a better prognosis. To achieve the best results, we need more data from more groups of individuals over a long period of time; thus, this is a problem of availability, patient permission, and privacy, which is currently not clearly defined. ML-based systems will continually improve if more data are supplied to their training set [35]. In many Asian and Middle Eastern countries, regulations related to data security and patient privacy are still nascent. In some cases, one country may have its own regulations for keeping patient-related records safely, either being used for sharing or for research purposes, so developing any new algorithm may require uniformity over the database and records; if this factor is not well addressed, it is a big challenge for better prognosis [36].

5.4 Patient-Based Risk

In 2001, the Institute of Medicine submitted a report on the issue of poor treatment of patients in superspecialty hospitals. The report was the outcome of long-term research in which several heterogeneous data were collected from various parts of the country and from various hospitals from different individuals i.e., medical practitioners, interns, medical experts, independent medical practitioners, registered physicians, specialist doctors, ward boys, and nurses [37]. This report raised a major question, are AI-based hospitals addressing the effect of the varying state of the disease if the demography of the patient varies? Do we really have a setup to record all these variations? In the pandemic phase, how many organizations were able to identify and study the different causative factors behind the varying parameters that ultimately cause the mutation in the virus? The organization must be equipped with AI-based services and must have facilities for this so that long-term research goals and better treatment can be achieved. However, several reports have created alert levels in this regard. A study conducted by 'Harris Interactive and ARiA Marketing, 2000' in the USA reported that 60% of US doctors have an advanced level of facility and services of patient care but do not report the cases that occurred because of medical errors and especially unsafe medical working conditions at the patient level. Another major issue that became the driving force behind the poor performance of patient care services is the lack of accommodation of patients' diverse demands and needs on hospital premises [38].

The National Center for Health Statistics study reported that most negligence and misdiagnosis occur when the patient is in a chronic condition. Doctors and researchers must make long-term plans with continuous to improve treatment when joint operations are required. Wagner *et al.* [39] stress in their research study the many factors why a multidisciplinary approach is needed to cure patients suffering from multiple diseases, and the diagnosis must be patient-centric where the patient is needed to stay for the long term in the n hospital itself for best result. Another challenge is the on-time reporting of disease spread by IoT devices if the patient has enabled it. In the USA, a serious concern has been raised over the alarming situation and its on-time reporting. A few wearables were able to send alerts in anthrax attacks; however, some wearables were not able to detect the issue and the cause behind them. In a survey conducted in the USA, statistics revealed that 25% of health staff workers were unable to find any alert from their linked patient in a biological weapon-based attack, in a separate controlled study [39]. These factors concluded that health environments must be more responsive to people with chronic diseases and focus on prevention, and health systems do not respond well to diverse cultural needs and different preferences of racial and ethnic groups [40].

5.5 Process-Based Risk

All IoT devices used in the healthcare industry had three categories (see Table 5.1).

Table 5.1 Different IoT devices and their use in healthcare.

S. no.	Type of IoT device	Related body part	Category of sensor used	Product name
1.	Pulse Sensor	Heart	Light sensor	Zacurate Pro Series 500DL
2.	Heartbeat Sensor	Heart	Light sensor/photo optic sensor	Garmin 010-12955-00 HRM-PRO
3.	Blood Pressure Sensor	Human veins	Pressure sensor	Vernier BPS-BTA
4.	Heart Rate Monitoring Sensor	Heart	Optical sensor	Polar H9 Heart Rate Sensor
5.	Respiratory Sensor Device	Lungs and ribcages	Girth sensor	SRP Respiratory sensor
6.	Nasal Airflow Sensor Device	Lungs/ Breathing	Temperature Sensor	ThermiSense Interface Box

(Continued)

Table 5.1 Different IoT devices and their use in healthcare. (*Continued*)

S. no.	Type of IoT device	Related body part	Category of sensor used	Product name
7.	IoT-coupled EEG sensor Device	Brain	Electrical sensor	NeuroSky MindWave Mobile 2 EEG Sensor
8.	IoT-based ECG Device	Heart	Wet sensor/ Electrical sensor	Robodo AD8232 Ecg Module AD8232
9.	IoT based EMG	Muscle	Wet sensor/ Electrical sensor	Robocraze EMGSEN EMG Sensor
10.	IoT-based Blood Glucose Monitoring device	Blood	Enzymatic Amperometric Glucose Biosensors	FreeStyle Libre Glucose Monitoring System
11.	Brain-wave Sensor IoT equipped	Brain	Electrical sensor	NeuroSky MindWave Mobile BrainWave
12.	IoT based Skin Sensor	Skin	Wet sensor/ Electrical sensor	Robocraze GSR skin current sensor
13.	Blood Saturation Monitoring Device/Pulse Oximeter	Blood vessel	Optical sensor	Phillips Oxy Sensor
14.	IoT based Body movement cum Motion Sensor	Body limb, eye pupil	Optical Sensor	Perenio wireless motion sensor
15.	Eye Movement Occular Communication Device	Eye	IR sensor	Robocraze Eyeblink sensor

(*Continued*)

Table 5.1 Different IoT devices and their use in healthcare. (*Continued*)

S. no.	Type of IoT device	Related body part	Category of sensor used	Product name
16.	Human Body Temperature Sensor—Contact Based	Skin	Thermal sensor	Thermal Sensor D6T-1A-01
17.	Human Body Temperature Sensor—Non-Contact Based	No Contact with the human body	Image sensor	BOSCH GTC 400 C – Thermal Camera
18.	Sleep Monitoring Finger Ring	Finger/Thumb	Pressure/Thermal sensor	GO2SLEEP Ring
19.	Stress Level Monitoring Finger Ring	Finger/Thumb	Pressure/Thermal sensor	Oura Ring
20.	Sleep Apnea Screening device	Finger/Thumb	Pressure/Thermal sensor	Philips Alice PDx Portable Sleep Diagnostic System
21.	Step Counter for Activity Tracking	Finger/Thumb	Pressure/Thermal sensor	ThreeH 3D Pedometer
22.	Finger Gloves IoT equipped	Fingers	Flex sensor/ Ultrasonic sensor	Neofect Smart Glove
23.	Smart IoT-based Socks	Leg	Thermal/Pressure sensor	Sensoria® Smart Socks
24.	Smart Helmet	Head	Thermal/Pressure sensor	Proxgy Smart Helmet
25.	Smart Chest Band	Chest	Thermal/Pressure sensor	Atlas chest band
26.	Smart Waist Band	Waist	Gyroscope sensor	TANTRA Zipper Smart Sports Running Waist Belt

(*Continued*)

Table 5.1 Different IoT devices and their use in healthcare. (*Continued*)

S. no.	Type of IoT device	Related body part	Category of sensor used	Product name
27.	Smart Clothes	Full Body	Thermal/Pressure/ Skin sensor	Fibocom smart cloths
28.	Smart Cap	Head	Thermal/Image sensor/Camera	Qualcomm Smart Cap
29.	Smart Jacket (health monitoring)	The upper part of the body	Thermal/Image sensor/ Gyroscope based sensor	Dainese D-air® airbag
30.	Smart Shoes	Foot	Thermal/Image sensor/ Gyroscope based sensor	Salted Smart Insole, IOT-Based Smart Wearable Shoes

a) **Connect:** This section identifies the approach to connect an IoT device to the human body and its other end to the Internet. Different types of IoT devices have different and standard ways of connecting such that data can be transferred smoothly [41]. The first part connects the device to the human body, and the following chart depicts the different devices and their ways of connecting to the human body.

b) **Care:** Data management was performed in this section. It deals with the following steps:

   a. **Collection of data:** In this process, the heterogeneous nature of the devices and the mode of receiving data invite risk while collecting the data. Billions of devices share private data. This sharing of data involves multiple stakeholders, such as the government, independent users, business organizations, and public authorities. Many times, the risk of loss of private data and loss of its attributes occurs because there is no standard protocol or guideline at the global level, which can bring homogeneity in the data collection method and minimize the risk. Other types of risks involve the transmission of data and encryption while uploading it to a third-party cloud. The data should not be transmitted as plain text. The third type of risk evolves with communication channels. Assaults can be launched by exploiting vulnerability using the channels that interface with IoT gadgets. This poses a security risk to the complete framework and makes the IoT device a potential contender for spoofing and denial-of-service (DoS) assaults. These threats lay the foundation for an unsteady-organized surface, and the risk is at the infrastructure level [42].

b. **Preprocessing of data:** Data preprocessing and data cleaning is necessary before making it ready for analysis to make any conclusions. To obtain a better insight into the data points, their distribution can only be determined if all flaws in the data are successfully completed [43]. Flaws such as missing data, distortion, redundancy, inconsistency, and other ambiguities must be removed before processing; otherwise, they may cause inherent vulnerabilities in the IoT system. Any IoT device can provide the best result when the imbibed algorithm learns from properly distributed data. The presence of flaws in the dataset can be rectified automatically using validation and authorization processing when the data are being generated. However, the following methods are used:

    i. **Data Transformation:** Risk may again rise in this step depending on how the IoT device collects the data. A healthcare IoT device may collect the data in an analogous format through its different sensors or transducers, so assurance of availability of all types of data that were collected must be ensured while transforming the data into digital format. Four cornerstones must be fulfilled: device type, strategy, objective, and method of collection of data, which refers to the type of device it is, i.e., the type of sensor used in that and what type of result we expect after processing the data collected from that device and initially what type of communication channel was used to receive the data (it ensures the sanctity of data while transforming). Considering all these factors, we can minimize the risk associated with this phase [44].

ii. **Data Reduction:** Depending on the size of the data, our algorithm and its learning ability data must be resized to ensure that each attribute of the data is present, and no null data should be recorded. Many methodologies must be analyzed before applying them for data reduction and ensuring that no small fraction of the data will be missed. In healthcare, very small deviation-based data points may be recorded, i.e., movement of the eye pupil in sleep monitoring devices; therefore, data reduction must ensure that the quality of the data is not compromised while lowering the risk through the reduction process.

iii. **Data Standardization:** Organizations must optimize the risk instead of lowering it if no standard policy is available for transforming the data into a standard format. In the market, many vendors are available with multiple products that are equipped with the ability to generate different types of data before storing the data locally or into cloud storage; data must be refined with the help of standard methods. In healthcare-based datasets, there may be many issues, i.e., artifacts, noise, bogus data, spikes, etc., so the risk is involved in analyzing these datasets if the quality of standard parameters is not improved. Data analysis can only provide the best results if standard data policies, rules, and standards are implemented, such as the use of standard encryption standards, hashing, authentication schemes, and other security mechanisms. The use of standard regulations to keep the data in its best form also helps in its further processing and usage in fog computing, cloud computing, etc. [45].

iv. **Data Cleaning:** Multiple vendors, different types of devices, different types of diseases and their related data, heterogeneity in data, complexity in the available data, dependency in the available data among several parameters, and their primary key deduced from attributes are among the several factors that must be addressed while cleaning the data so that it can be used for better analysis and making it ready for the next process. To overcome these challenges, standard models must be used to clean the data, which further minimizes the risk. To avoid risk in the future, the IoT device must have a mechanism to receive data in clean form while collecting it from the human body. It may include error detection and error correction, and in some advanced IoT devices, error correction is also possible so that the occurrence can be minimized. Some common issues that were addressed at the primary level to minimize the risk are Missing Data, Partial Values, Null Values, Redundant Duplicate Data, Outliers Present in Data, Erroneous Data, and the Presence of Irrelevant Data.

v. **Data Integration:** Machine cannot learn in the same way how the human learns, so there are two types of challenges observed here—first is the collection of data from the primary device in a standard form, and the second challenge is making the data ready for the second process in an interoperable format so that it can be used in the cloud, fog, or other setups.

c. **Storage of the Data:** What should be the standard way to store health-related data, what should be the most scientific way to segregate the data according to its pattern, what should be the appropriate authentication scheme, and how should multi-authentication be deployed? These are certain questions for which a long-term research-based study is required and no objective answers can be provided. In most cases, the data are not directly stored in the main devices; instead, data are stored at the sub-system level, where it may be a cloud or fog computing device. Edge computing-based services and other third-party companies do not directly communicate with storage; sometimes, third- and fourth-party applications are used for communication and file exchange. Therefore, lack of standard protocols poses the risk of data leakage, third-party insecurity, and lack of appropriate encryption standards. A good example of a third-party service is the service of a certificate authority (CA) for third-party validation of all types of data that are being exchanged. The data may be signed with a secure certificate [46].

d. **Normalization of Data:** All relevant data must be ingested well after a transaction for better data analytics, and for a successful transaction, data must be normalized properly. Alert and notification must be available with the system in case of any failure or anomalous behavior observed in any transaction. To minimize the risk related to data behavior, a reverse engineering approach must be used for the inspection of tampered data, errant activity, missing values, corrupted data, or any rogue device, which is a source of that type of data.

e. **Processing of Data:** To make a sensible decision, the data collected from different sensors that are being generated at a very high pace must be processed at the same pace. A high volume of raw data must be processed.

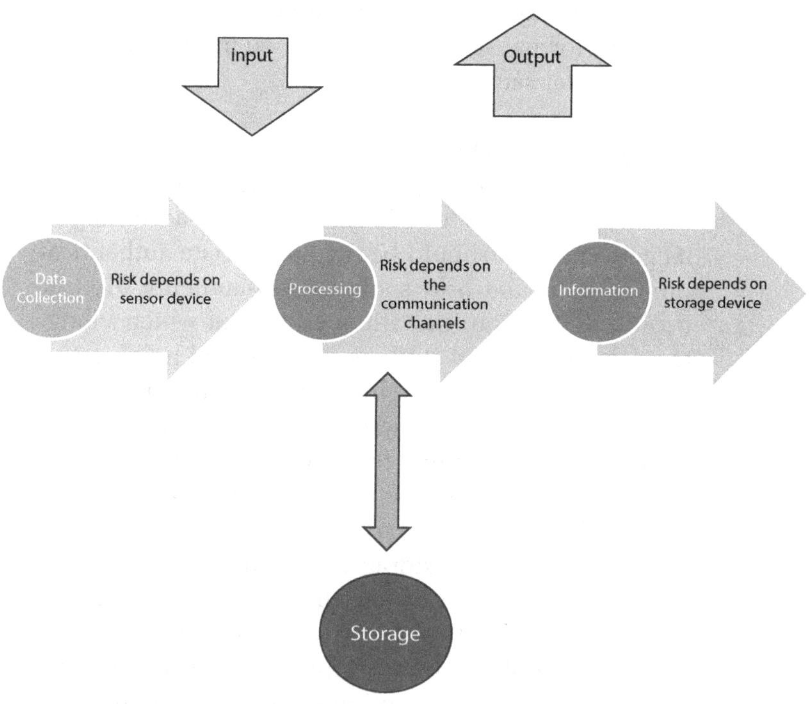

Figure 5.4 Processing in IoT devices.

Raw data are available in many forms, so the risk lies here. All data must be properly preprocessed to ensure uniformity in type. Let us see how data processing works (see Figure 5.4)

In the above diagram, the processing phase of IoT devices is depicted, where the first stage is the collection of data. Data are collected or received in raw format, after which they are transformed into the required format as per the channel being used. Multiple types of sensors collect data, i.e., temperature and pressure sensors, and the risk lies in these devices, as discussed earlier. The second phase involves the transfer of data through different communication channels. In some IoT devices, data are stored first in a compressed format, and the risk lies here. Depending on the type and media, different compression algorithms are used, which may cause insecurity in data storage, i.e., NRZ and RZ. format. In the last phase, the output is received, and the decision for detection and prediction is made. The output must be in a readable format so that the medical consultant/doctor can make the correct decision. In some automated devices where there is no need for a consultant, the output must be presented in such a manner that the end user can reach the correct conclusion. The major risks that lie in this phase are as follows:

1. Cost Management
2. Data Management
3. Insecure environment
4. Insecure channel
5. Incompetent data storage
6. Fragile Data Recovery
7. Poor quality
8. Non-uniform data format
9. Leaky Deployment Process
10. Third-party services.

5.6 Technology-Based Risk

As reported by different studies, the risk in the healthcare industry and in medicine can be classified as "technology-based risk."

1. **Technology-Based Risk:** When the Internet was not readily available, traditional healthcare management struggled with

its inherent problems and challenges, such as the availability of instruments, availability of doctors, updating of knowledge with current ongoing research for better diagnosis, and proper implementation. However, the healthcare industry uses different types of devices that involve the two major elements of IT. All healthcare-based devices supporting the Internet of Things (IoT) have enabled remote medical monitoring through the use of server-based technology, keeping patients safe and healthy and expanding the possibilities and opportunities for doctors to deliver world-class care. By facilitating quicker and more effective interactions between patients and doctors, the integration of IoT and AI into healthcare services has also increased patient involvement and happiness [47]. Remote patient health monitoring can also assist in reducing hospital stays and avoiding readmissions. The Internet of Things will also have a significant influence on lowering healthcare costs and increasing patient outcomes. According to all research studies and reviews, IoT is unquestionably changing the healthcare sector while reshaping the working relationships between its stakeholders, including those between doctors and patients.

Technology-based risks can be classified into the following categories:

1. **Data Security-Related Risks:** When discuss data security-based risk in IoT devices, data must be secured first in all Internet-enabled devices. These can be classified into two categories:
   a. **Privacy-Based Risk:** Privacy is a major issue in the case of medical devices as many malefactors may attack devices to steal the private data of patients. Strong privacy-compliant acts must be enforced to protect the personal data of users on devices. i.e., HIPAA and HITEC. Different types of attacks have been reported to steal confidential data from hospitals and data common to many devices. In a very famous TV show 'Homeland' which was aired in the USA, a hacker described anonymously that once he had a plan to disrupt the working of the pacemaker of a former vice president of UA as a part of the plan in assassination attack. If an investigation is done, it simply reveals that the confidential information

related to the vice president's health was leaked somewhere, which must be stopped. Either from devices or hospital staff, privacy is always under attack, considering both outsider and insider attacks. A new term was coined last decade 'Medjacking' about a process in which hackers tamper with medical devices to harm an individual by mis-utilizing private data. Some major recent cases have been reported related to privacy attacks on IoT devices in the healthcare industry [48].

i. **Mirai Botnet attack:** A botnet-based attack was used to exploit the vulnerabilities in digital cameras and DVR players in hospital premises in 2016 in the USA reported by Cyber Management Alliance Group. This attack searches for devices in which the default passwords are not changed to either a standalone PC or a PC in the network [49].
ii. **Verkada Hack:** Verkada, the name of cloud-based surveillance was exploited using credential theft over the network in the year 2012 reported by many news channels. The live feed of more than 10,000 cameras was captured unethically, and later, data were available for sale on the dark web [50].
iii. **HIMSS ARMIS Case:** Armis, the leading asset security company in the USA, reported in the year 2022 that in many hospitals, IoMT devices are vulnerable to malicious activity in clinical environments. Nurse call, infusion pump, medication dispensing, and VOIP devices are the most vulnerable systems. These figures provide a clear picture of the difficulties that healthcare organizations face worldwide. As healthcare businesses struggle with a lack of fully trained healthcare professionals in all in-house services, technological advancements are crucial for enhancing the speed and quality of medical care delivery for patients. However, as healthcare becomes more linked, there is greater potential for an attack on data and related items [51].
iv. **Infusion Pump Vulnerability Case:** The Food and Drug Administration (FDA) reported that most infusion pumps have one or more of the 70 additional IoT device vulnerabilities and 40 known inherent

security flaws induced by manufacturing companies. More than 50% of the infusion pumps under analysis were exposed to two serious flaws that were made public in 2019. Additionally, infusion pumps and other medical equipment are even more vulnerable to exploitation due to insufficient network segmentation and lack of application of fundamental security best practices.

v. **Wannacry Attack:** In 2017, a ransomware attack was reported, which encrypted data on at least 75,000 systems across 99 nations. Payments were required for access to be granted. Russia and other European nations have suffered the most. The threat is still present even if it looks like the spread of the ransomware known as WannaCry, and its variations have halted [52].

From various studies, there are six major devices that have been classified as the most vulnerable:

i. Infusion and Insulin Pumps
ii. Security Cameras
iii. Smart Pens
iv. Implantable Cardiac Devices
v. Wireless Vital Monitors
vi. Wearable Devices
vii. Thermometers and Temperature Sensors

Different types of attacks have been reported in this category:

i. Routing Attack
ii. Router Attack
iii. Brute Force Attack
iv. Dictionary Attack
v. DoS Attack
vi. DDoS Attack
vii. Replay Attack
viii. Select and Forward Attack
ix. Medjacking Attack
x. Fingerprint Attack

xi. Location-based Attack.
xii. Sensor Attack

b. **Infrastructure-Based Risk:** Lack of standardization in IoT is a major security issue. There is no standard policy or protocol on how a particular device will be deployed in a healthcare-related environment or in hospital premises. Many vendors have their own standards that are not approved and validated by any third party at the global level. It is challenging to guarantee the compatibility and interoperability among them because there are many various devices, protocols, and platforms. Attackers may be able to exploit these vulnerabilities. The industry standards for IoT platforms, protocols, and devices can aid in ensuring compatibility and interoperability. Standards for communication protocols, data privacy, and device security may fall under this category. IoMT systems and AI-enabled devices in the healthcare industry may be able to achieve certain security requirements with the aid of certification from a global standard company or regulatory authority. This can assist organizations in discovering devices that may be more vulnerable to attacks and increase their trust in the security of the devices they use.

2. **Network Security-Related Risks:** Either it is a wired or wireless network, and vulnerabilities at the network level pose a major scope of exploitation in case of an attack launched over it. When data are transmitted encrypted from sensor to sensor or from a sensor to a private location, the wireless network is unable to identify new security concerns. IoT devices frequently use unprotected networks to connect to the Internet, leaving them open to assault. For instance, a hacker may acquire sensitive information by intercepting interactions between an IoT device and the internet [53].

In addition, unprotected networks can be exploited to target other networked devices. The common risks are as follows:

i. Unsecure communications
ii. Lack of encryption

iii. Lack of awareness
iv. Lack of digital divide
v. Lack of proper training
vi. Lack of mock drills
vii. Lack of economical products
viii. Unsecure devices
ix. Use of old devices
x. Lack of deployment strategy

Solutions: The following solutions to improve the security controls in IoMT devices at a better network level are:

i. **Use of Secure Network Protocol:** By adopting secure network protocols such as VPN and HTTPS, data transfer on many devices via various protocols may be rendered safe, resilient, and vulnerability-free. Virtual private networks (VPNs) may be used to encrypt communication between IoT devices and the Internet, making it more difficult for hackers to steal sensitive data. Hospitals must have a solid policy that is strictly adhered to, with the aim of enabling VPN-based services and communications.
ii. **Use of Firewall:** The implementation of secure network protocols such as VPN and HTTPS can help to ensure safe data transport. To make it more difficult for hackers to steal data, virtual private networks (VPNs) may be used to encrypt connections between IoT devices and the Internet.
iii. **Use of Better Identity and Access management:** These days, many businesses need two-factor authentication for network logins, as well as for email logins and other log-in-required devices. To join a system or Wi-Fi network, users might also need to enter a code they receive by text message or another manner in addition to their login and password.
iv. **Use Automation and Analysis Tools:** The system collects data from network devices, endpoint logs, and threat intelligence feeds to identify security events, policy violations, fraudulent activity, and other risks. Security specialists can immediately detect and respond to these solutions because of a high level of automation, which accelerates the reaction time.

Non-Technology-Based Risks: Cyber security and data protection are not always about technology, but also cover issues that can be termed as non-technology affairs. Non-compliance-based risks can be categorized as such. There are several issues that are not directly related to core computing-related items, regardless of whether IoT devices are implemented, usage patterns, lack of strict policy, compliance with rules and regulations, lack of global standards and ordinances, and enforcement of acts formed by government agencies. In the case of data security, compliance with the local laws of the country, awareness of staff, lack of a plan, and lack of business continuity planning. These major areas must be addressed immediately by different bodies that work in the field of IoT in the healthcare industry [54]. In some cases, social engineering has been reported as a major technique for stealing personal data in the healthcare network industry. Non-technology-based security risks in IoT devices can be categorized as follows:

a. **Compliance-Based Risks:** Compliance deals with the law that must be followed for each entity, either a device or an individual who is involved with IoT devices in healthcare organizations. Depending on the environment and country, many regulations and laws must be enforced when the compliance term comes into the picture. Compliance-based risks can be categorized into the following:

i. **Policy-Based Risks:** Almost all major developed countries in the world have a policy document for implementing any IoT device for medical organizations, manufacturing companies have to follow these policy guidelines. Many nations, including the US, South Korea, and China, have taken the lead in getting ready to benefit from the policies drafted, especially for the Internet of Things. The objectives of the "Value Up" and "Cost Down" models should be the only ones on which the Internet of Things strategy should be based. There must be a policy for monitoring patients' vital signs, such as subtle changes in heart rate, breathing, temperature, and heart condition, as well as for preventive warnings on the early onset of life-threatening conditions such as pneumonia (in young children), as well as inside hospitals and at remote patient locations such as nursing homes and ambulances. In short, these are the different major areas in which each organization should implement policy documents for the better success of IoT devices:

i. Standardization Policy of instruments
ii. Policy for Use of standard communication and protocols
iii. Standards for internal and external cloud communication
iv. Policy for International standards for data generation, collection, and data traceability.
v. Policy for Standard for energy consumption by each device
vi. Policy for Standards for safety (for instance, if gadgets or sensors are applied to people for the collection of data)
vii. Policy Security standards data storage and data use by external and internal users.
viii. Policy for use of open-source technology.
ix. Policy for Architecture Technology–IoT architecture, platform interoperability.
x. Policy for Material Technology—Silicon, semiconductor manufacturing, etc.

ii. Operation Risk

b. **Non-Compliance-Based Risks:** Protecting personal data and protected health information (PHI) is essential for preserving healthcare cybersecurity, especially as cyberattacks continue to grow in size and sophistication. However, Operational Technology (OT) systems are also ubiquitous, from hospital parking lot gates to devices within the building, and they must be given the same priority. Operational technology systems in healthcare facilities, which regulate, monitor, and safeguard equipment, processes, and operational environments, especially IoT devices while they are at work, are sometimes disregarded; however, they are just as important for maintaining data security, building a positive reputation, and even ensuring staff safety. A white paper by the International Society of Automation (ISA) outlined the primary reasons why IT and OT security were traditionally seen as distinct. First, because OT systems are not often connected to the Internet, IT environments have been the primary target for cyber threat actors. Additionally,

OT settings were historically disconnected from networks, and IT prioritized data security over the availability of physical devices [55]. The majority of cases can be classified into two categories:

i. **Physical Security-Based Risks:** The physical security of IoT devices deployed in the healthcare industry must be ensured by organizations, including prohibiting access to hardware components and ensuring that only authenticated access is permitted. The physical security sector is also being improved through technological advancements in the field of surveillance-based devices, such as integrated sensors, cameras, and access systems. Hardware and network infrastructure security issues have driven the market's evolution. Growth is also being stimulated by the usage of the cloud and a rise in investments in hybrid solutions for real-time monitoring is observed; however, we are still far behind in terms of robust security. For example, although 802.1x is frequently advocated and used as a secure IoT solution for communication in many healthcare organizations; it has been reported by many independent surveying security firms that in 802.1x, the right and appropriate deployment is more important than whether or how 802.1x is being used. Any networked system anywhere in the organization is vulnerable to intrusion at any moment. For a short time, some in-house access control-based security controls may safeguard that data and take control of their relationship with IoT, which can only be achieved by employing a dedicated security company that manages and protects physical security using smart technology, as opposed to allowing the spread of IoT to govern the assets of the organization. These are the areas that must be considered for better physical security:

   i. Building Infrastructure
   ii. IT Infrastructure
   iii. Inventory Management Equipment

   Individual components of traditional security systems can be programmed to communicate freely and used to develop automated incident responses to carry out remote administrative tasks and ensure that teams always have access to actionable system data that are being communicated so that we make the security robust in IoT-based devices.

ii. **Lack of Emergency Response Team (ERT):** All healthcare organizations must have an emergency response team on hand given their ability to improve public safety and crisis management initiatives in case of any emergency. They contribute to lowering the risk to residents and minimizing the effects of calamities on all important assets of organizations. Additionally, by facilitating improved coordination and better communication between various agencies, the integration of IoT devices and systems can enhance the overall efficiency and efficacy of emergency services in that health setup. In an independent study, Damasevicius *et al.* [55] reported the following benefits of ERT:

    i. Early detection of the disasters
    ii. Automated response in observed issues
    iii. Minimizing the minor risks in follow-up schedules
    iv. Improvement in the Reliability of the devices
    v. Improved communications
    vi. Availability of instantaneous technical expertise
    vii. Improvement in the overall performance of organizations.

The emergency response team concentrates on five scenarios: industrial accidents, medical emergencies, public safety, and disaster response.

5.7 Conclusion

To ensure that no systems are neglected and exposed to possible risks in healthcare-based organizations and to provide better services to patients by minimizing all types of risks, all IoT devices must first be tracked and regularly monitored. To reduce the chance of credentials being stolen, the internal staff must update and maintain all devices, and passwords must be regularly reviewed and altered. To lessen the possibility of human mistakes resulting in significant data breaches at any layer of device communication or at the human resource level, staff training should be consistent and required. Additionally, sophisticated cyber security measures, such as network segmentation, data encryption, multi-factor authentication, and continuous data protection, should be implemented, and they should be regularly checked in a timely manner. All modern healthcare organizations are quickly adopting IoT security systems as a necessary component because they offer IT and security teams efficient, informed safeguards against typical physical and cyber threats while also enhancing incident reaction times and streamlining operations in most services; thus, at any point in time, security should not be weak. The year 2023 brings a wide range of issues for cyber security globally, reported in all organizations dealing with IoT services in medical-related operations. Organizations must prioritize and invest in thorough cybersecurity plans to protect their digital assets, because cyberattacks are becoming more complicated, IoT devices are proliferating, there is a skills shortage, and regulatory compliance and data privacy are essential.

References

1. Ghosh, A., Chakraborty, D., Law, A., Artificial intelligence in the Internet of Things. *CAAI Trans. Intell. Technol.*, 3, 4, 208–218, 2018, https://doi.org/10.1049/trit.2018.1008.
2. What is IoT Security? Definition and Challenges of IoT Security. (n.d.). Fortinet. https://www.fortinet.com/resources/cyberglossary/iot-security retrived on January 14, 2024.
3. Di Pascale, E., Macaluso, I., Nag, A., Kelly, M.C., Doyle, L., The Network As a Computer: A Framework for Distributed Computing Over IoT Mesh Networks. *IEEE Internet Things J.*, 5, 3, 2107–2119, 2018, https://doi.org/10.1109/jiot.2018.2823978.
4. Xu, T., Wendt, J.B., Potkonjak, M., Security of IoT systems: Design challenges and opportunities, in: *2014 IEEE/ACM International Conference on Computer-Aided Design (ICCAD)*, 2014, https://doi.org/10.1109/iccad.2014.7001385.
5. Chiang, M. and Zhang, T., Fog and IoT: An Overview of Research Opportunities. *IEEE Internet Things J.*, 3, 6, 854–864, 2016, https://doi.org/10.1109/jiot.2016.2584538.
6. Khan, M.A. and Salah, K., IoT security: Review, blockchain solutions, and open challenges. *Future Gener. Comput. Syst.*, *82*, 395–411, 2018, https://doi.org/10.1016/j.future.2017.11.022.
7. Al-Fuqaha, A., Guizani, M., Mohammadi, M., Aledhari, M., Ayyash, M., Internet of Things: A Survey on Enabling Technologies, Protocols, and

Applications. *IEEE Commun. Surv. Tutorials*, *17*, 4, 2347–2376, 2015, https://doi.org/10.1109/comst.2015.2444095.

8. Mohanta, B.K., Jena, D., Satapathy, U., Patnaik, S., Survey on IoT security: Challenges and solution using machine learning, artificial intelligence and blockchain technology. *Internet Things*, *11*, 100227, 2020, https://doi.org/10.1016/j.iot.2020.100227.
9. Zhang, H., Li, J., Wen, B., Xun, Y., Liu, J., Connecting Intelligent Things in Smart Hospitals Using NB-IoT. *IEEE Internet Things J.*, *5*, 3, 1550–1560, 2018, https://doi.org/10.1109/jiot.2018.2792423.
10. Hussain, A., Wenbi, R., Da Silva, A.L., Nadher, M., Mudhish, M., Health and emergency-care platform for the elderly and disabled people in the Smart City. *J. Syst. Softw.*, *110*, 253–263, 2015, https://doi.org/10.1016/j.jss.2015.08.041.
11. Yang, Y., Wu, L., Yin, G., Li, L., Zhao, H., A Survey on Security and Privacy Issues in Internet-of-Things. *IEEE Internet Things J.*, *4*, 5, 1250–1258, 2017, https://doi.org/10.1109/jiot.2017.2694844.
12. Kumar, S.A., Vealey, T., Srivastava, H., Security in Internet of Things: Challenges, solutions and future directions, in: *2016 49th Hawaii International Conference on System Sciences (HICSS)*, Koloa, HI, USA, pp. 5772–5781, 2016, doi: 10.1109/HICSS.2016.714.
13. Catarinucci, L., De Donno, D., Mainetti, L., Palano, L., Patrono, L., Stefanizzi, M.L., Tarricone, L., An IoT-Aware Architecture for Smart Healthcare Systems. *IEEE Internet Things J.*, *2*, 6, 515–526, 2015, https://doi.org/10.1109/jiot.2015.2417684.
14. Kang, S., Baek, H., Jung, E., Hwang, H., Yoo, S., Survey on the demand for adoption of Internet of Things (IoT)-based services in hospitals: Investigation of nurses' perception in a tertiary university hospital. *Appl. Nurs. Res.*, *47*, 18–23, 2019, https://doi.org/10.1016/j.apnr.2019.03.005.
15. Zhang, H., Na, J., Zhang, B., Autonomous Internet of Things (IoT) data reduction based on adaptive threshold. *Sensors (Basel)*, 23, 23, 9427, 26 Nov 2023. doi: 10.3390/s23239427. PMID: 38067800; PMCID: PMC10708721.
16. Perera, C., Liu, C.H., Jayawardena, S., Chen, M., A Survey on Internet of Things from Industrial Market Perspective. *IEEE Access*, *2*, 1660–1679, 2014, https://doi.org/10.1109/access.2015.2389854.
17. de Souza Cimino, L. *et al.*, IoT and HPC integration: Revision and perspectives, in: *2017 VII Brazilian Symposium on Computing Systems Engineering (SBESC)*, Curitiba, PR, Brazil, pp. 132–139, 2017, doi: 10.1109/SBESC.2017.24.
18. Dang, L.M., Piran, M.J., Han, D., Min, K., Moon, H., A Survey on Internet of Things and Cloud Computing for Healthcare. *Electronics*, *8*, 7, 768, 2019, https://doi.org/10.3390/electronics8070768.
19. Das, R., Tuna, A., Demirel, S.T., Yurdakul, M.K., A Survey on the Internet of Things Solutions for the Elderly and Disabled: Applications, Prospects, and

Challenges. *Int. J. Comput. Netw. Appl.*, *4*, 3, 1, 2017, https://doi.org/10.22247/ijcna/2017/49023.
20. Shanin, F. *et al.*, Portable and centralised e-Health record system for patient monitoring using Internet of Things (IoT), in: *2018 International CET Conference on Control, Communication, and Computing (IC4), Thiruvananthapuram,* India, pp. 165–170, 2018, doi: 10.1109/CETIC4.2018.8530891.
21. Riad, K., Hamza, R., Huang, T., Sensitive and Energetic IoT Access Control for Managing Cloud Electronic Health Records. *IEEE Access*, *7*, 86384–86393, 2019, https://doi.org/10.1109/access.2019.2926354.
22. Verma, P. and Sood, S., Cloud-centric IoT based disease diagnosis healthcare framework. *J. Parallel Distrib. Comput.*, *116*, 27–38, 2017, https://doi.org/10.1016/j.jpdc.2017.11.018.
23. Abdulkareem, K.H., Mohammed, M.A., Zaki, S.A., Arif, M., Geman, O., Gupta, D., Khanna, A., Realizing an Effective COVID-19 Diagnosis System Based on Machine Learning and IoT in Smart Hospital Environment. *IEEE Internet Things J.*, *8*, 21, 15919–15928, 2021, https://doi.org/10.1109/jiot.2021.3050775.
24. Haleem, A., Javaid, M., Khan, I., Internet of things (IoT) applications in orthopaedics. *J. Clin. Orthop. Trauma*, *11*, S105–S106, 2020, https://doi.org/10.1016/j.jcot.2019.07.003.
25. Islam, S.K., Kwak, D., Kabir, M.H., Hossain, M., Kwak, K.S., The Internet of Things for Health Care: A Comprehensive Survey. *IEEE Access*, *3*, 678–708, 2015, https://doi.org/10.1109/access.2015.2437951.
26. Darwish, S., Nouretdinov, I., Wolthusen, S.D., Towards Composable Threat Assessment for Medical IoT (MIoT). *Proc. Comput. Sci.*, *113*, 627–632, 2017, https://doi.org/10.1016/j.procs.2017.08.314.
27. Safi, M., Dadkhah. S., Shoeleh, F., Mahdikhani, H., Molyneaux, H., Ghorbani, A.A., A survey on IoT profiling, fingerprinting, and identification. *ACM Trans. Internet Things,* 3, 4, Article 26 (November 2022), 39 pages, 2022. https://doi.org/10.1145/3539736
28. Abdul-Ghani, H.A., Nijdam, N.A., Collen, A., Konstantas, D., A Study on Security and Privacy Guidelines, Countermeasures, Threats: IoT Data at Rest Perspective. *Symmetry*, *11*, 6, 774, 2019, https://doi.org/10.3390/sym11060774.
29. Sundaravadivel, P., Kougianos, E., Mohanty, S.P., Ganapathiraju, M.K., Everything you wanted to know about smart health care: Evaluating the different technologies and components of the Internet of Things for better health. *IEEE Consum. Electron. Mag.*, 7, 1, 18–28, Jan. 2018, doi: 10.1109/MCE.2017.2755378.
30. Nock, M.K., Borges, G., Bromet, E.J., Cha, C.B., Kessler, R.C., Lee, S., Suicide and Suicidal Behavior. *Epidemiol. Rev.*, *30*, 1, 133–154, 2008, https://doi.org/10.1093/epirev/mxn002.
31. Wulz, A.R., Law, R., Wang, J., Wolkin, A.F., Leveraging data science to enhance suicide prevention research: A literature review. *Inj. Prev.: Journal*

of the International Society for Child and Adolescent Injury Prevention, 28, 1, 74–80, 2022. https://doi.org/10.1136/injuryprev-2021-044322
32. Farouk, A., Alahmadi, A.A., Ghose, S., Mashatan, A., Blockchain platform for industrial healthcare: Vision and future opportunities. *Comput. Commun.*, *154*, 223–235, 2020, https://doi.org/10.1016/j.comcom.2020.02.058.
33. Dimitrov, D.S., Medical Internet of Things and Big Data in Healthcare. *Healthcare Inf. Res.*, *22*, 3, 156, 2016, https://doi.org/10.4258/hir.2016.22.3.156.
34. Kruskal, J.B., Berkowitz, S.A., Geis, J.R., Kim, W., Nagy, P., Dreyer, K.J., Big Data and Machine Learning—Strategies for Driving This Bus: A Summary of the 2016 Intersociety Summer Conference. *J. Am. Coll. Radiol.*, *14*, 6, 811–817, 2017, https://doi.org/10.1016/j.jacr.2017.02.019.
35. Pathinarupothi, R.K., Durga, P., Rangan, E.S., IoT-Based Smart Edge for Global Health: Remote Monitoring with Severity Detection and Alerts Transmission. *IEEE Internet Things J.*, *6*, 2, 2449–2462, 2019, https://doi.org/10.1109/jiot.2018.2870068.
36. Thibaud, M., Chi, H., Zhou, W., Piramuthu, S., Internet of Things (IoT) in high-risk Environment, Health and Safety (EHS) industries: A comprehensive review. *Decis. Support Syst.*, *108*, 79–95, 2018, https://doi.org/10.1016/j.dss.2018.02.005.
37. Dwivedi, A.D., Srivastava, G., Dhar, S., Singh, R., A Decentralized Privacy-Preserving Healthcare Blockchain for IoT. *Sensors*, *19*, 2, 326, 2019, https://doi.org/10.3390/s19020326.
38. Van Hee, K.M., Schonenberg, H., Serebrenik, A., Sidorova, N., Van Der Werf, J.M.E.M., Adaptive Workflows for Healthcare Information Systems, in: *Springer eBooks*, pp. 359–370, 2008, https://doi.org/10.1007/978-3-540-78238-4_37.
39. Wagner, B., Liable, but not in control? Ensuring meaningful human agency in automated decision-making systems. Policy & Internet, 11, 1, 104–122, 2019. https://doi.org/10.1002/poi3.198
40. Piwek, L., Ellis, D., Andrews, S., Joinson, A., The Rise of Consumer Health Wearables: Promises and Barriers. *PloS Med.*, *13*, 2, e1001953, 2016, https://doi.org/10.1371/journal.pmed.1001953.
41. Leminen, S., Westerlund, M., Rajahonka, M., Siuruainen, R., Towards IOT ecosystems and business models. In: S. Andreev, S. Balandin, Y. Koucheryavy (eds), Internet of Things, Smart Spaces, and Next Generation Networking, ruSMART 2012 NEW2AN 2012. *Lecture Notes in Computer Science,* vol. 7469. Springer, Berlin, Heidelberg, 2012. https://doi.org/10.1007/978-3-642-32686-8_2
42. Deogirikar, J. and Vidhate, A., Security attacks in IoT: A survey, in: *2017 International Conference on I-SMAC (IoT in Social, Mobile, Analytics and Cloud) (I-SMAC)*, 2017, https://doi.org/10.1109/i-smac.2017.8058363.
43. Ruta, M., Scioscia, F., Loseto, G., Pinto, A., Di Sciascio, E., Machine learning in the Internet of Things: A semantic-enhanced approach. *Semant. Web*, *10*, 1, 183–204, 2018, https://doi.org/10.3233/sw-180314.

44. Singh, A., Ramirez-Gonzalez, G., Abu-Elnasr, O., Shawkat, S.A., Arunkumar, N., Farouk, A., Secure Medical Data Transmission Model for IoT-Based Healthcare Systems. *IEEE Access, 6*, 20596–20608, 2018, https://doi.org/10.1109/access.2018.2817615.
45. Sicari, S., Rizzardi, A., Grieco, L.A., Coen-Porisini, A., Security, privacy and trust in Internet of Things: The road ahead. *Comput. Netw., 76*, 146–164, 2015b, https://doi.org/10.1016/j.comnet.2014.11.008.
46. Cai, H., Xu, B., Jiang, L., Vasilakos, A.V., IoT-Based Big Data Storage Systems in Cloud Computing: Perspectives and Challenges. *IEEE Internet Things J., 4*, 1, 75–87, 2017, https://doi.org/10.1109/jiot.2016.2619369.
47. Islam, M.R., Kabir, M.M., Mridha, M.F., Alfarhood, S., Safran, M., Che, D., Deep learning-based IoT system for remote monitoring and early detection of health issues in real-time. *Sensors (Basel, Switzerland)*, 23, 11, 5204, 2023. https://doi.org/10.3390/s23115204
48. Ahmed, M. and Pathan, A.K., False data injection attack (FDIA): An overview and new metrics for fair evaluation of its countermeasure. *Complex Adapt. Syst. Model.*, 8, 1, 2020. https://doi.org/10.1186/s40294-020-00070-w
49. Kambourakis, G., Kolias, C., Stavrou, A., The Mirai botnet and the IoT zombie armies, in: *MILCOM 2017 - 2017 IEEE Military Communications Conference (MILCOM)*, Baltimore, MD, USA, pp. 267–272, 2017, doi: 10.1109/MILCOM.2017.8170867.
50. Hackers breach 150,000 Verkada surveillance cameras. *Biom. Technol. Today, 2021*, 4, 2–3, 2021, https://doi.org/10.1016/s0969-4765(21)00041-2.
51. Baker, M., Real, Unreal, and Hacked. *IEEE Pervasive Comput., 17*, 1, 104–112, 2018, https://doi.org/10.1109/mprv.2018.011591069.
52. Ehrenfeld, J.M., WannaCry, cybersecurity and health information technology: A time to act. *J. Med. Syst.*, 41, 7, 2017. https://doi.org/10.1007/s10916-017-0752-1
53. Kimani, K., Oduol, V.K., Langat, K., Cyber security challenges for IoT-based smart grid networks. *Int. J. Crit. Infrastruct. Prot., 25*, 36–49, 2019, https://doi.org/10.1016/j.ijcip.2019.01.001.
54. Jaigirdar, F.T., Rudolph, C., Bain, C., Risk and compliance in IoT-health data propagation: A security-aware provenance based approach. In S.I. Ahamed, N. Atukorala, C.K. Chang, E. Damiani, G. De Pietro, L. Liu, Z. Wang, J. Zhang, & F. Zulkernine (Eds.), *Proceedings - 2021 IEEE International Conference on Digital Health, ICDH 2021*, IEEE, Institute of Electrical and Electronics Engineers, pp. 27–37, 2021. https://doi.org/10.1109/ICDH52753.2021.00015
55. Holstein, D.K., and Stouffer, K., Trust but verify critical infrastructure cyber security solutions, in: *2010 43rd Hawaii International Conference on System Sciences*, Honolulu, HI, USA, pp. 1–8, 2010, doi: 10.1109/HICSS.2010.410.

6

A Hybrid Deep Learning Framework to Diagnose Sleep Apnea Using Electrocardiogram Signals for Smart Healthcare

Sampoorna Poria[1], Ahona Ghosh[1], Biswarup Ganguly[2] and Sriparna Saha[1]*

[1]*Department of Computer Science & Engineering, Maulana Abul Kalam Azad University of Technology, West Bengal, India*
[2]*Department of Electrical Engineering, National Institute of Technology Silchar, Assam, India*

Abstract

Sleep apnea is a global health problem that requires early diagnosis and intervention to treat and prevent the associated symptoms. This study presents a new hybrid deep learning framework to identify and classify sleep apnea from single-channel electrocardiogram (ECG) signals into four classes. The ECG signals were preprocessed using a discrete wavelet transform to remove noise and unwanted signals. Furthermore, the filtered signals are fed to a proposed relational autoencoder for relevant feature extraction, where it can automatically identify the most relevant features of a dataset by compressing it into a lower-dimensional representation. A bidirectional long short-term memory network was incorporated to learn the trained feature set for the necessary sleep apnea diagnosis. The comparative results illustrate the efficacy of the proposed sleep apnea diagnosis method by considering its performance metrics. Moreover, a cost-effective low-power embedded device was developed and implemented in the laboratory for smart healthcare applications. The developed module could be a potential contender in any computer-aided diagnosis systems with increased performance.

Keywords: Computer-aided diagnosis, deep learning, electrocardiogram, feature extraction, healthcare application

**Corresponding author*: sahasriparna@gmail.com

Neha Sharma, Korhan Cengiz and Prasenjit Chatterjee (eds.) Intelligent Data Analytics for Bioinformatics and Biomedical Systems, (145–162) © 2024 Scrivener Publishing LLC

6.1 Introduction

Sleep apnea (SA) is a potentially consequential condition when the upper respiratory airway is blocked multiple times during sleep, resulting in abnormal breathing patterns, or worse, if the brain cannot activate and send signals to unblock the airway [1]. Usually, patients with SA require continuous monitoring to detect such events and appropriately diagnose their condition. SA can be classified into four major types: Obstructive SA (OSA) is the most common, occurring when the throat muscles relax and airflow to the lungs is blocked; Central SA (CSA) occurs when the brain is unable to transmit proper signals to the muscles controlling breathing; Hypopnea (HPA) is characterized by abnormally slow or shallow breathing; and Mixed Apnea (MXA), which includes symptoms of both OSA and CSA [2].

Considerable research has been conducted to detect and classify sleep apnea events. These include continuous recording accelerations of the diaphragm, monitoring of polysomnogram (PSG) records, and use of a respiratory effort belt to measure tension. These studies require continuous monitoring over a long period [3]. Furthermore, non-invasive techniques for such conditions are preferred using sensors and probes inside the body that can be uncomfortable and increase the risk of complications. In addition, such monitoring can be performed outside a medical facility [4], allowing patients to undergo testing anywhere and improving compliance with the testing protocol [5].

Electrocardiogram (ECG) signal monitoring is a nonintrusive method for detecting cardiac disorders. ECG signals that capture the heart's electrical activity provide more comprehensive and accurate information about a person's heart activity and breathing patterns than physiological monitoring techniques [6].

After going through several state-of-the-art studies, this section analyses their contributions and limitations, which motivated us to consider this area of research and address the existing research challenges. Yuzer *et al.* [7] employed a micro-electro-mechanical system-based acceleration sensor to develop a system that detects sleep apnea in real-time. Many parameters related to sleep apnea are detected, such as total sleep time, apnea times, low signal, information regarding the lying position, and total number of apnea events. However, accelerator vibrations are unsuitable for different age groups. Nassi *et al.* [8] utilize a single respiratory effort belt and a WaveNet architecture to detect the four classes of SA. A capacitively coupled sensor with capacitively coupled ECG and capacitively coupled bio-impedance data was by Deviaene *et al.* [9] to detect sleep apnea. The device utilized a random-forest-based backward wrapper. The only limitation is the loss of some ccBioz data due to sensor failure. Bernardini *et al.* [10] developed a neural network architecture that is capable of assessing OSA severity and tagging apnea events at one-second granularity utilizing deep learning (DL) frameworks such as convolutional neural network (CNN) and long short-term memory (LSTM) architecture with depthwise separable convolutions. Another study [11] employed a cost-effective respiration belt to detect SA using a CNN classifier. The only limitation is that the EEG sensors cannot perform arousal-based scoring. A supervised learning scheme has been proposed for the detection of SA [12], where an encoder is used for data representation and a classifier is used for fine-tuning as well as classification. Sudhamathy *et al.* [13] presented a hybrid DL model, where various sleep stages are analysed via CNN, LSTM, and CNN-LSTM models. Chen *et al.* [14] presented an electronic model for diagnosis of obstructive sleep apnea using two Transformers model. It is found from the above-mentioned literature that feature extraction has been carried out by classical signal processing tools or deep learning-aided algorithms followed by classification. However, none of the methods analyze or fine-tune the features before feeding them to the proposed classifier to perform multiclass sleep apnea classification. In this study, a dataset of 25 PSGs was collected overnight from adults with suspected sleep disorders and abnormal breathing patterns. Signal pre-processing was conducted using the wavelet transform approach, followed by feature extraction and classification. The salient features of this chapter are as follows:

1. A hybrid deep learning framework was proposed to identify and classify sleep apnea from single-channel ECG signals into four classes to develop a smart healthcare system.
2. The ECG signals were preprocessed via a discrete wavelet transform to remove noise and unwanted signals. Furthermore, the filtered signals are fed to a relational autoencoder (RAE) for relevant feature extraction, which can automatically identify the most important features of a dataset by compressing it into a lower-dimensional representation.
3. A bidirectional long short-term memory network was incorporated to learn the trained feature set obtained from the RAE. A two-layer bi-LSTM was constructed for the diagnosis of sleep apnea. The comparative findings demonstrate

the effectiveness of the proposed classification approach in terms of the five-performance metrics.
4. A cost-effective smart healthcare system was developed by integrating a microcontroller unit with an AD8232 sensor module to extract real-time data for developing a computer-aided diagnostic system for Internet of Things applications. Moreover, to judge the robustness of the developed system, different signal-to-noise ratios were added to the raw signals.

The remainder of this chapter is organized into four sections. *Section 6.2* outlines the proposed methodology and framework. *Section 6.3* presents the description of the experiment and its findings, and *Section 6.4* draws the conclusion and future work.

6.2 Proposed Methodology

The proposed framework involves four steps: data acquisition from the ECG, preprocessing using DWT, feature extraction using an autoencoder, and classification using bi-LSTM. A synopsis of the framework is presented in Figure 6.1.

6.2.1 Introduction to the Data Acquisition Device

The proposed work involves Holter ECG [5] as the data acquisition device, which noninvasively records the electrical activity of the heart for 24–48 h. Electrodes were attached to certain points on the chest and abdomen, and were connected by wires to a small, portable recording device.

6.2.2 Preprocessing Using Discrete Wavelet Transform

To extract relevant features from the raw signal, the discrete wavelet transform (DWT) [15] can decompose the ECG signals, as it provides a multiresolution signal analysis. The frequency bands obtained through the DWT correspond to different physiological phenomena related to sleep apnea, such as changes in heart rate variability and respiratory patterns. By decomposing the ECG signal into different frequency bands, DWT can help identify SA patterns that may not be apparent in the raw signal. Here, the DWT was incorporated to preprocess the raw ECG signals. R-peak annotations, which are the maximum amplitudes in the R-wave of the ECG

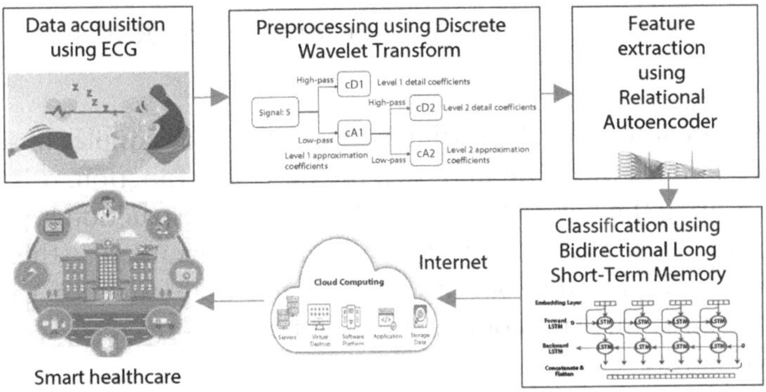

Figure 6.1 Overview of the proposed architecture for sleep apnea detection.

signals, were detected. An iterative algorithm can be applied to the raw signals to perform the DWT. The components with low-frequency $L_{j,k}$ and high-frequency $H_{j,k}$ after the decomposition of the signal with multilevel filter banks are:

$$L_{j,k} = \Sigma_l \, \mathrm{h}(1-2\mathrm{k}) L_{j-1,m} \tag{6.1}$$

$$H_{j,k} = \Sigma_l \, \mathrm{g}(1-2\mathrm{k}) L_{j-1,m} \tag{6.2}$$

Here, j is the parameter that affects the DWT scaling, h (.) and g (.) are low-pass and high-pass filters, respectively, l is the number of levels, and k is the translation at each level of the wavelet function.

6.2.3 Feature Extraction Using Auto Encoder

Autoencoders [16] are neural networks that can learn the underlying features of unlabeled data. It generates latent variables sampled from a multivariate Gaussian distribution, considering the means and standard deviations. In this study, the autoencoder architecture comprises an encoder to extract observable latent variables of decreased dimensions compared to the original input. While conventional autoencoders minimize the reconstruction loss of the data, the relational autoencoder does the same for the data as well as the relationships among the data. The objective function of a relational autoencoder can be expressed as:

$$\theta = (1-\alpha)\min_{\theta} L(S,S') + \alpha\, \min_{\theta} L\big(R(S),R(S')\big) \tag{6.3}$$

where $R(S)$ denotes the relationship between the data samples in signals S, and $R(S')$ denotes the same in S', i.e., the decoding function. α is responsible for scaling the network by controlling its reconstruction loss weights and relationships, and θ is the neural network parameter. The rectifier function was employed in our model as an activation function to manage similar weights, increase computational efficiency and remove unnecessary associations.

6.2.4 Classification Using Bidirectional LSTM

LSTM is a special variation of recurrent neural network (RNN), that can capture both short-term and long-term dependencies in sequential data. They are designed with feedback connections that enable them to learn the time dependencies in a long data series. A bi-LSTM network is a sequence processing model containing two LSTM networks [17] that simultaneously processes the input's time-series sequence in two opposite directions.

Out of both LSTM networks (refer to Figure 6.2), the first unit processes the temporal sequence in the forward direction, while the second unit processes the reverse. The resultant outputs were combined to evaluate the classification performed using the bi-LSTM network. Each LSTM unit comprises an input gate, a memory cell, an output gate, and a forget gate. In this study, a feature-induced bi-LSTM was proposed for bidirectionally learning features in the temporal domain extracted from the relational autoencoder. Bi-LSTM models are more effective as their output depends

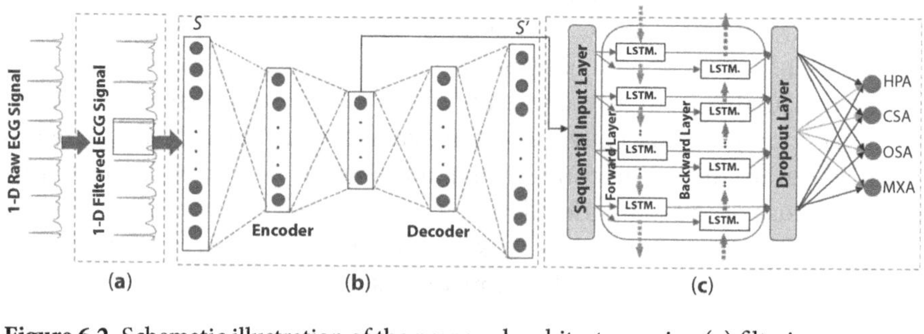

Figure 6.2 Schematic illustration of the proposed architecture using (a) filtering operation, (b) feature extraction and (c) classifiation.

on both the previous and following segments, capable of utilizing information from either side.

Consider the input to the bi-LSTM as $S = [s_1, s_2, \ldots s_{t-1}, s_t, s_{t+1}, \ldots, s_T]$ and the output set $Y = [y_1, y_2, \ldots y_{t-1}, y_t, y_{t+1}, \ldots, y_T]$ for $t = [1, T]$ time steps. The same input, S, is processed by each baseline LSTM unit in the given approach. Using the current input s_t, the output of the previous hidden layer h_{t-1}, and the forget gate f_t at time t, the memory cell of each LSTM determines which information of the previous state to keep or which to forget.

$$f_t = sig(W_{fs}.s_t + W_{fh}.h_{t-1} + b_f) \tag{6.4}$$

where W_{ab} is the weight vector representing the connection between layers a and b, and b_f is the bias of the forget gate. Based on i_t, i.e., the input gate information, previous cell state c_{t-1}, and next cell state, the memory cell calculates the amount of information that needs to be stored to c_t as:

$$i_t = sig(W_{is}.s_t + W_{ih}.h_{t-1} + b_i) \tag{6.5}$$

$$\hat{c}_t = tanh(W_{cs}.s_t + W_{ch}.h_{t-1} + b_c) \tag{6.6}$$

$$c_t = i_t.\hat{c}_t + f_t.c_{t-1} \tag{6.7}$$

Ultimately, the output gate o_t plays a vital role in propagating information from the current cell to the next cell, represented by h_t. The equations describing these parameters are as follows.

$$o_t = sig(W_{os}.s_t + W_{oh}.h_{t-1} + b_o) \tag{6.8}$$

$$h_t = o_t.\tanh(c_t) \tag{6.9}$$

The two nonlinear functions utilized are sigmoid (*sig*) and *tanh*, defined as $sig(f) = \frac{1}{1+e^{-f}}$ and $tanh(f) = \frac{2}{2+e^{-2f}} - 1$.

All weight matrices and biases were trained by back-propagation over time. Unlike vanilla LSTMs, bi-LSTMs, have forward sequences $(\overrightarrow{h_t})$ and backward sequences $(\overleftarrow{h_t})$, in the hidden layers at time t as follows:

$$\overrightarrow{h_t} = \tanh(G_{\vec{h}} \, . \, s_t + W_{\vec{h}} \, . \, \vec{h}_{t-1} + b_{\vec{h}}) \tag{6.10}$$

$$\overleftarrow{h_t} = \tanh(G_{\overleftarrow{h}} \, . \, s_t + W_{\overleftarrow{h}} \, . \, \overleftarrow{h}_{t-1} + b_{\overleftarrow{h}}) \tag{6.11}$$

where G is the weight matrix that combines the input and hidden layers. At the same time, the output layer of the bi-LSTM, h_t, at time t, is restricted as the combined effect of both the forward and backward sequences and is given by the equation below.

$$h_t = \tanh(U_{\vec{h}} \, . \, \overrightarrow{h_t} + U_{\overleftarrow{h}} \, . \, \overleftarrow{h_t} + b_y) \tag{6.12}$$

where U is another weight matrix connecting the hidden and output layers. In this work, two bi-LSTM layers with 16 hidden units were used with one drop-out layer. The classification layer contains a *softmax* activation function, which produces the class probability in the classification layer.

6.3 Experiment Results and Discussions

This section first describes the dataset and then presents the experimental outcomes of the various phases of our proposed model. Finally, a statistical validation was conducted to analyze the suitability of the proposed framework for real-time applications.

6.3.1 Dataset Details

The ECG signals were obtained from the St. Vincent's University Hospital/University College Dublin Sleep Apnea Database [18]. The database was compiled by monitoring subjects selected randomly over six months to diagnose OSA, CSA, or potentially snoring. A total of 25 adults (21 males and four females) aged between 28 and 68 years with a body mass index (BMI) range of 25.1–42.5 kg/m^2 were chosen for analysis. The Apnea–Hypopnea Index (AHI) was between 1.7 and 90.9 (mean AHI: 24.1 ± 20.3).

PSGs were conducted using the Jaeger-Toennies system (Erich Jaeger GmbH, Germany). The recorded signals encompassed the ECG signal of

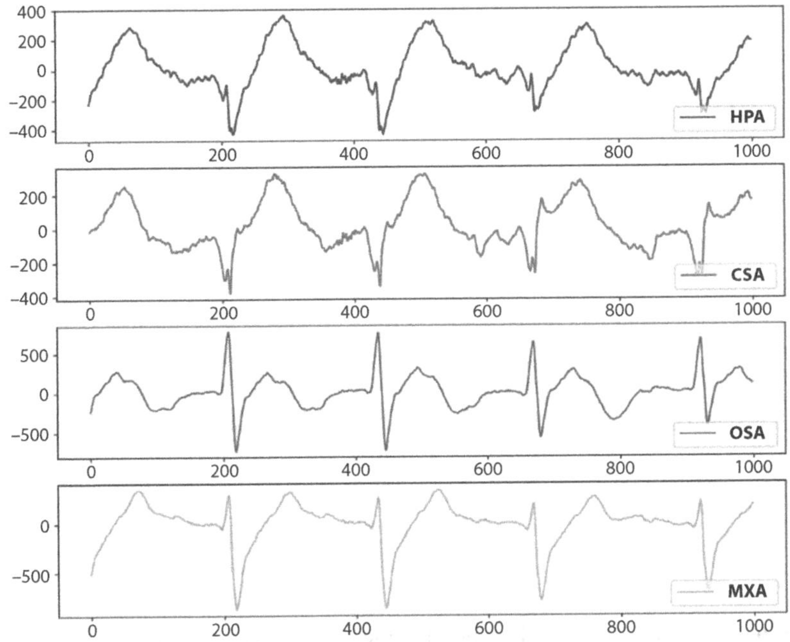

Figure 6.3 Waveforms belonging to HPA, CSA, OSA, and MXA respectively.

the modified lead, V2. A sleep technologist annotated the onset time and duration of respiratory events, i.e., HPA, CSA, OSA, and MXA. The waveforms for the four classes are shown in Figure 6.3.

6.3.1.1 *Preprocessing Outcomes*

The ECG signals undergo segmentation into heartbeats, which is performed by considering 179 samples following the R-peaks and 75 samples preceding the R-peaks. Each extracted heartbeat was subjected to subsequent processing, involving the division of the beat into 16 segments with a 50% overlap between consecutive segments. These segmented portions were subsequently utilized as inputs for the relational autoencoder for feature extraction. This section illustrates the outcome of the proposed filtering technique, shown in Figure 6.4 for a particular channel. It assesses the performance by displaying the signal amplitude with respect to time before and after applying the DWT. From the pictorial view, the proposed filtering method can successfully remove noise from raw data.

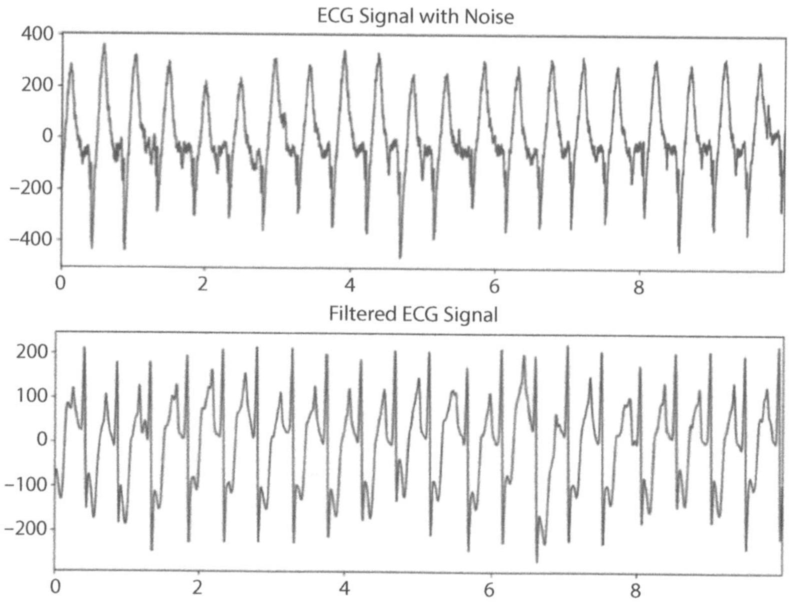

Figure 6.4 Signal amplitude with respect to time before and after filtering.

6.3.2 Feature Extraction Outcomes

The feature extraction approach was also compared with existing competitors, such as temporal, frequency domain, and time-frequency domain features. Table 6.1 displays that the proposed RAE-based feature extraction technique outperforms contemporary feature extractors in terms of Mean Absolute Error (MAE), Mean Square Error (MSE), and R^2 score [19].

Table 6.1 Comparison of proposed feature extractor with existing approaches.

Feature extractor	MAE	MSE	R^2 score
RAE-based features	**0.23**	**0.21**	**0.19**
Time based features	0.34	0.42	0.25
Frequency based features	0.29	0.36	0.29
Time-frequency based features	0.25	0.23	0.27

6.3.3 Classification Results

The classification outcome was evaluated by tuning the hyperparameters of our proposed bi-LSTM in terms of the learning curve, confusion matrix, and Receiver Operating Characteristics (ROC) curve [20]. Figure 6.5 shows the learning curves generated by varying the batch size to 50, 100, 150, and 200. In these plots, if we look for the inflection point for which the validation loss no longer increases and only the training time increases, we can conclude that a batch size of 100 outperforms the others.

Figure 6.6 presents the comparison of ROC curves generated by varying the number of epochs to 100, 200, 300, and 400. The performance over 200 epochs was remarkable showing the ROC with an area under convergence (AUC) value of 0.96. Figure 6.7 shows the variation in the True Positive Rate (TPR) and False Positive Rate (FPR) [21] in the confusion matrix by varying the learning rates to 0.1, 0.2, 0.3, and 0.4. The combination of 100, 200, and 0.2 respectively as batch size, number of epochs, and learning rate, respectively, achieved the best performance; thus, it was finally chosen for the proposed bi-LSTM model.

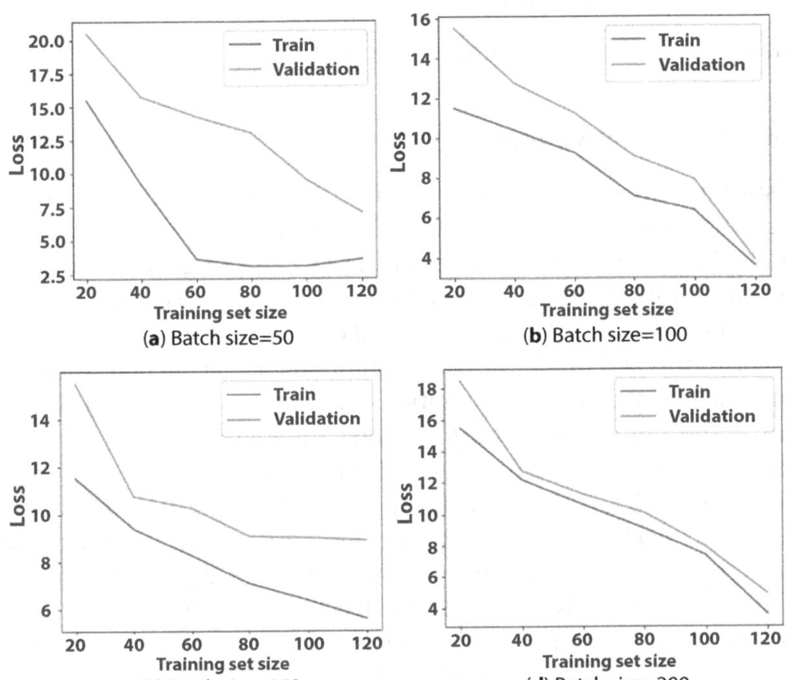

Figure 6.5 Illustrations of learning curves by hyper-tuning batch size.

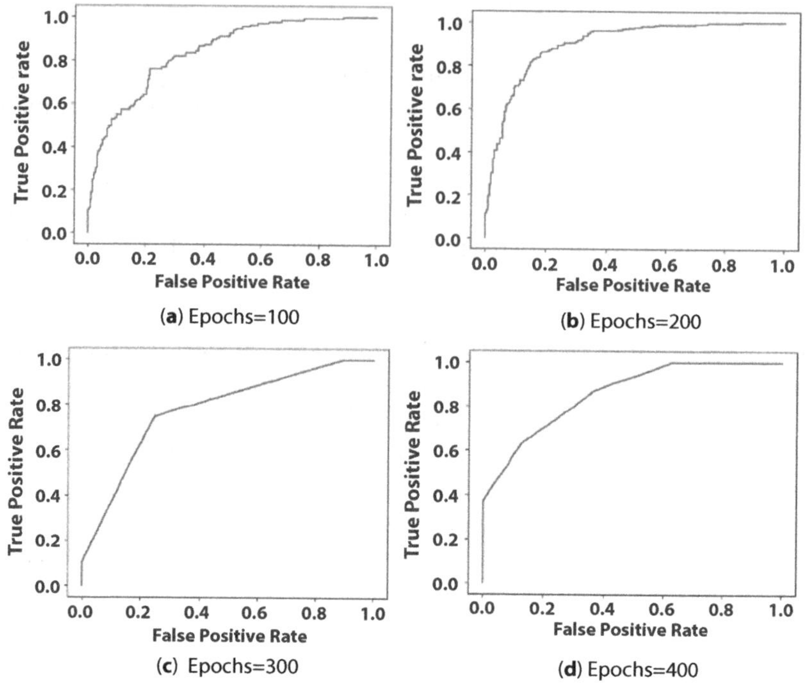

Figure 6.6 ROC curves for variable number of epochs.

6.3.4 Statistical Validation

Statistical validation of the proposed classification task was also performed using McNemar's test [22]. Let algorithms A and B be fed into a standard training dataset of features obtained from ECG readings collected for sleep apnea detection. If the number of readings wrongly classified using A but not using B is n_{10} and n_{01} is the number of compensations wrongly classified by algorithm B and not by A. Let p_1 denote the experimental result's marginal probability when compensations are wrongly classified using algorithm A and not using B, and p_2 denotes the marginal probability of the experimental results when compensations are wrongly classified by algorithm B but not by A. Then, according to the null hypothesis of McNemar's test denoted by H_0, p_1 and p_2 are equal. The alternative and null hypotheses, denoted by h_1 and h_0, respectively, can be represented by h_1: $p_1 \neq p_2$ and h_0: $p_1 = p_2$. From this, it is clearly stated that the errors in running both the algorithms are the same, and McNemar's statistics Z follows χ^2, having the degree of freedom equal to 1 and can be represented by

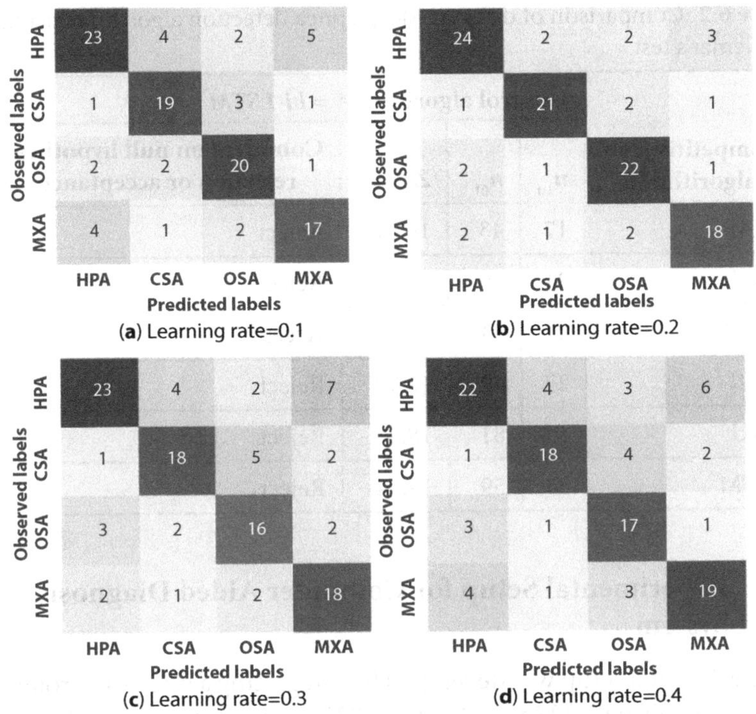

Figure 6.7 Confusion matrix of the proposed SA diagnosis for variable learning rate.

$$Z = \frac{(|n10 - n01| - 1)^2}{n10 + n01} \tag{6.13}$$

Suppose that *A* is our proposed bi-LSTM and *B* represents the six competitors, i.e., support vector machine (SVM), k nearest neighbor (kNN), back propagation neural network (BPNN), RNN, gated recurrent unit (GRU), and traditional LSTM. In this case, $Z = Z_1$–Z_6 was evaluated. The comparative statistics of the wrong classification between algorithm *M* and the *i*th competing algorithm among the six mentioned in the first column of Table 6.2, and *i* represents the *i*th row in the table. The null hypothesis gets rejected if $Z_i > Z_i > \chi^2_{1,\alpha=0.05} = 3.84$ when $\chi^2_{1,\alpha=0.05} = 3.84$ is the χ^2 distribution's critical value for one degree of freedom at a probability value of 0.05.

A close analysis of the results of McNemar's test, shown in Table 6.2 has indicated that the bi-LSTM model has remained consistently better than the existing competitors in a statistically significant way.

Table 6.2 Comparison of different sleep apnea detection algorithms using McNemar's test.

Competitive algorithm *B*	Control algorithm A = *bi-LSTM*			
	n_{10}	n_{01}	Z_i	Comment on null hypothesis rejection or acceptance
SVM	17	43	10.41	Reject
kNN	21	70	27.47	Reject
BPNN	21	34	2.61	Accept
RNN	27	62	12.98	Reject
GRU	34	81	18.4	Reject
LSTM	23	59	14.94	Reject

6.3.5 Experimental Setup for Computer Aided Diagnosis System

An experimental setup was developed by integrating a microcontroller unit (MCU), i.e., ATmega328p, with an AD8232 sensor module for the acquisition of real-time data. For the proposed setup, 10 subjects (six males and four females) with an average age of 30–50 years were chosen to validate the proposed hybrid DL algorithm. Figure 6.8 depicts the experimental prototype for a computer-aided diagnosis system, where the data captured by the developed module has been sent to a local server for Internet of Things (IoT) applications. The developed low-power embedded device is provided with three electrodes connected to the subject to receive the requisite electrical signals.

6.3.6 Performance Evaluation

Moreover, in the testing session, white Gaussian noise with various signal-to-noise ratios (SNR) was added to the raw signals of each category to determine the applicability of the proposed architecture under contamination of noise. In addition to the raw signal, the SNR of six different levels, i.e., 10, 20, 30, 40, 50, and 60 dB, were considered for this purpose. Table 6.3 presents the performance comparison regarding precision, accuracy, recall, error rate (ER), and F1-score. The results show that the performance

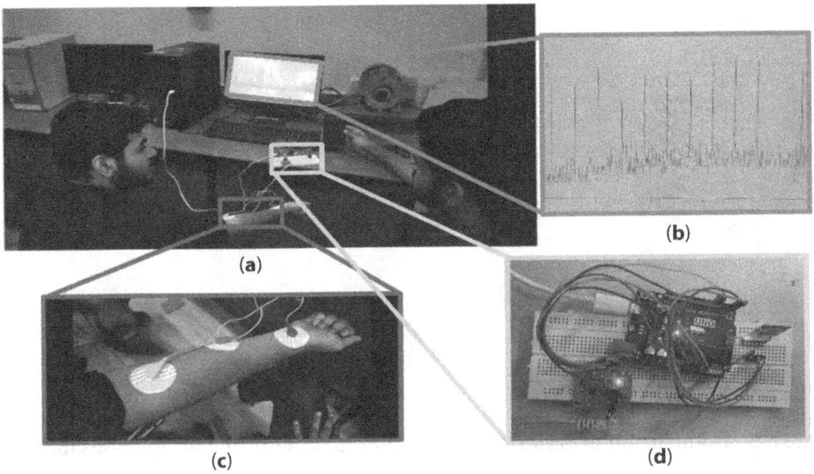

Figure 6.8 (a) Experimental setup, (b-d) zoomed versions of signal acquisition, electrode setting, and developed IoT module, respectively.

Table 6.3 Performance of the proposed method on considered noise with variable SNRs.

SNR (dB)	Accuracy	Precision	Recall	F1 score	ER
10	95.62	93.52	89.67	96.03	2.44
20	94.34	95.06	91.52	94.56	1.67
30	92.36	94.37	92.48	93.42	3.58
40	91.73	95.45	88.56	93.43	4.63
50	94.27	92.34	93.37	95.37	3.83
60	93.12	92.85	92.45	94.34	4.67

is satisfactory, and that the proposed hybrid DL framework is immune to noise up to a certain limit.

The effectiveness of the proposed hybrid architecture was evaluated by comparing it with recent methods. The comparative analysis in Figure 6.9 shows that the proposed work best suits the related domain.

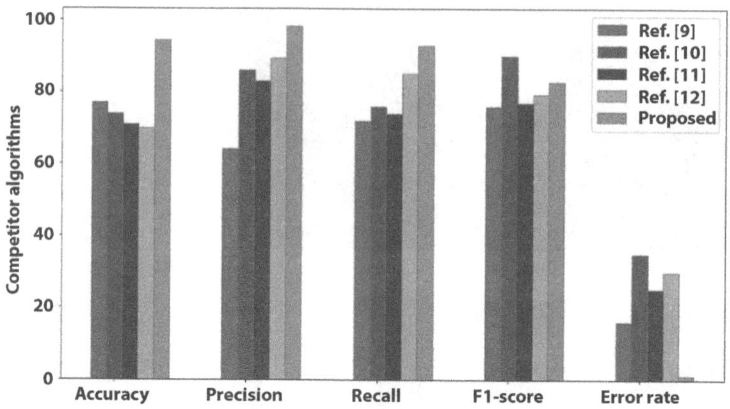

Figure 6.9 Comparison of performance metrics with state-of-the-art methods for SA diagnosis.

6.4 Conclusion and Future Scope

The current research deals with the detection of sleep apnea, a serious health problem that causes fatigue, sleepiness, and irritation even after night sleep. The combination of discrete wavelet transform, relational autoencoder, and bidirectional LSTM with an acceptable performance (accuracy = 95%) has been able to classify sleep apnea efficiently, and based on its remarkable performance, a prototype of the system has also been developed in our laboratory to check its applicability in a real-world scenario where early detection and treatment can ease the diagnosis.

Acknowledgments

A. Ghosh is thankful to the university for providing the AICTE Doctoral Fellowship, with appointment letter Ref. No.2.2.1/Regis./Appt.(AG)/ Ph.D(ADF)/ 2021 dated 01.02.2021, and S. Saha is grateful for the UGC Start-up Grant under the scheme of Basic Scientific Research, File No. F.30-449/2018(BSR) dated 21.11.2019.

References

1. Beebe, D.W. and Gozal, D., Obstructive sleep apnea and the prefrontal cortex: towards a comprehensive model linking nocturnal upper airway obstruction to daytime cognitive and behavioral deficits. *J. Sleep Res.*, *11*, 1, 1–16, 2002.

2. Sateia, M.J., International classification of sleep disorders. *Chest*, *146*, 5, 1387–1394, 2014.
3. Penzel, T., Schöbel, C., Fietze, I., New technology to assess sleep apnea: wearables, smartphones, and accessories. *F1000Research*, *7*, 413, 2018.
4. Ganguly, B., Das, A., Ghosal, A., Das, D., Chatterjee, D., Rakshit, D., Das, E., A Non-Invasive Approach for Fetal Arrhythmia Detection and Classification from ECG Signals, in: *2020 IEEE VLSI Device Circuit and System (VLSI DCS)*, IEEE, pp. 84–88, 2020, July.
5. Patel, K. and Suh-Lailam, B.B., Implementation of point-of-care testing in a pediatric healthcare setting. *Crit. Rev. Clin. Lab. Sci.*, *56*, 4, 239–246, 2019.
6. Ganguly, B., Ghosal, A., Das, A., Das, D., Chatterjee, D., Rakshit, D., Automated Detection and Classification of Arrhythmia from ECG Signals using Feature Induced Long Short-Term Memory Network. *IEEE Sensors Lett.*, 4, 8, 1–4, 2020.
7. Yüzer, A.H., Sümbül, H., Polat, K., A novel wearable real-time sleep apnea detection system based on the acceleration sensor. *IRBM*, 41, 1, 39–47, 2020.
8. Nassi, T.E., Ganglberger, W., Sun, H., Bucklin, A.A., Biswal, S., van Putten, M.J., Thomas, R.J., Westover, M.B., Automated Scoring of Respiratory Events in Sleep with a Single Effort Belt and Deep Neural Networks. *IEEE Trans. Biomed. Eng.*, 69, 6, 2094–2104, 2021.
9. Deviaene, M., Castro, I.D., Borzée, P., Patel, A., Torfs, T., Buyse, B., Testelmans, D., Van Huffel, S., Varon, C., Capacitively-coupled ECG and respiration for the unobtrusive detection of sleep apnea. *Physiol. Meas.*, 42, 2, 024001, 2021.
10. Bernardini, A., Brunello, A., Gigli, G.L., Montanari, A., Saccomanno, N., AIOSA: An approach to the automatic identification of obstructive sleep apnea events based on deep learning. *Artif. Intell. Med.*, *118*, 102133, 2021.
11. Kristiansen, S., Nikolaidis, K., Plagemann, T., Goebel, V., Traaen, G.M., Øverland, B., Akerøy, L., Hunt, T.E., Loennechen, J.P., Steinshamn, S.L., Bendz, C.H., A clinical evaluation of a low-cost strain gauge respiration belt and machine learning to detect sleep apnea. *Smart Health*, 27, 100373, 2023.
12. Kumar, C.B., Mondal, A.K., Bhatia, M., Panigrahi, B.K., Gandhi, T.K., Self-Supervised Representation Learning-Based OSA Detection Method Using Single-Channel ECG Signals. *IEEE Trans. Instrum. Meas.*, 72, 1–15, 2023, Art no. 2511915, doi: 10.1109/TIM.2023.3261931.
13. Sudhamathy, G., Valliammal, N., Subashini, P., Dhivyanrabha, T.T., Sneha, R.G., Hybrid Convolutional Neural Network - Long Short-Term Memory Model for Automated Detection of Sleep Stages. *2023 International Conference on Intelligent Systems for Communication, IoT and Security (ICISCoIS)*, Coimbatore, India, pp. 510–515, 2023, doi: 10.1109/ICISCoIS56541.2023.10100489.
14. Chen, Z., Siltala-Li, L., Lassila, M., Malo, P., Vilkkumaa, E., Saaresranta, T., Virkki, A.V., Predicting Visit Cost of Obstructive Sleep Apnea using Electronic Healthcare Records with Transformer. *IEEE J. Transl. Eng. Health Med.*, 11, 2023.

15. Chervyakov, N., Lyakhov, P., Nagornov, N., Analysis of the quantization noise in discrete wavelet transform filters for 3D medical imaging. *Appl. Sci.*, *10*, 4, 1223, 2020.
16. Meng, Q., Catchpoole, D., Skillicom, D., Kennedy, P.J., May. Relational Autoencoder for feature extraction, in: *2017 International joint conference on neural networks (IJCNN)*, IEEE, pp. 364–371, 2017.
17. Ghosh, L., Saha, S., Konar, A., Bi-directional Long Short-Term Memory model to analyze psychological effects on gamers. *Appl. Soft Comput.*, 95, 106573, 2020.
18. PhysioBank, P., Physionet: components of a new research resource for complex physiologic signals. *Circulation*, *101*, 23, e215–e220, 2000.
19. Mitra, A., Jain, A., Kishore, A., Kumar, P., A Comparative Study of Demand Forecasting Models for a Multi-Channel Retail Company: A Novel Hybrid Machine Learning Approach. *Oper. Res. Forum*, 3, 4, 58, Springer International Publishing, Cham, 2022, September.
20. Prasetya, R. and Ridwan, A., Data mining application on weather prediction using classification tree, naïve bayes and K-nearest neighbor algorithm with model testing of supervised learning probabilistic brier score, confusion matrix and ROC. *J. Appl. Commun. Inf. Technol.*, *4*, 2, 25–33, 2020.
21. Ghosh, A. and Saha, S., Suppression of positive emotions during pandemic era: a deep learning framework for rehabilitation. *Int. J. Model. Identif. Control*, *41*, 1-2, 143–154, 2022.
22. Konar, A. and Saha, S., Type-2 Fuzzy Classifier Based Pathological Disorder Recognition, in: *Gesture Recognition: Principles, Techniques and Applications*, pp. 135–194, 2018.

7

Deep Ensemble Feature Extraction Based Classification of Bleeding Regions Using Wireless Capsule Endoscopy Images

Srijita Bandopadhyay[1]*, Kyamelia Roy[2], Sheli Sinha Chaudhuri[2], Soumen Banerjee[3] and Korhan Cengiz[4,5]

[1]*Department of Electronics and Communication Engineering, University of Engineering and Management, Kolkata, West Bengal, India*
[2]*Department of Electronics and Tele-Communication Engineering, Jadavpur University, Kolkata, West Bengal, India*
[3]*Narula Institute of Technology, Kolkata, West Bengal, India*
[4]*Department of Computer Engineering, Istinye University, Istanbul, Turkey*
[5]*Department of Information Technologies, Faculty of Informatics and Management, University of Hradec Kralove, Kralove, Czech Republic*

Abstract

Wireless capsule endoscopy (WCE) is a minimally invasive medical imaging technique that provides real-time visual information about the digestive system, enabling the detection and diagnosis of various gastrointestinal disorders. It offers a patient-friendly alternative to traditional endoscopic procedures, providing valuable insights into the digestive system's health with minimal discomfort and invasive procedures. However, accurate classification of bleeding and normal WCE images is challenging due to varying lighting conditions, artifacts, and the presence of bleeding regions. In this study, an ensemble feature extraction approach utilizing the ResNet 50, VGG 16, and Inception V3 neural networks was proposed for the classification of bleeding and normal WCE images. The proposed framework incorporates image processing, augmentation, data preprocessing, and feature extraction, thereby enhancing the accuracy of classification. Furthermore, an autoencoder was employed to reconstruct the extracted features, and a Support Vector Machine classifier was integrated to differentiate and classify bleeding and normal images. The experimental results demonstrated an impressive average

**Corresponding author*: srijitabando30@gmail.com

Neha Sharma, Korhan Cengiz and Prasenjit Chatterjee (eds.) Intelligent Data Analytics for Bioinformatics and Biomedical Systems, (163–194) © 2024 Scrivener Publishing LLC

accuracy of 99% with a precision of 99.5%, showcasing the efficacy of the proposed method. This study contributes to improving the timely diagnosis and treatment planning of gastrointestinal disorders using WCE imaging.

Keywords: Wireless capsule endoscopy, bleeding, ensemble feature extraction, convolutional neural network (CNN)

7.1 Introduction

Gastrointestinal (GI) disorders in the gastrointestinal tract lead to various diseases and associated problems. Wireless Capsule Endoscopy (WCE) has emerged as a valuable tool for the detection of a wide range of diseases throughout the GI tract, from the mouth to the anus. It allows for the examination of the entire GI tract using a small, swallowable capsule comprising four LEDs, CMOS imager lens, color camera, batteries, antennas, and RF transmitter. The primary purpose of endoscopy is to capture images of disorders in the upper digestive system, allowing for visual examination and collection of tissue samples (biopsy) to diagnose conditions such as anemia, bleeding, inflammation, or diarrhea. Among digital imaging techniques, endoscopy plays a pivotal role in obtaining detailed gastrointestinal images that reveal the presence of diseases. Advanced machine-learning and deep-learning approaches [1] have been employed to address the challenge of anomaly detection within the GI tract.

Accurate detection of diseases such as polyps [2], ulcers [3], bleeding [4], Crohns disease [5–7], and tumors [8, 9] are of utmost importance in effectively treating gastrointestinal disorders. Gastrointestinal bleeding [10, 11] represents a severe condition within the digestive tract, where blood may be present in the stool or vomit but is not always visible. In contrast, although capsule endoscopy is relatively more expensive, it offers distinct advantages as a noninvasive procedure capable of capturing images of the entire GI tract.

7.2 Related Works

Deep Learning-based models have demonstrated superior performance in multiple lesion recognition compared to conventional algorithms [12]. In [13], a hybridized ensemble stacking method combining machine learning and deep learning was utilized. Authors in [14] presented an intelligent approach integrating empirical wavelet transform (EWT) and convolutional neural network (CNN) to classify alimentary disorders such as esophagitis, polyps, hemorrhoids, and ulcerative colitis. Disease classification in medical diagnosis utilizing a CNN was explored in [15]. Transfer learning [16], another technique for classifying and detecting different anomalies in health monitoring systems, has shown improved accuracy over conventional machine learning algorithms. Recent detection methods have also incorporated meta-learning [17] for anomaly detection using fundus images, which requires a more balanced dataset for computation. In [18], a contrastive lifelong learning model employing vision transformers (VIT) is implemented for image anomaly detection, with the visualization extracted by the model. The combination of feature encoders, deep learning, and machine learning in machine health surveillance systems [19] facilitates better data analysis for anomaly detection Convolutional Neural Networks find application across various domains for both object classification and detection purposes, as highlighted in references [20–22]. In [23], the authors addressed the combination of a two-stage CNN and autoencoder for anomaly detection. To enhance the effectiveness of the proposed CNN compared to the conventional CNN and autoencoder methods, the proposed methodology was implemented. The study in [24] demonstrated the application of CNNs to an image dataset for diabetes diagnosis using an iris dataset. In addition, signal processing operations are executed by employing pre-trained CNN models such as ResNet-101, Xception, and EfficientNet [25] for the classification of various time-series data. In [26], a time-frequency analysis technique was presented that utilizes a high-precision CNN model for classifying biomedical health disorders, specifically cardiac arrhythmia. Furthermore, CNN and BiLSTM [27] networks have been extensively employed to assess the quality of ECG signals.

Ensemble feature extraction techniques have gained significant attention for biomedical image classification owing to their improved accuracy and robustness in disease diagnosis. In [28], the bagging ensemble technique was employed with support vector machines (SVM) for breast cancer diagnosis. The ensemble of SVM classifiers demonstrated improved accuracy compared with individual classifiers. The boosting ensemble technique was utilized with a deep CNN for malarial parasite detection [29]. The ensemble of CNN models showed enhanced performance in detecting malaria parasites in blood smear images. The stacking ensemble technique was applied for brain tumor classification. Multiple classifiers are stacked [30], and their predictions are combined using a meta-classifier, resulting in improved accuracy in identifying brain tumor types. The random subspace method was employed to combine the texture features for lung nodule classification [31]. Multiple deep-learning models were trained, and their predictions were combined, leading to improved accuracy in classifying skin lesions [32].

The integration of segmentation and classification methods in medical imaging is crucial for accurately analyzing different anomalies [33]. Significant advancements have been made in [34] for polyp, tumor, and ulcer detection, emphasizing automated prediction using video frames. Texture- and color-based descriptors for the segmentation of pathologies in WCE images are discussed in [35]. The integration of machine learning with computer vision [36] has provided additional advantages for investigating diseases with high precision and recall scores. The remainder of this study is organized as follows: Section 7.3 demonstrates the methodology used in the study. Section 7.4 represents the experiments conducted in the proposed study and Section 7.5 comprises of a detailed discussion of the findings. Finally, Section 7.6 concludes the study by summarizing the key points and highlighting the contributions made.

7.3 Methodology

Deep neural networks have become a crucial area of research for classification, localization, and detection. The integration of Deep CNN with machine learning algorithms for classifying and detecting bleeding WCE images was demonstrated by the authors in [37]. The integrated system enhances the speed of data acquisition but also improves the quality of digital images, providing researchers with a more efficient pathway to conduct their experiments.

The study introduces a novel technique for classifying bleeding regions in WCE images. The overall framework of the proposed method involves several stages, including data acquisition, image processing, data augmentation, data preprocessing, feature extraction, and classification, as illustrated in Figure 7.1. The key highlights of the proposed approach are outlined below:

- This work focuses on classical image processing techniques such as histogram equalizer, denoising, and adaptive filtration to enhance the quality of WCE bleeding images.
- The most important part of the framework involves with the extraction of features using an Ensemble Convolutional Neural Network. Three different CNNs, namely ResNet50,

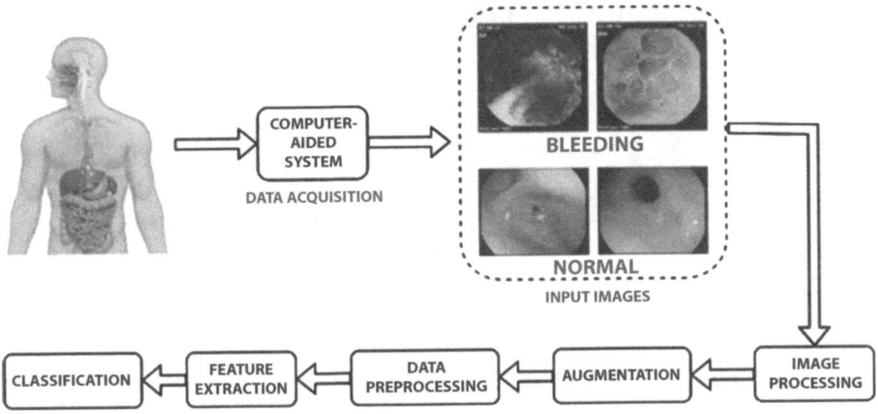

Figure 7.1 Workflow diagram.

VGG 16, and Inception V3, were used, and their features were concatenated for further processing.

- Feature extraction is followed by feature reconstruction and classification of bleeding and normal WCE images. Feature reconstruction is achieved by utilizing an autoencoder combined with a Support Vector Machine (SVM) for the purpose of classification. Their work generated an average classification accuracy of 99% and a precision score of 99.5%.
- In conclusion, the entire experiment was also conducted by extracting features using a single deep neural architecture and feeding them into several classifiers, such as Support Vector Machine (SVM), K-Nearest Neighbor (KNN), Decision Tree (DT), and Random Forest (RF). This method aids in understanding the importance of ensemble feature extraction over a single deep architecture.

7.3.1 Dataset

Endoscopy plays a crucial role in aiding medical practitioners and researchers in the diagnosis of various diseases. In the case of GI tract disorders, the detection and classification of these diseases are particularly important because of their significant impact on individuals' health. To achieve effective detection, a diverse and well-curated dataset is essential for training the automated detection systems. The dataset used in this study was obtained from [38] wherein the images inside the dataset were categorized into different groups based on specific

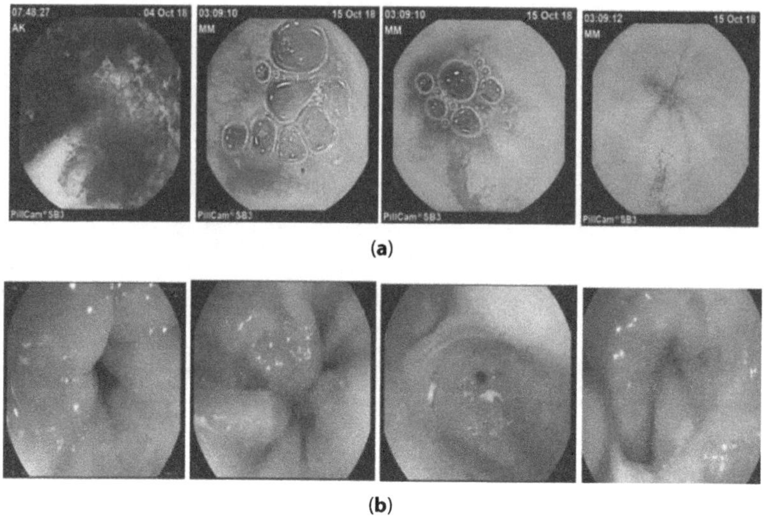

Figure 7.2 Dataset (a) bleeding images, (b) normal images.

diseases. In the context of the present research, the primary focus is on two classes within the dataset: bleeding and normal; some of the samples are shown in Figure 7.2. These images offer valuable information regarding the visual aspects and attributes of gastrointestinal bleeding. They play a crucial role in the examination and understanding of endoscopic observations, contributing to precise diagnosis and formulation of effective treatment strategies.

7.3.2 Image Processing

Image processing encompasses a wide range of tasks including image restoration, enhancement, denoising, compression, and segmentation. Using image processing, meaningful insights can be extracted to improve the quality of analysis. In the present framework, several image processing techniques were implemented to quantify the dataset. Three different techniques, namely histogram equalizer, de-noising and adaptive filtering, are utilized to improve the standard of the dataset collected. Figure 7.3 depicts the entire pipeline of the image processing framework used in this study. In biomedical imaging, image processing is a vital aspect because it helps in filtering the accurate images required for computation. The following methods were used in this study:

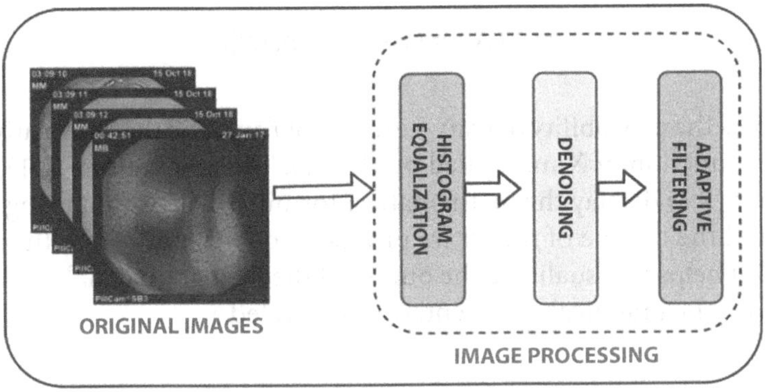

Figure 7.3 Image processing.

7.3.3 Histogram Equalizer

The histogram of an image represents the distribution of pixel intensities, with darker regions represented by lower intensity values and brighter regions represented by higher intensity values. Let *f* be a given image represented as an $m_r \times m_c$ matrix of integer pixel intensities ranging from 0 to L – 1; where L is the number of possible intensity values (often 256). Let p_n be the normalized histogram of *f* with a bin for each possible intensity. So

$$p_n = \frac{Number\ of\ pixels\ with\ intensity}{total\ numbers\ of\ pixel}\ \mathrm{n} = 0,1,2,3,4\ldots\ldots \quad (7.1)$$

The histogram equalized image H can be defined by

$$H_{ij} = floor\ ((L-1)\textstyle\sum_{n=0}^{f_{ij}} p_n) \quad (7.2)$$

where floor () is rounded down to the nearest integer. This is analogous to transforming the pixel intensities *k*, *f* by the function

$$\mathrm{T(k)} = floor\ ((L-1)\textstyle\sum_{n=0}^{f_{ij}} p_n) \quad (7.3)$$

The provocation for this transformation comes from thinking of the intensities of *f* and *g* as continuous random variables X, Y on [0, L-1] with Y defined by

$$Y = T(X) = (L-1)\int_0^X p_x(x)dx \tag{7.4}$$

where p_x is the probability density function of *f* and T is the cumulative distributive function of X multiplied by (L – 1). Thus, Equations (7.1), (7.2), (7.3), and (7.4) display the mathematical formulations behind using histogram, and the outline of the entire process is depicted in Algorithm (7.1). Figure 7.4 helps in visualizing the output of the histogram equalized image, along with the graphical representation generated.

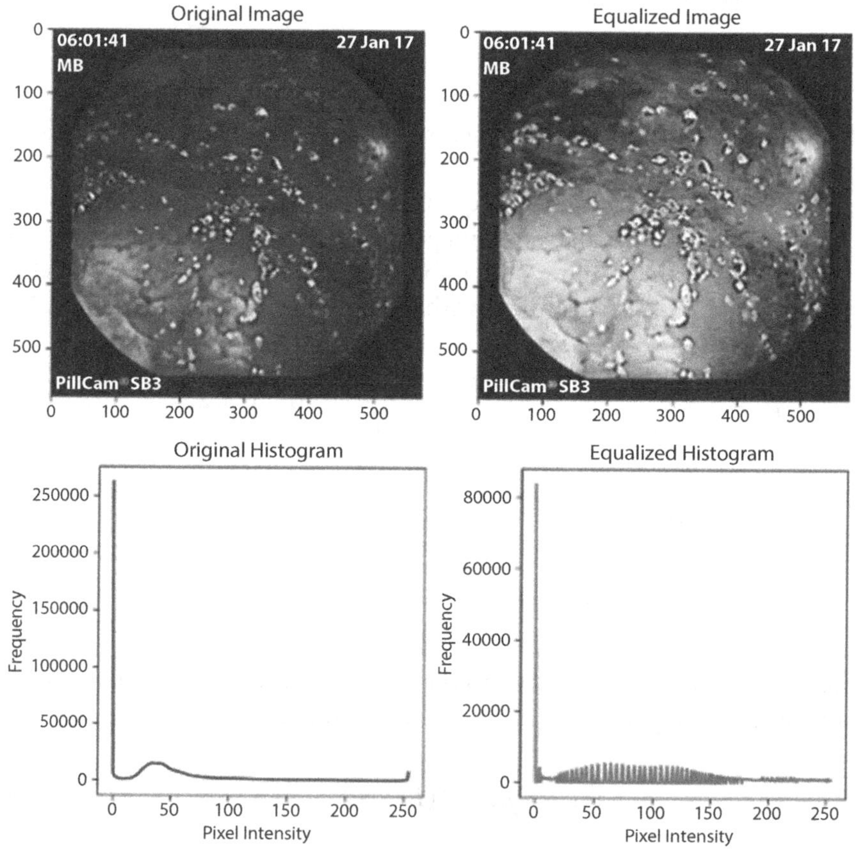

Figure 7.4 Histogram equalized image.

Algorithm 7.1: Histogram Equalization Algorithm

```
Input: An image with intensity values ranging from 0 to L – 1, where L is the maximum intensity level.
Output: The equalized image.
Initialize an array H of size L, where each element is initialized to zero.
for i← 0 to L – 1 do//Traverse it from i to L – 1
    H[i]← 0
end for
Calculate the histogram of the input image
for each pixel (x, y) in the image do
    intensity← getIntensityValue(x, y) // Retrieve the intensity value of the current pixel
    H[intensity] +← 1 // Increment the corresponding bin in the histogram
end for
return H
Calculate the total number of pixels N in the image.
N ← totalNumberOfPixels(image)// Initialize total number of pixels
Normalize the Histogram
for i ←0 to L – 1 do// Traverse each bin i in the histogram
    H[i] /← N
end for
Calculate the Cumulative Distribution Function (CDF)
C[0]←H [0]// Initialize an array C of size L with the first element C[0] set to H[0].
for i← 1 to L – 1 do// Traverse each bin i from 1 to L – 1
    C[i] ← C[i – 1] + H[i]
end for
Calculate the Transformation Function T(k)
Initialize an array T of size L.
for i← 0 to L – 1 do
    T[i] ← round((L – 1) * C[i])
end for
newImage ← createImageWithSameSize(image)// Create a new image
for each pixel (x, y) in the image do
```

Intensity ← *getIntensityValue*(**x, y**) // *Retrieve the intensity value of the current pixel*

newIntensity ← **T[intensity]** // *Get the new intensity value from the transformation function*

setIntensityValue(newImage, x, y, newIntensity) // *Assign the new intensity value to the corresponding pixel in the new image*

end for

return newImage// *Return the new equalized image*

7.3.4 Denoising

Noise is the unwanted random variations in brightness or color that occur due to factors such as sensor limitations, low-light conditions, or transmission. In a WCE, different sensors and LEDs are incorporated within the capsule; hence, there is a chance that the data extracted from it might contain noise. Therefore, denoising algorithms aim to provide the underlying structure and details of an image while suppressing noise. Previously, a histogram equalization method was used to understand the contrast and intensities of images; hence, this process might induce some noise, and denoising the same is a major requirement for this work. In this study, the wavelet transformation technique was used to denoise the bleeding and WCE images as shown in Figure 7.5.

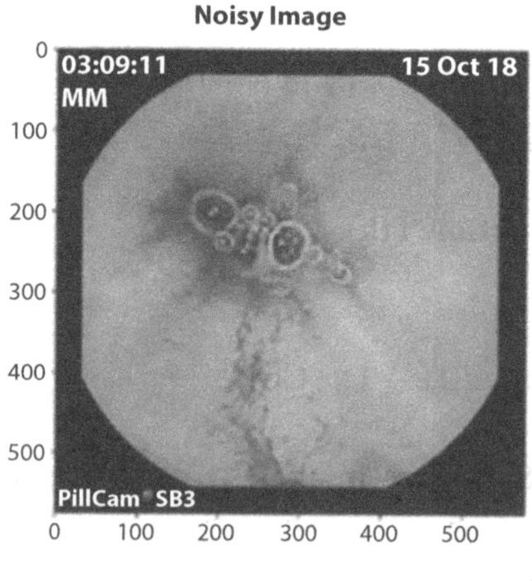

Figure 7.5 Denoised images.

7.3.5 Adaptive Filtering

Gaussian adaptive filtering plays a significant role in the ensemble feature extraction and classification of bleeding and normal WCE images. This preprocessing step, combined with ensemble feature extraction techniques, helps extract relevant features from the enhanced images, enabling the classification algorithms to effectively distinguish between bleeding and normal regions. The incorporation of Gaussian adaptive filtering as part of the ensemble feature extraction and classification pipeline enhanced the overall accuracy and reliability of the diagnostic system, ultimately aiding medical professionals in making informed decisions regarding the presence or absence of gastrointestinal bleeding based on WCE images. Some samples of the adaptive filtering image-processing technique are shown in Figure 7.6.

7.3.6 Augmentation

In the biomedical domain, the greatest challenge is to obtain sufficient images for computation. Thus, image augmentation plays a crucial role in increasing the diversity of the datasets. The original dataset contains only 46 bleeding WCE images and 160 normal images, which are insufficient for computation. In the present study, variations such as rotation, shifts, flips, and shear ranges were implemented to augment the bleeding and normal WCE images, respectively. The modifications were performed using an Image Data Generator library. Some of the images that are generated after applying the code are depicted in Figure 7.7 and Table 7.1 illustrates the parameters that are specified for image augmentation. Table 7.2 shows the increased amount of bleeding and the normal images after augmentation.

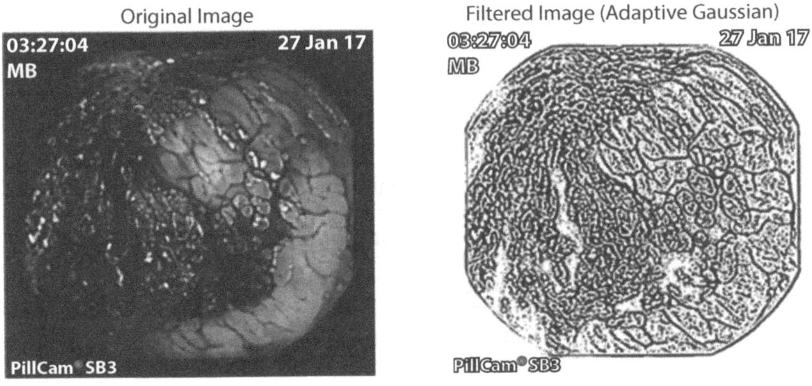

Figure 7.6 Adaptive filtered image.

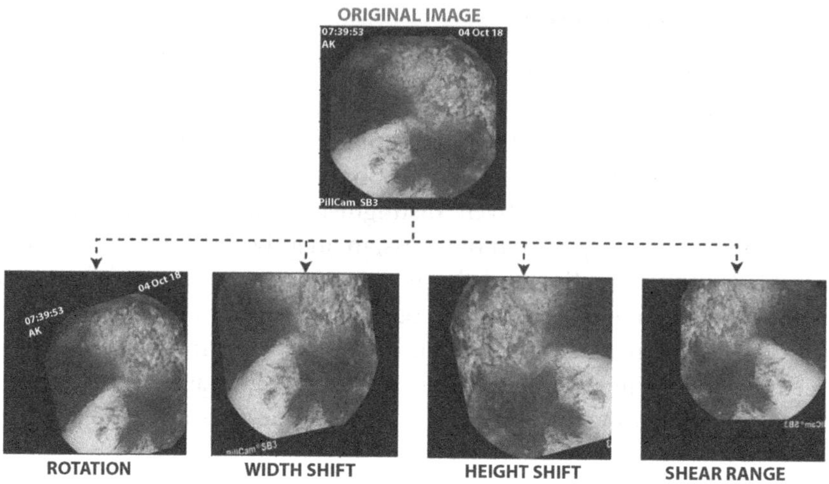

Figure 7.7 Samples of the augmented images.

Table 7.1 Parameters for image augmentation.

Parameters	Values
Rotation	20^0
Width Shift	0.2
Height Shift	0.2
Shear	0.2

Table 7.2 Original dataset.

Classes	Total images
Bleeding	1,091
Normal	1,064

7.3.7 Data Processing

Model development involves partitioning data into training and test sets. In this study, the augmented data were divided into training and testing sets using the k-fold validation method. This approach, involving K-fold cross-validation, enhances the robustness of evaluating model performance. The dataset was segmented into K subsets (folds), with each fold acting as a validation set. while the remaining folds were utilized for training. This iterative process was repeated K times, and the performance metrics were averaged across all instances. Employing K-fold cross-validation diminishes the reliance on a specific data split, thereby mitigating the risk of bias in the assessment of model performance.

7.3.8 Convolutional Neural Network

Convolutional Neural Networks have revolutionized feature extraction in various fields including computer vision and image processing. One key advantage of CNNs is their ability to capture local spatial dependencies within an image. By applying convolutional filters, these networks can detect low-level features such as edges, corners, and textures. As the network layers deepen, higher-level features such as shapes, objects, and even abstract concepts can be extracted. In this study, three different CNN models were utilized to extract the features discussed in the following subsections:

7.3.8.1 ResNet 50

ResNet-50 is a widely used CNN architecture that has made significant advancements in terms of feature extraction. The architecture of ResNet-50 possesses 50 layers, with a combination of convolutional, pooling, fully connected, and identity-mapping layers. The initial layers perform typical operations such as convolution, batch normalization, and activation functions. However, the core building blocks of ResNet-50 are residual blocks, specifically, bottleneck residual blocks. Each bottleneck residual block in ResNet-50 included three convolutional layers with 1×1, 3×3, and 1×1 filter sizes. The 1×1 convolutions are used for lowering and restoring the dimensionality of the feature maps, whereas the 3×3 convolution applies nonlinearity to learn more complex features. Additionally, batch normalization and activation functions were applied after each convolutional layer to enhance training stability and model performance. The overall

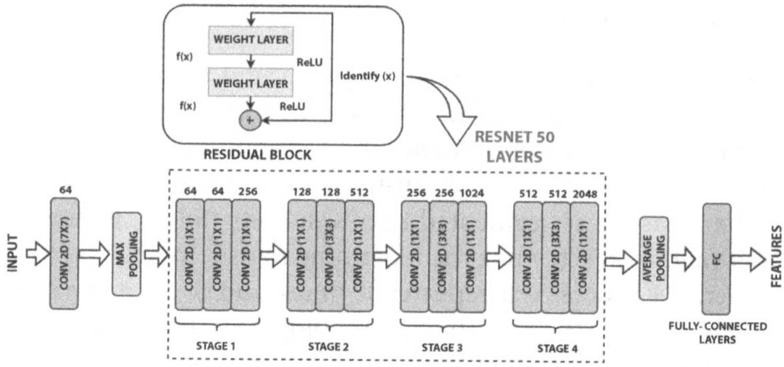

Figure 7.8 Block diagram of ResNet50 architecture.

architecture of ResNet-50 with its deep layers and residual blocks is shown in Figure 7.8.

7.3.8.2 VGG 16

The architecture of VGG-16 was identified by its deep stack of convolutional neural layers. Comprising 16 layers, the structure includes 13 convolutional layers and three fully connected layers. The convolutional layers were organized into distinct blocks, where each block incorporated multiple convolutional layers featuring compact 3 × 3 filters, followed by subsequent max pooling. The initial layers of VGG-16 perform basic operations, such as convolution, activation functions (usually ReLU), and pooling. The primary objective of these layers is to capture fundamental features at a lower level, encompassing elements, such as edges, textures, and corners. The repeated use of small 3 × 3 filters allows the network to capture finer details in images, leading to a rich feature representation. After several convolutional blocks, VGG-16 incorporated fully connected layers for classification. The fully connected layers serve as classifiers that take the flattened feature maps from the preceding convolutional layers and produce the final predictions.

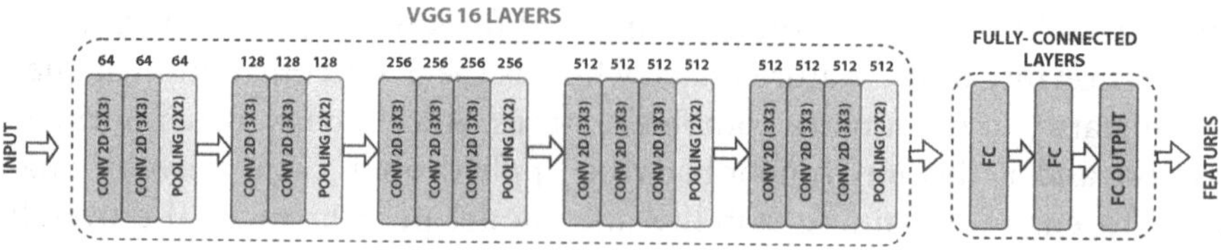

Figure 7.9 Block diagram of VGG 16 architecture.

These layers systematically decreased the dimensionality of the features while capturing the overall context essential for classification. Figure 7.9 depicts the block diagram of VGG 16 used for feature extraction in the proposed work.

7.3.8.3 Inception V3

InceptionV3 architecture is a popular CNN model that has been widely utilized for feature extraction in computer vision tasks. The key idea behind InceptionV3 is the utilization of "Inception modules," which allows the network to capture features at different spatial scales while minimizing computational complexity. InceptionV3 incorporates various types of convolutional filters within each inception module, including 1 × 1, 3 × 3, and 5 × 5 filters. The utilization of 1 × 1 convolutions aids in diminishing the dimensionality of the feature maps, serving as a bottleneck, and effectively lowering computational expenses. Larger filters (3 × 3 and 5 × 5) capture more spatial context and allow the network to learn complex patterns and structures. Inception V3 also incorporates max pooling and average pooling layers to downsample the feature maps and extract the most salient information. These pooling layers help reduce spatial dimensions, increase translation invariance, and improve computational efficiency. A diagrammatic representation of the Inception V3 model used for ensemble feature extraction is shown in Figure 7.10.

7.3.9 Feature Extraction

Ensemble feature extraction can improve feature representation and boost predictive accuracy in various computer vision tasks by leveraging the complementary capabilities of different models, such as ResNet-50, VGG-16, and InceptionV3. The proposed method introduces an ensemble feature extraction technique by concatenating the features of the three different CNN models. The block diagram representation is shown in Figure 7.11, which provides a clear idea of the method developed. The concatenated

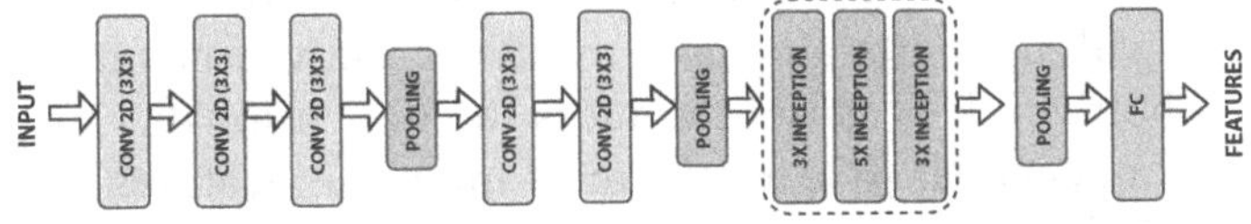

Figure 7.10 Block diagram of Inception V3 architecture.

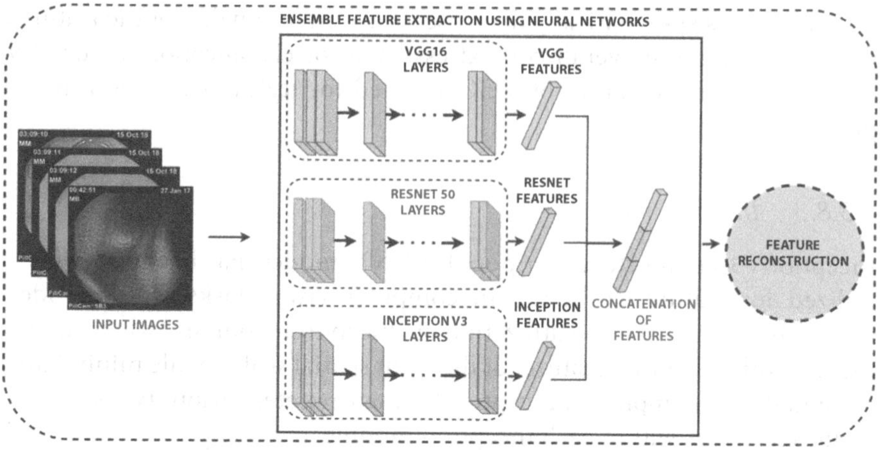

Figure 7.11 Diagrammatic representation of the ensemble feature extraction technique.

features were further used for the classification of the bleeding and normal images. This method is predominately better when extracting features that provides raw insights into the data. By combining ResNet-50, VGG-16, and InceptionV3 into an ensemble, we can leverage the unique characteristics of each model. This ensemble approach allows models to compensate for each other's limitations and capture a broader range of features.

7.3.10 Feature Reconstruction

Feature reconstruction using an autoencoder aims to reconstruct the original input data from a compressed representation obtained through an encoder–decoder architecture. In this model, the input features are processed through two dense layers that incorporate ReLU activation functions. The initial dense layer comprised 64 units and the second dense layer further reduced the dimensionality to 32 units.

$$Y = \max(0, j) \tag{7.5}$$

Equation (7.5) represents the working of the ReLU, where Y is the output generated. The bottleneck layer, also known as the latent space, is a dense layer with 16 units and uses the ReLU activation function. This serves as a bottleneck because it reduces the dimensionality of the data, forcing the autoencoder to learn the most important features and discard unnecessary information. The decoder part of the autoencoder model aims

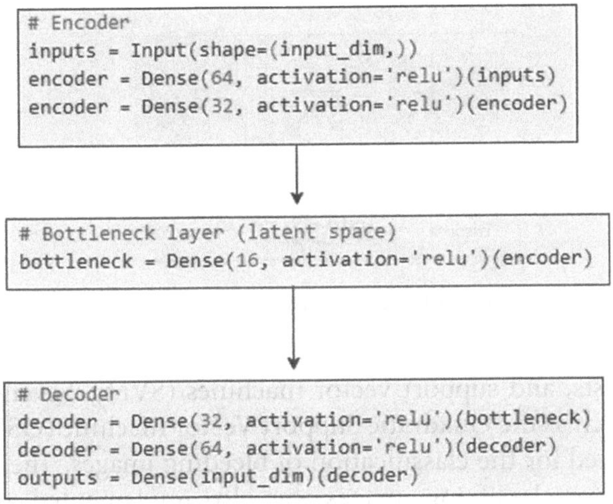

Figure 7.12 Specification for the autoencoder.

to reconstruct input features from the bottleneck layer. It comprises two dense layers that integrate ReLU activation functions. The earliest dense layer had 32 units, serving as the initial step in expanding the dimensionality back to the original size. The second fully connected layer has 64 units, further expanding its dimensions. The final output layer of the autoencoder had the same dimensionality as the input features, representing the reconstructed features. The training of the autoencoder model involves minimizing the loss, specifically the mean squared error (MSE), between the original input features and reconstructed output features. The specifications and arrangement of the autoencoder for the feature reconstruction are shown in Figure 7.12.

7.3.11 Classification

In the world of machine learning, classification is a fundamental undertaking in which predefined labels or categories are assigned to input data according to their inherent characteristics or features. Classifications can also be performed using deep neural networks, as in [39], where a technique that infuses high-level Inception-ResNet-V2 and low-level CNN was employed. Several other methods involving Mobile Net [40] have been implemented to classify gastrointestinal bleeding diseases. In the process of classification, the model is trained to distinguish different classes by determining the decision boundaries or decision rules in the feature space. Popular classification algorithms include logistic regression, decision trees,

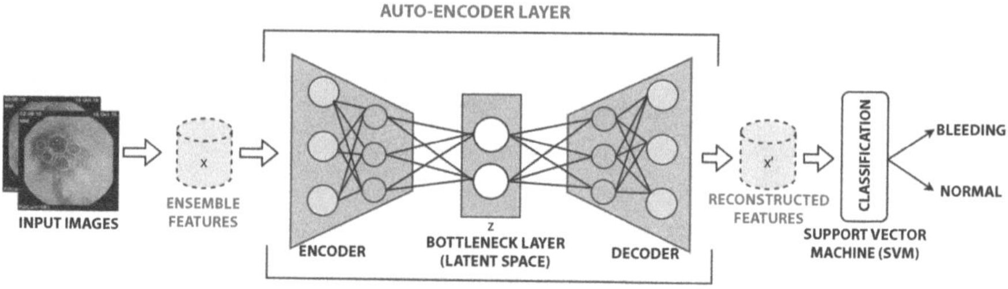

Figure 7.13 Proposed framework architecture.

random forests, and support vector machines (SVM). Several integrated classifiers, such as the Quadratic Support Vector Machine (QSVM) in [41], are also applied for the classification of bleeding images. The morphological process for classifying images was also implemented and reported in [42]. In the proposed work, an SVM integrated with an auto-encoder layer was implemented for classification. The SVM classifier was initialized using a Python library called sckit-learn. Overall, the classification process combines the power of autoencoders to reconstruct meaningful features and the SVM for performing the classification task, as shown in Figure 7.13. This approach can be effective in scenarios where the original feature space is high dimensional or contains complex patterns, allowing for improved classification accuracy.

7.4 Results and Discussion

A detailed and extensive validation process was conducted to compute the overall process for classifying WCE bleeding and normal classes. The model training was performed using Google Collaboratory. The implementation of the model is performed out using Keras and TensorFlow libraries in the Python programming language.

A comprehensive experiment is performed using the proposed framework. This study evaluated the classification of bleeding and normal disease. This study was performed using a deep feature extraction method. This involves the concatenation of feature vectors from three different deep neural network models. The ensemble features were subjected to a comprehensive validation process involving 50 epochs to reconstruct the features using an autoencoder. The autoencoder model was defined and compiled using the Adam optimizer and mean binary loss to ensure effective feature reconstruction.

Figures 7.14a and b show the accuracy and loss graphs, respectively, which provide insight into the performance of the autoencoder throughout the training process. This study evaluated different performance parameters in terms of accuracy, precision, recall, F1-score, AUC-score, Matthew's correlation coefficient, false positive rate (FPR), and false negative rate (FNR). The parameters were as follows:

$$Accuracy(ACC) = \frac{T_p + T_n}{T_P + T_n + F_p + F_n} \tag{7.6}$$

$$Precision(PPV) = \frac{T_p}{T_p + F_p} \tag{7.7}$$

$$Recall(Sensitivity) = \frac{T_p}{T_p + F_n} \tag{7.8}$$

$$F1 - Score = \frac{2T_P}{2T_p + F_p + F_n} \tag{7.9}$$

$$MCC = \frac{(T_p * T_n) - (F_p * F_n)}{\sqrt{(T_p + F_p) * (T_p + F_n) * (T_n + F_p) * (T_n + F_n)}} \tag{7.10}$$

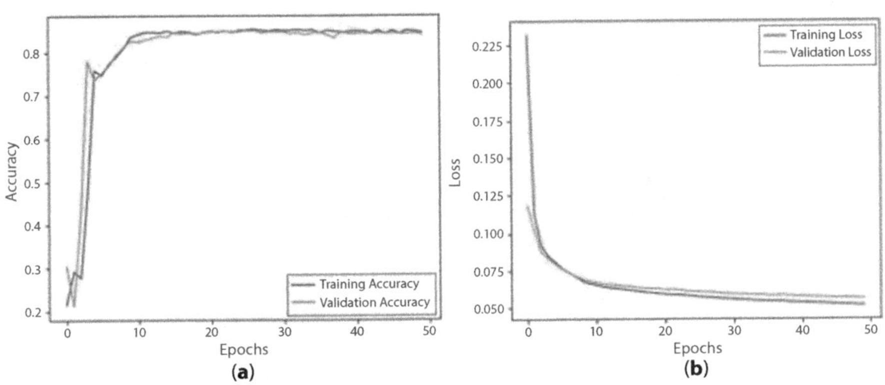

Figure 7.14 (a) Accuracy graph for the autoencoder classifier, (b) loss graph for the autoencoder classifier.

$$FPR = \frac{F_p}{F_p + T_n} \tag{7.11}$$

$$FNR = \frac{F_n}{F_n + T_p} \tag{7.12}$$

The reconstructed features obtained from the autoencoder are then utilized as inputs for a machine learning classifier, namely, a Support Vector Machine. This classifier further classifies the features into bleeding and normal classes, aiding the identification of anomalies within the examined images. To assess the performance of the SVM classifier, confusion matrices of 5-fold cross validation were generated, as shown in Figure 7.15. This matrix provides a visual representation of the classifier's ability to correctly classify instances as true positives, true negatives, false positives, or false negatives. To evaluate the overall performance of the classifier, various performance metrics were calculated. These metrics, listed in Table 7.3, provide a comprehensive understanding of the classifier's ability to classify bleeding and normal images accurately. Table 7.4 illustrates the hyperparameters used while validating the machine learning algorithms

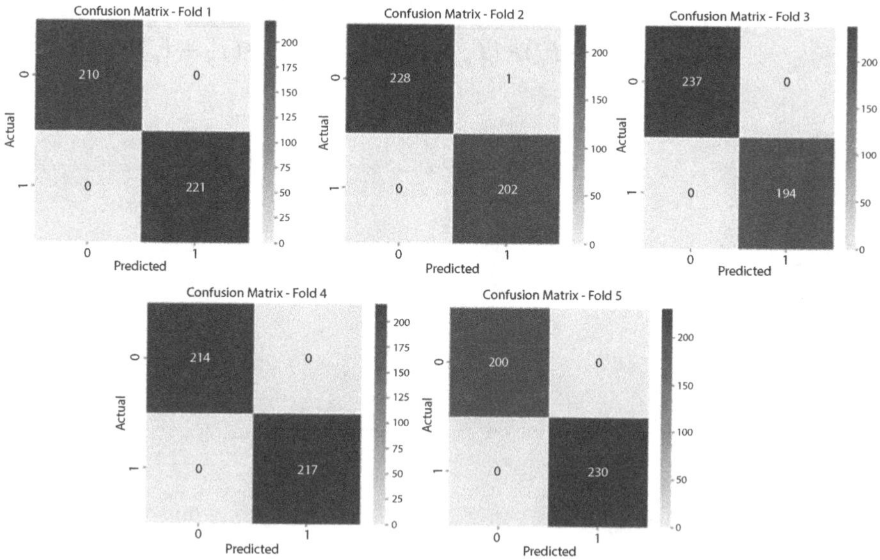

Figure 7.15 Confusion matrix for the proposed classifier using 5-fold validation.

Table 7.3 Performance results generated from encoder-SVM classifier using 5-fold validation.

Ensemble feature extractor	K-folds	Accuracy	Precision.	Recall	F1-score	AUC-score	MCC	FPR	FNR
ResNet50 + VGG16 + Inception V3	1	1.00	1.00	1.00	1.00	1.00	1.00	0.0045	0.0048
ResNet50 + VGG16 + Inception V3	2	0.995	0.9952	0.9952	0.9952	0.99	0.99	0.0045	0.0048
ResNet50 + VGG16 + Inception V3	3	1.00	1.00	1.00	1.00	1.00	1.00	0.0045	0.0048
ResNet50 + VGG16 + Inception V3	4	1.00	1.00	1.00	1.00	1.00	1.00	0.0045	0.0048
ResNet50 + VGG16 + Inception V3	5	1.00	1.00	1.00	1.00	1.00	1.00	0.0045	0.0048

Table 7.4 Hyperparameters of the machine learning models.

Support Vector Machine (SVM)	**Kernel = radial basis function**
K-Nearest Neighbor (KNN)	Leaf_size = 5, p = 1, neighbors = 7
Decision Tree (DT)	Max_depth = 200
Random Forest (RF)	n_estimators = 200, random_state = 5, max_depth = 200

corresponding to 5-fold cross validation. The table demonstrates that, for the SVM, the radial basis function kernel is utilized for classification. The K-Nearest Neighbor algorithm was implemented with three hyperparameters: leaf size, probability value, and n neighbors. A maximum depth value of 200 was incorporated into the decision tree. Under the Random Forest algorithm, an n-estimator value of 200 signifies the creation of a 200-decision tree.

The study was further compared by using a single different Deep Feature extractor for feature extraction and then classifying the normal and bleeding images using ML algorithms. Figure 7.16 illustrates the ROC curve obtained after validating different ML classifiers using the ResNet 50 feature extractor. The ROC curve for the VGG 16 feature extractor is depicted in Figure 7.17, and that for Inception v3 it is shown in Figure 7.18. ROC graphs were plotted against the overall AUC generated by the 5-fold validation method. In Table 7.5, a detailed report of the performance parameters.

This study work highlights valuable methods for classifying bleeding and normal WCE classes in the gastrointestinal tract. The entire method comprises several steps, including Data Acquisition, Image Processing, Augmentation, Data pre-processing, Feature Extraction and Classification. The impact of ensemble feature extraction on the proposed method is profound, as it significantly contributes to the generation of highly accurate results. The entire framework was developed utilizing three deep neural networks, namely ResNet50, VGG 16, and Inception V3, which were used to extract features from the pre-processed augmented images. The features were concatenated and used to feed the Encoder-SVM classifier for smooth classification. The autoencoder comprises an encoder layer, a bottleneck layer, and a decoder channel to reconstruct the ensemble features extracted from the three deep neural networks. A k-fold validation of five folds was performed to assess the scores. The overall framework generates an average

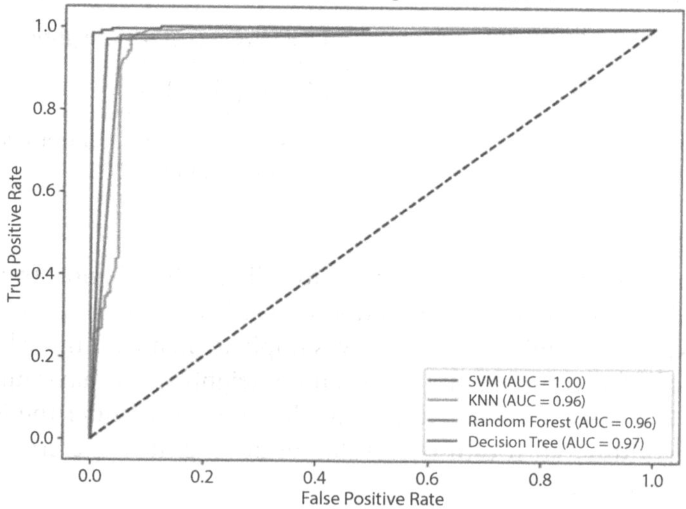

Figure 7.16 Receiver operating characteristic (ROC) curve for the classifiers using ResNet features.

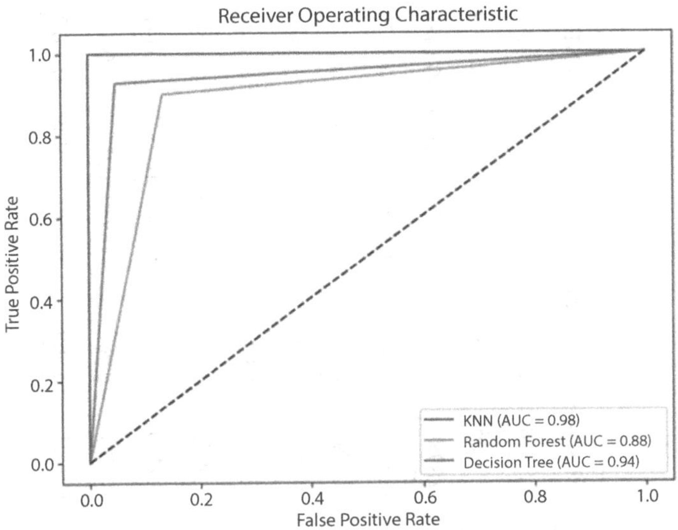

Figure 7.17 Receiver operating characteristic (ROC) curve for the classifiers using VGG features.

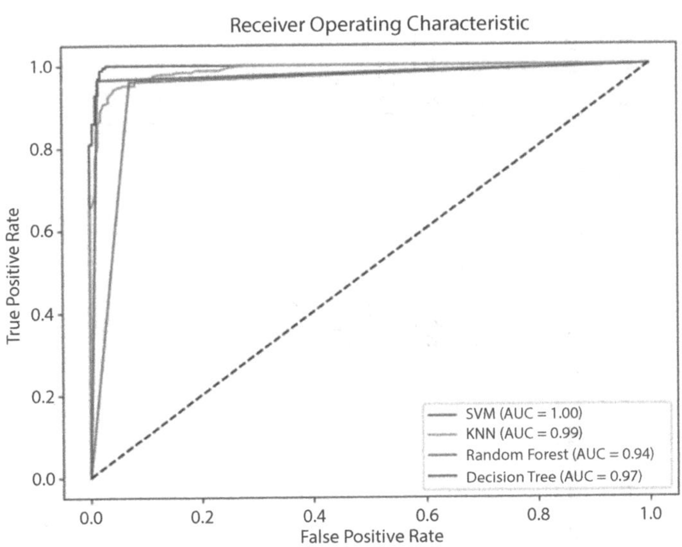

Figure 7.18 Receiver operating characteristic (ROC) curve for the classifiers using inception features.

Table 7.5 Comparison table using different feature extractor.

Ensemble feature extractor	Classifier	K-folds	Accuracy.	Precision.	Recall	F1-score	AUC-score	MCC	FPR	FNR
ResNet50	SVM	5	0.9861	0.9905	0.9811	0.9858	0.99	0.9722	0.0091	0.0189
	RF	5	0.9652	0.9524	0.9756	0.9636	0.96	0.9306	0.0442	0.0244
	KNN	5	0.8956	0.9524	0.8511	0.8989	0.96	0.7970	0.0510	0.1489
	DT	5	0.9722	0.9762	0.9670	0.9716	0.97	0.9443	0.0228	0.0330
VGG16	RF	5	0.884	0.8667	0.8922	0.8792	0.88	0.7680	0.1233	0.107
	KNN	5	0.877	0.7952	0.9435	0.8630	0.98	0.7620	0.1693	0.0565
	DT	5	0.9397	0.9524	0.9259	0.9390	0.94	0.8797	0.0465	0.0741
Inception. V3	SVM	5	0.9861	0.9905	0.9811	0.9858	0.99	0.9722	0.0091	0.0189
	RF	5	0.9443	0.9286	0.9559	0.9420	0.94	0.8888	0.0661	0.0441
	KNN	5	0.9490	0.9571	0.9393	0.9481	0.987	0.8980	0.0415	0.0607
	DT	5	0.9745	0.9857	0.9628	0.9741	0.969	0.9492	0.0139	0.0372

accuracy, precision, recall, F1-score, AUC-score, Matthew's correlation coefficient (MCC), false positive rate (FPR), and false negative rate (FNR) of 99.5%, 99.51%, 99.51%, 99.51%, 99%, 99%, 0.0045, and 0.0048, respectively. Ensemble feature extraction has a significant impact. The ensemble approach showed potential for synergy among different methods, leading to a more comprehensive and discriminative representation of WCE images. Through the generation of highly accurate results, the ensemble feature extraction proved its value in advancing the field of image classification and contributed to the overall success of the proposed method.

In the experimentation phase, the features extracted from the ResNet model were utilized to classify bleeding and normal WCE images. The ResNet model, renowned for its exceptional performance in image recognition tasks, was employed with specific weights and incorporated a fully connected layer at the top of the network. These ResNet features served as input for four distinct machine learning classifiers: SVM, DT, KNN, and RF. The purpose of this evaluation was to understand the proficiency of these classifiers in precisely categorizing WCE images based on ResNet features. Additionally, an array of performance metrics, including accuracy, precision, recall, and F1-score, are generated to evaluate the classifiers' performance. By comparing the results obtained from the four classifiers, using 5-fold validation process, it becomes possible to discern their strengths and weaknesses in classifying bleeding and normal WCE images. Among the SVM, DT, KNN, and RF, the SVM classifier generated the highest accuracy of 98.61%. The findings of this study have the potential to guide future research endeavors and facilitate the development of more accurate and efficient classification models tailored for WCE applications.

In this study, experiments were conducted to investigate the classification of bleeding and normal WCE images using the features extracted from the VGG model. The VGG model is widely recognized for its exceptional performance in image-recognition tasks, making it a suitable choice for research. The use of specific weights and fully connected layers in the network enhances its capabilities. The features extracted from the VGG 16 model served as the input for three prominent machine learning classifiers: DT, KNN, and RF. A comparative analysis of these models was conducted to determine the efficacy of the eminent classifier. The entire study proved that the decision tree resulted in generating the top accuracy of 93.97% for the VGG-based feature extraction process. In contrast, K-nearest Neighbor and Random Forest had average accuracies of 87.7% and 88.4%, respectively. Thus, this analysis provides a comprehensive understanding of the strengths and weaknesses of each classifier in handling the WCE image classification task using VGG features.

Classification is a major problem in the biomedical domain, and an investigation using Inception features was conducted in this study. Features were extracted using a single deep neural network named Inception V3 with specific alterations in the model. Different classifiers, such as SVM, DT, KNN, and RF, were fed into the pipeline to classify the bleeding and normal images. The comparative report displayed various performance scores in the form of accuracy, precision, recall, F1-score, AUC-score, Matthew's correlation coefficients, etc. The detailed analysis provides a thorough perspective that SVM resulted in the highest accuracy of 98.61% among all the classifiers using Inception features.

The proposed work also contains an overall comparison based on the different state-of-the-art approaches presented in the literature, as listed in Table 7.6. The analysis showed that the novel framework utilizing ensemble features outperformed any other illustrated technique. In summary, the experimentation and analysis conducted in this study demonstrate the superiority of ensemble feature extraction over single deep neural network features in the classification of WCE images. By combining the features extracted from multiple deep models, namely ResNet 50, VGG16, and InceptionV3, the ensemble approach outperformed state-of-the-art techniques and achieved the best results. A comparison of different machine learning classifiers, such as SVM, DT, KNN, and RF, further validated the effectiveness of the ensemble feature extraction approach. The ensemble features provide a more comprehensive representation of the WCE images, enabling the classifiers to make more accurate and robust predictions. This study contributes to advancing the field of WCE image classification by

Table 7.6 Comparison of the proposed work with other state-of-the-art works reported in the literature.

Reference	Accuracy	Precision.	Recall	F1-score	AUC-score
SVM-based Pipeline [39]	–	98.11%	–	–	–
Inception-ResNet-V2 [40]	98.5%	98.5%	98.5%	–	–
MobileV2-BiLSTM [37]	99.6%	–	–	–	–
BIR Model [41]	99.3%	100%	99.4%	99.7%	–
Quadratic SVM [42]	95.8%	80%	95%	85%	–
CNN(BIR) [22]	99.3%	100%	99.4%	99.4%	99.5%
Proposed Model	99%	99.5%	99.5%	99.5%	99%

highlighting the importance of ensemble feature extraction. The ensemble approach surpasses the limitations of single deep neural network architectures and harnesses the power of multiple models, leading to improved classification performance and diagnostic accuracy.

7.5 Conclusion

The proposed work successfully demonstrated the effectiveness of ensemble feature extraction for the classification of WCE images. By combining features extracted from multiple deep models, namely ResNet, VGG, and InceptionV3, the ensemble approach achieves superior performance compared to single deep neural network architectures and outperforms state-of-the-art techniques. An accuracy of 99% was achieved when validating the ensemble features using 5-fold validation process. The utilization of multiple models allows diverse and complementary information to be captured. However, it is essential to address the limitations of this study. First, this study focused on bleeding and normal WCE image classification, and the performance of other GI tract diseases has not been explored. Future learning could extend this study to encompass a wider range of GI tract pathologies. Additionally, although ensemble feature extraction yields promising results, the computational cost associated with combining multiple models and training an ensemble should be considered. Future research could explore more efficient ensemble techniques to mitigate computational complexity while maintaining or even improving the performance. Furthermore, the current study used pre-trained deep models and focused on the extraction of high-level features. Exploring the potential of fine-tuning models specifically for WCE image classification could lead to even better results. Finally, the proposed ensemble feature extraction approach is evaluated on a specific dataset. Subsequent research efforts should focus on confirming the conclusions using more extensive and diverse datasets, thereby ensuring the approach's generalizability and robustness.

References

1. Wahab, H., Mehmood, I., Ugail, H., Sangaiah, A.K., Muhammad, K., Machine learning based small bowel video capsule endoscopy analysis: Challenges and opportunities. *Future Gener. Comput. Syst.*, 143, 191–214, 2023.

2. Tanwar, S., Vijayalakshmi, S., Sabharwal, M., Kaur, M., AlZubi, A.A., Lee, H.N., Detection and Classification of Colorectal Polyp Using Deep Learning. *BioMed. Res. Int.*, 1, 2805607, 2022.
3. Masmoudi, Y., Ramzan, M., Khan, S.A., Habib, M., Optimal feature extraction and ulcer classification from WCE image data using deep learning. *Soft Comput.*, 26, 1–14, 2022.
4. Muruganantham, P. and Balakrishnan, S.M., Attention aware deep learning model for wireless capsule endoscopy lesion classification and localization. *J. Med. Biol. Eng.*, 42, 2, 157–168, 2022.
5. Marin-Santos, D., Contreras-Fernandez, J.A., Perez-Borrero, I., Pallares-Manrique, H., Gegundez-Arias, M.E., Automatic detection of crohn disease in wireless capsule endoscopic images using a deep convolutional neural network. *Appl. Intell.*, 53, 10, 1–15, 2022.
6. Klang, E., Grinman, A., Soffer, S., Yehuda, R.M., Barzilay, O., Amitai, M.M., Konen, E., Ben-Horin, S., Eliakim, R., Barash, Y., Kopylov, U., Automated detection of Crohn's disease intestinal strictures on capsule endoscopy images using deep neural networks. *J. Crohn's Colitis*, 15, 5, 749–756, 2021.
7. de Maissin, A., Vall´ee, R., Flamant, M., Fondain-Bossiere, M., Le Berre, C., Coutrot, A., Normand, N., Mouchère, H., Coudol, S., Trang, C., Bourreille, A., Multi-expert annotation of Crohn's disease images of the small bowel for automatic detection using a convolutional recurrent attention neural network. *Endosc. Int. Open*, 9, 07, E1136–E1144, 2021.
8. Falin, Z., Haihua, L., Ning, P., Gastrointestinal Polyps and Tumors Detection Based on Multi-scale Feature-fusion with WCE Sequences, 2022, arXiv preprint arXiv:2204.01012.
9. Ellahyani, A., Jaafari, I.E., Charfi, S., Ansari, M.E., Fine-tuned deep neural networks for polyp detection in colonoscopy images. *Pers. Ubiquitous Comput.*, pp. 1–13, 2022.
10. Kundu, A.K., Fattah, S.A., Rizve, M.N., An automatic bleeding frame and region detection scheme for wireless capsule endoscopy videos based on interplane intensity variation profile in normalized RGB color space. *J. Healthcare Eng.*, 1, 9423062, 2018.
11. Pogorelov, K., Suman, S., Hussin, F.A., Malik, A.S., Ostroukhova, O., Riegler, M., Halvorsen, P., Ho, S.H., Goh, K.L., Bleeding detection in wireless capsule endoscopy videos—Color versus texture features. *J. Appl. Clin. Med. Phys.*, 20, 8, 141–154, 2019.
12. Jiang, H., Diao, Z., Shi, T., Zhou, Y., Wang, F., Hu, W., Zhu, X., Luo, S., Tong, G., Yao, Y.D., A review of deep learning-based multiple-lesion recognition from medical images: classification, detection and segmentation. *Biol. Med.*, 157, 106726, 2023.
13. Sivari, E., Bostanci, E., Guzel, M.S., Acici, K., Asuroglu, T., ErcelebiAyyildiz, T., A New Approach for Gastrointestinal Tract Findings Detection and Classification: Deep Learning-Based Hybrid Stacking Ensemble Models. *Diagnostics*, 13, 4, 720, 2023.

14. Mohapatra, S., Pati, G.K., Mishra, M., Swarnkar, T., Gastrointestinal abnormality detection and classification using empirical wavelet transform and deep convolutional neural network from endoscopic images. *Ain Shams Eng. J.*, 14, 4, 101942, 2023.
15. Satyanarayana, G., Naidu, P.A., Desanamukula, V.S., Rao, B.C., A mass correlation based deep learning approach using deep Convolutional neural network to classify the brain tumor. *Biomed. Signal Process. Control*, 81, 104395, 2023.
16. Pan, Q., Bao, Y., Li, H., Transfer learning-based data anomaly detection for structural health monitoring. *Struct. Health Monit.*, 22, 5, 14759217221142174, 2023.
17. Matta, S., Lamard, M., Conze, P.H., Guilcher, A.L., Ricquebourg, V., Benyoussef, A.A., Massin, P., Rottier, J.B., Cochener, B., Quellec, G., Meta learning for anomaly detection in fundus photographs, in: *Meta-Learning with Medical Imaging and Health Informatics Applications*, pp. 301–329, Academic Press, 2023.
18. Fan, W., Shangguan, W., Bouguila, N., Continuous image anomaly detection based on contrastive lifelong learning. *Appl. Intell.*, 53, 1, 1–15, 2023.
19. Ahmed, I., Ahmad, M., Chehri, A., Jeon, G., A Smart-Anomaly-Detection System for Industrial Machines Based on Feature Autoencoder and Deep Learning. *Micromachines*, 14, 1, 154, 2023.
20. Bandopadhyay, S., Ray, I.J., Mondal, S., Manna, S., Mitra, S., Roy, K., Banerjee, S., Chaudhuri, S.S., Drowsy Driving Detection Based on Deep Neural Network for Accident Avoidance, in: *Proceedings of International Conference on Computational Intelligence, Data Science and Cloud Computing, Algorithms for Intelligent Systems*, Springer, Singapore, 2022.
21. Roy, K., Chaudhuri, S.S., Frnda, J., Bandopadhyay, S., Ray, I.J., S.Banerjee, J., Nedoma, Detection of Tomato Leaf Diseases for Agro-Based Industries Using Novel PCA DeepNet. *IEEE Access*, 11, 14983–15001, 2023, doi: 10.1109/ACCESS.2023.3244499.
22. Goel, S. and Shah, A.K., CNN-based Classification over Wireless Capsule Endoscopy Bleeding Images, in: *2022 Second International Conference on Advanced Technologies in Intelligent Control, Environment, Computing Communication Engineering (ICATIECE)*, IEEE, pp. 1–5, 2022.
23. Wang, Z., Wang, Z., Zeng, C., Yu, Y., Wan, X., High-quality image compressed sensing and reconstruction with multi-scale dilated convolutional neural network. *Circuits Syst. Signal Process.*, 42, 3, 1593–1616, 2023.
24. Yin, C., Zhang, S., Wang, J., Xiong, N.N., Anomaly Detection Based on Convolutional Recurrent Autoencoder for IoT Time Series. *IEEE Trans. Syst. Man Cybern.: Syst.*, 52, 1, 112–122, 2022.
25. Onal, M.N., Guraksin, G.E., Duman, R., Convolutional neural network-based diabetes diagnostic system via iridology technique. *Multimed. Tools Appl.*, 81, 1, 173–194, 2023.

26. Lopac, N., Hržić, F., Vuksanović, I.P., Lerga, J., Detection of Non-Stationary GW Signals in High Noise from Cohen's Class of Time–Frequency Representations Using Deep Learning. *IEEE Access*, 10, 2408–2428, 2022, doi: 10.1109/ACCESS.2021.3139850.
27. Zhang, Y., Yi, J., Chen, A., Cheng, L., Cardiac arrhythmia classification by time–frequency features inputted to the designed convolutional neural networks. *Biomed. Signal Process. Control*, 79, 104224, 2023.
28. Jin, Y., Li, Z., Qin, C., Liu, J., Liu, Y., Zhao, L., Liu, C., A novel attentional deep neural network-based assessment method for ECG quality. *Biomed. Signal Process. Control*, 79, 104064, 2023.
29. Yang, J. *et al.*, Bagging ensemble of support vector machines for improved ac- curacy in breast cancer diagnosis. *J. Med. Syst.*, 42, 8, 141, 2018.
30. Rajaraman, J. *et al.*, Boosting ensemble of deep convolutional neural networks for malaria parasite detection. *Comput. Biol. Med.*, 102, 223–235, 2018.
31. Ahn, M. *et al.*, Stacking ensemble of multiple classifiers for brain tumor classification. *BMC Med. Inf. Decis. Making*, 17, 1, 155, 2017.
32. Popuri, M. *et al.*, Random subspace ensemble of texture features for lung nodule classification. *J. Med. Imaging*, 3, 4, 044506, 2016.
33. Kavitha, S. *et al.*, Deep ensemble learning for skin lesion classification. *Comput. Methods Programs Biomed.*, 194, 105518, 2020.
34. Sharma, N., Gupta, S., Koundal, D., Alyami, S., Alshahrani, H., Asiri, Y., Shaikh, A., U-Net Model with Transfer Learning Model as a Backbone for Segmentation of Gastrointestinal Tract. *Bioengineering*, 10, 1, 119, 2023.
35. Rahim, T., Usman, M.A., Shin, S.Y., A survey on contemporary computer-aided tumor, polyp, and ulcer detection methods in wireless capsule endoscopy imaging. *Comput. Med. Imaging Graphics*, 85, 101767, 2023.
36. Tuba, E., Tuba, M., Jovanovic, R., An algorithm for automated segmentation for bleeding detection in endoscopic images, in: *2017 International Joint Conference on Neural Networks (IJCNN)*, 2017, May, IEEE, pp. 4579–4586, 2017.
37. Padmavathi, P. and Harikiran, J., Wireless Capsule Endoscopy Infected Images Detection and Classification Using MobileNetV2-BiLSTM Model. *Int. J. Image Graphics*, 23, 5, 2350041, 2022.
38. Mandal, S., Adhikari, M., Banerjee, S., Chaudhuri, S.S., Novel Adaptive Statistical Method-CNN Synergism Based Two-Step WCE Image Segmentation, in: *2019 International Conference on Intelligent Computing and Control Systems (ICCS)*, IEEE, pp. 1024–1029, May, 2019.
39. Goyal, A., Kaur, J., Dhatarwal, J., Handa, P., Goel, N., Automatic detection of WCE bleeding frames using hybrid features and machine learning algorithms, in: *2022 IEEE India Council International Subsections Conference (INDISCON)*, pp. 1–7, 2022.

40. Garbaz, A., Lafraxo, S., Charfi, S., El Ansari, M., Koutti, L., Bleeding classification in wireless capsule endoscopy images based on inception-resnet-v2 and CNNs, in: *2022 IEEE Conference on Computational Intelligence in Bioinformatics and Computational Biology (CIBCB)*, IEEE, pp. 1–6, 2022.
41. Rustam, F., Siddique, M.A., Siddiqui, H.U.R., Ullah, S., Mehmood, A., Ashraf, I., Choi, G.S., Wireless capsule endoscopy bleeding images classification using CNN based model. *IEEE Access*, 9, 33675–33688, 2021.
42. Mamun, A.A., Hossain, M.S., Em, P.P., Tahabilder, A., Sultana, R., Islam, M.A., Small intestine bleeding detection using color threshold and morphological operation in WCE images. *Int. J. Electr. Comput. Eng.*, 11, 4, 3040, 2021.

8

Advances in Brain Tumor Detection and Localization: A Comprehensive Survey

Krishnangshu Paul, Arunima Patra and Prithwineel Paul*

Department of Computer Science & Engineering, Institute of Engineering & Management, Kolkata, University of Engineering & Management, Kolkata, West Bengal, India

Abstract
Brain tumors present a formidable challenge in modern medicine. These diverse growths require early detection and precise localization for effective treatment. Recent medical imaging innovations, including magnetic resonance images (MRI) and computed tomography scan (CT) scans, offer detailed insights into the tumor characteristics. Various algorithms, such as K-means and convolutional neural networks (CNNs), enhance the detection and localization accuracy. Support vector machine (SVM) have emerged as effective classifiers and innovative approaches such as the Fractional Harley transformation show promise. Multi-CNN architectures improve accuracy, while combining algorithms such as K-means and Fuzzy K-means enhance segmentation. Moreover, Convolutional Neural Networks consistently excel in brain tumor detection. Deep learning, particularly CNNs, offers superior performance, although complexities and resource constraints should be considered. This survey highlights the evolving landscape of brain tumor detection and localization, highlighting the power of deep learning in improving diagnostics and treatment planning.

***Keywords*:** MRI, CT scans, K-Means, CNNs, SVM, fractional harley transformation, fuzzy K-Means, segmentation

8.1 Introduction

Brain tumors represent a complex and formidable challenge in modern medicine [18]. According to the American Cancer Society, approximately

**Corresponding author*: prithwineel.paul@iem.edu.in

Neha Sharma, Korhan Cengiz and Prasenjit Chatterjee (eds.) Intelligent Data Analytics for Bioinformatics and Biomedical Systems, (195–212) © 2024 Scrivener Publishing LLC

24,810 malignant tumors of the brain or spinal cord have been recorded for the year 2023 [19]. The abnormal growth of cells within the brain can manifest in various forms, each posing unique diagnostic and therapeutic dilemmas. Brain tumors exhibit remarkable diversity in terms of their histology, location, and clinical presentation. Understanding the nature of glioblastomas [1, 2], the most aggressive form of brain cancer, to benign tumors like meningiomas is crucial for effective management. These tumors can cause cognitive deficits and motor impairments, further emphasizing the need for their early detection and localization [3–5]. Timely and accurate detection, as well as precise localization, are paramount for ensuring optimal patient outcomes. The last decade has witnessed a notable surge in research and technological innovations aimed at enhancing brain tumor detection and localization. This introduction sets the stage for a comprehensive exploration of this critical area, underscored by the analysis of several recent brain tumor cases. Recent advancements in medical imaging technologies have played a pivotal role in transforming the landscape of brain tumor diagnosis. MRI and CT have become indispensable tools, that enable clinicians to visualize the brain in detail. These high-resolution images not only aid in identifying the presence of tumors but also provide vital information about their size, shape, and closeness to vital structures of the brain. Over the decades, several methods have been developed to detect brain tumors [6]. The segmentation process begins by employing the k-means algorithm to partition the image based on its gray-level intensity. Subsequently, the distance between the cluster data points and the cluster centroid is computed using the Fuzzy C-means algorithm.

In [7], the authors demonstrated enhancements in image quality using contrast enhancement techniques. Subsequently, they applied an optimized Fuzzy C-means algorithm with a genetic algorithm to perform feature extraction using the GLRLM and GLCM. The classification task involved distinguishing between images of normal brains and those with tumors, achieving an accuracy rate of 94.8%. Due to the inherent complexities in the analysis of medical images, an elaborate methodology combining CNN and SVM was extensively discussed in [8]. In [9], the authors conducted a comparative analysis of various machine learning classifiers to distinguish between benign and malignant brain cancer MRIs. The evaluated classification algorithms included support SVM, neural network, naive Bayes, and K-nearest neighbors. The findings of this study indicate that the SVM model is the most efficient approach for tumor detection. Nagabushanam *et al.* [10] proposed a study of the two-phased approach. After enhancing the image contrast, they used the fractional Harley transformation method to pre-process the MRI scans. The coefficients of the transformation were classified into normal and abnormal based on adaptive neuro fuzzy inference (ANFIS) approach. The accuracy without the clinical dataset was 99.3%; however, with the Brain Tumor Image Segmentation (BRAT) 2015 clinical dataset, the accuracy was 97.54%. However, the entire process was evaluated using several metrics, such as sensitivity, specificity, classification rate, and accuracy. An article focusing on the low accuracy of traditional brain tumor detection has shown the use of multi-CNN as an effective measure [11]. The normalization layer added between the convolutional layers and pooling layers reduces the problem of overfitting. The accuracy improved significantly compared to 2D detection networks. Moreover, the accuracy improved significantly in comparison to the single-mode brain tumor detection methods.

In [12], a combination of four algorithms, i.e., K-means, Fuzzy K-means, Gaussian Hidden Markov Random Field (GHMRF), and Gaussian Mixture Model (GMM), has been proposed for brain tumor segmentation. Although various methods have been explored for brain tumor detection and localization, Convolutional Neural Networks (CNNs) have been widely acknowledged as the most effective and accurate approach. In [13], a Convolutional Neural Network (CNN) was used to segment tumors in seven types of brain diseases: glioma, Alzheimer's disease, Alzheimer's plus, meningioma, pick, Huntington, and sarcoma. In [14], Abd-Ellah *et al.* introduced a two-phase approach in which the first phase showed how CNN was used for feature extraction, and Error-correcting Outputs (ECO-SVM) were used for feature classification. This phase focuses on detecting and classifying MRI images into normal and abnormal images. The next phase focused on localization within abnormal MRIs using a region-based Convolutional Neural Network. In [15], an automatic segmentation method based on a CNN was proposed by the second-place holder of the onsite BRATs 2015 challenge. It explores small kernels, as they provide a deeper architecture and have positive results for overfitting. They also focused on the use of intensity normalization during preprocessing, resulting in the enhancement of the regions. In [16], a methodology using deep convolutional activation features was proposed, where the challenge of limited data for training and the large dimensions of the image were tackled by transferring the features extracted from CNNs activations trained using ImageNet.

Machine Learning algorithms continue to serve as effective tools for brain tumor detection and localization. However, Deep Learning algorithms, such as CNNs, have significantly narrowed the gap by delivering superior performance. This was achieved through automatic feature learning and their ability to process extensive datasets. Nonetheless, DL's heightened complexity, computational demands, and interpretability challenges should be thoughtfully considered, particularly in medical contexts with resource constraints. A detailed overview of the various ML and DL models used was presented in [17]. The choice between ML and DL depends on specific task requirements, available resources, and desired accuracy levels. Although ML remains relevant, DL, exemplified by CNNs, has become a powerful ally in the quest for precise brain tumor detection and localization, offering a pathway to improve diagnostic capabilities and treatment planning.

8.2 Background Study on Various Methods

To enhance brain tumor detection and precise localization, several cutting-edge methods, including machine learning and deep learning techniques, have emerged as powerful contenders. This comparative analysis delves into the effectiveness of these methods, shedding light on their strengths, limitations, and real-world applications.

8.2.1 SVM [24]

Support Vector Machines belong to the category of supervised learning algorithms. It was used for classification and regression. The SVM helps us to find a hyperplane that separates the data into different classes. The mathematical formulation for a linear SVM in a binary classification can be summarized as a minimization problem, i.e.,

$$minimize\ ||w_1||^2 \quad subject\ to\ y_i'(w_1{}^T.x_i' - b') \geq 1\,;\, i \in \{1,2,\ldots,n\}$$

where $(x_i', y_i')\,(i = 1,2,\ldots,n)$ represents the training dataset and w represents the normal vector to the hyperplane $w_1{}^T\ x_i - b' = 0$. Moreover, the classifier is based on the values of w_1 and b'.

8.2.1.1 Advantages

SVMs effectively handle both linear and non-linear classification in complex medical image data. They are ideal for high-dimensional medical images (e.g., MRI with thousands of pixels). SVMs minimize overfitting, which is crucial for small, noisy datasets. They maximize class separation by finding optimal hyperplanes, making them suitable for moderately sized datasets, which is essential when obtaining large labeled data is challenging.

8.2.1.2 Limitations

Traditional SVMs are binary classifiers suited for tasks such as binary brain tumor detection (present/absent). For complex tasks such as tumor type or grading, SVMs may require extensions. They handle nonlinearity but struggle with highly complex data, where deep learning, such as CNNs, may perform better. Imbalanced datasets can bias SVMs toward the majority class, requiring techniques such as class weight adjustment or resampling. Tuning the SVM hyperparameters for peak performance can be computationally expensive, e.g., with grid search or cross-validation.

8.2.2 KNN [24]

K-Nearest Neighbors (KNN) is a simple and intuitive supervised machine-learning algorithm. It has also been used for classification and regression. We use KNN to predict the assignment of the label of an unknown data point. More specifically, based on the training data, an unknown data point is assigned a label that is either assigned or most common to its k-nearest neighbors.

8.2.2.1 Advantages

KNN is predicted by a majority vote of K-nearest neighbors, making it user friendly. It handles nonlinear data, which are vital for complex tasks such as brain tumor detection. The KNN relies on the local context for predictions and is valuable for medical imaging. This is a lazy learning algorithm that does not build an explicit training model. Furthermore, it stores the entire dataset for predictions, is useful with limited labeled data and avoids complex model building.

8.2.2.2 Limitations

KNN's computational demands increase with larger datasets and high-dimensional spaces. K parameter choice is vital. Small K values yield noise, and large K values yield overly smooth boundaries. Distance metric selection impacts performance and often requires experimentation. KNN is sensitive to class imbalance, which is common in the medical imaging of rare tumor samples. This is addressed through resampling or class-weight adjustment.

8.2.3 Logistic Regression [24]

Logistic Regression is a popular statistical method used for binary classification in data analytics. The logistic function (also known as the sigmoid function) is a key component of the logistic regression equation. Logistic regression is primarily used for binary classifications. Moreover, a logistic function (sigmoid function) transforms the input variables into values between 0 and 1. The Sigmoid function is represented mathematically in the following manner: $f(z)=\frac{1}{1-e^{-z}}$. An important observation of the sigmoid function is that $f(z)\rightarrow 1$ whenever $z\rightarrow\infty$ and $f(z)\rightarrow 0$ whenever $z\rightarrow-\infty$.

8.2.3.1 Advantages

Logistic regression is well-suited for binary brain tumor detection (present or absent) and can be adapted for multiclass classification. It has a lower risk of overfitting, which is crucial in medical imaging for the generalization to new data. Logistic regression provides probabilities, aiding medical decision-making and confidence assessment. L1 or L2 regularization can be applied to prevent overfitting and enhance the model generalization.

8.2.3.2 Limitations

Logistic regression assumes a linear decision boundary, limiting its ability to capture complex nonlinear patterns in the imaging features. Medical imaging datasets can be high-dimensional, posing efficiency challenges for logistic regression. Feature selection or dimensionality reduction is required. Logistic regression is sensitive to outliers, which are common in medical imaging data and potentially lead to biased model results. Logistic regression may not harness the full potential of deep learning techniques such as CNNs, which have excelled in image-based tasks, including medical imaging.

8.2.4 CNN [24]

Convolutional Neural Networks (CNNs) are well-known deep learning architectures. It is can process structured grid data, i.e., images.

The components of the CNNs are (1) convolutional layers, (2) pooling layers, and (3) fully connected layers.

8.2.4.1 *Advantages*

CNNs are ideal for grid-like data, which are crucial for identifying structures in brain scans by effectively capturing the spatial relationships. They learn features at different levels of detail by adapting to various tumor characteristics. Transfer learning from ResNet-trained models enhances the performance by leveraging prior knowledge. CNNs are robust to tumor position and orientation variations and recognize patterns across images. CNNs require less sequential data, which is crucial in situations where labeled sequences are scarce and expensive. They benefit from parallel processing, accelerated training, and inference for large medical image datasets.

8.2.4.2 *Limitations*

To achieve high performance, a large amount of labeled data is required by CNNs for training. In medical imaging, collecting extensive and accurately labeled datasets is challenging and time consuming. A graph of validation loss and iterations has been shown in Figure 8.1. CNNs are often considered as *"black-box"* models. It is challenging to interpret how CNNs perform predictions. This lack of interpretability can be a drawback in medical contexts, where understanding the reasoning behind a diagnosis is important.

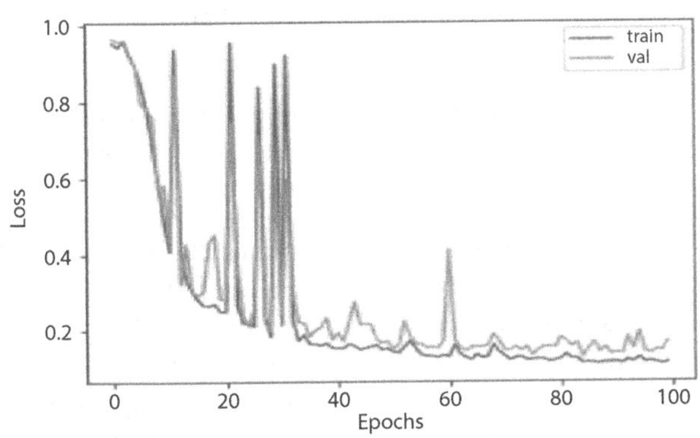

Figure 8.1 Graph of validation loss vs. iterations.

8.3 Methodology

Convolutional Neural Networks (CNNs) have demonstrated exceptional capabilities for the detection and localization of brain tumors. Unlike traditional machine learning methods, such as SVM, KNN, and Logistic Regression, CNNs excel at automatically extracting intricate features and patterns from medical images, particularly MRI scans (see Table 8.1). This inherent ability to discern subtle distinctions between tumor and non-tumor regions enables CNNs to precisely localize tumors within the brain. By leveraging CNN-based models, healthcare professionals can expedite the diagnosis process, aid in timely treatment planning, and improve patient outcomes. In summary, CNNs have emerged as a transformative

Table 8.1 Comparison of machine learning algorithms.

Method	Advantage	Limitations	References
SVM	Nonlinearity Handling High Dimensionality Robustness to Overfitting Clear Margin and Decision Boundary Effective on Small Datasets	Limited to Binary Classification Limited Handling of Imbalanced Data Handling Complex Data Computationally Intensive Parameter Tuning	[20]
KNN	Nonlinearity Handling Local-context Consideration No need for model training	Computational intensity Sensitivity to the Value of K Sensitivity to Distance Metric Data Imbalance	[21]
Logistic Regression	Low Overfitting Risk Probabilistic Output Regularization	Linear Assumption High-Dimensional Data Limited Deep Learning Use	[22]
CNN	Hierarchical Feature Extraction Spatial Information Pretrained Models Translation Invariance Data Efficiency	Requires a large amount of training data. Complex model architecture may lead to longer training times. Model interpretability can be challenging.	[23]

tool, surpassing conventional machine learning techniques in the realm of brain tumor detection and localization. In this study, we provide a detailed methodology for tumor detection and localization using a CNN. CNNs, or Convolutional Neural Networks, are deep learning models specifically designed for image-related tasks. They excel at learning hierarchical features from images and have been highly successful in several computer vision tasks, including medical image analysis.

Transfer learning is a technique in which a pretrained neural network, usually trained on a large dataset for a different task, is fine-tuned for a specific problem or domain. In the context of brain tumor detection and localization, transfer learning can be beneficial due to the limited availability of medical imaging data. The ResNet-50 model is a deep CNN architecture with 50 layers. ResNet-50 is primarily used for image-classification tasks. This model can classify an input image into one or several predefined classes or categories. It has been pretrained on large datasets, such as ImageNet, which makes it particularly useful for a wide range of image classification problems. ResBlock is a fundamental component of ResNet-based architecture. It comprises multiple convolutional layers with skip connections. Skip connections allow gradients to flow more effectively during training, making it easier to train deep networks. In ResBlock, the main path consists of convolutional layers, whereas the short path is a direct connection from the input to the output. This direct connection facilitates the gradient flow during training. The kernel-size parameter specifies the size of the convolutional kernel (filter). In this case, the matrix is 1×1. The stride parameter determines how the convolutional filter moves across input data. Here, a 1×1 matrix indicates that the filter moves one pixel at a time, both horizontally and vertically. In this configuration, there was no downsampling of the input. The kernel initializer parameter specifies the setting of the initial values of the convolutional filter weights. It is designed to work well with Rectified Linear Unit (ReLU) activation functions and helps train deep neural networks. A Conv2D layer that performs 2D convolution with 16 filters of size 3×3 applies the ReLU activation function to the output, uses uniform padding to maintain spatial dimensions, and initializes the filter weights with the kernel initializer. This layer is applied to the input tensor in the neural network architecture. To downsample the spatial dimensions of the input data, we used a max-pooling layer. More specifically, MaxPool2D was used, which worked as a 2D max-pooling layer. Max-pooling is a type of operation that selects the maximum value from a group of values within a defined region of the input feature map. The pool size determines the size of the pooling window. In this case, (2, 2) indicates that the pooling window is a 2×2 matrix. During the max-pooling operation, this 2 × 2 window slides over the input feature map and selects the maximum value from each 2 × 2 block. Next, we add the Output from the Main Path and Short Path Together. In ResBlock, we combined the output from the main path and the short path by element-wise addition. This combination enhances the feature learning. Depending on the architecture, particularly in U-Net-like models for image segmentation, we need to upscale and concatenate feature maps from earlier layers to capture both high- and low-level details, such as the part with an anomaly in the image and the rest of the image. To build our CNN model, we referred to the ResBlock function and Conv2D layers in stages. The Conv2D layers perform convolution operations, whereas ResBlocks introduce residual connections. To address the challenge of data imbalance in medical image segmentation during the compilation process, we employed a custom loss function derived from the Tversky index. This tailored loss function effectively balances the trade-off between precision and recall, particularly when dealing with small structures such as lesions. In our evaluation, we enhanced the attention U-Net model by integrating an image pyramid approach to retain important contextual features. Kernel convolution is a fundamental image-processing technique that involves the application of a small numerical matrix, referred to as a kernel or filter, across an input image. This process transforms the image based on values within the filter. To compute the values of the resulting feature map, we utilized the following formula, where x_1 represents the input image and y_1 is the kernel. The indices for rows and columns in the resulting matrix are denoted as 'b' and 'c,' while the function's boundaries are indicated by 'I' and 'j.'

$$A_1[b,c] = (x_1.y_1)[b.c]\sum_i \sum_j y_1[i,j]x_1[b-i,c-j] \tag{8.1}$$

To create a generative tumor localization model, we used a custom loss function based on the Tversky Loss index. It addresses the class imbalance issues in segmentation tasks. Tversky loss allows us to balance precision and recall by adjusting hyperparameters. This corresponds to the Dice coefficient, which is a common segmentation metric. The Tversky index is defined as:

$$X(A_1,B_1;\alpha_1,\beta_1) = |A_1B_1|/[|A_1B_1| + \alpha_1|A_1/B_1| + \beta_1|B_1/A_1|] \tag{8.2}$$

Let A_1 and B_1 be the sets of predicted and ground-truth binary labels, respectively. The magnitude of the penalties for false positives (FPs) is

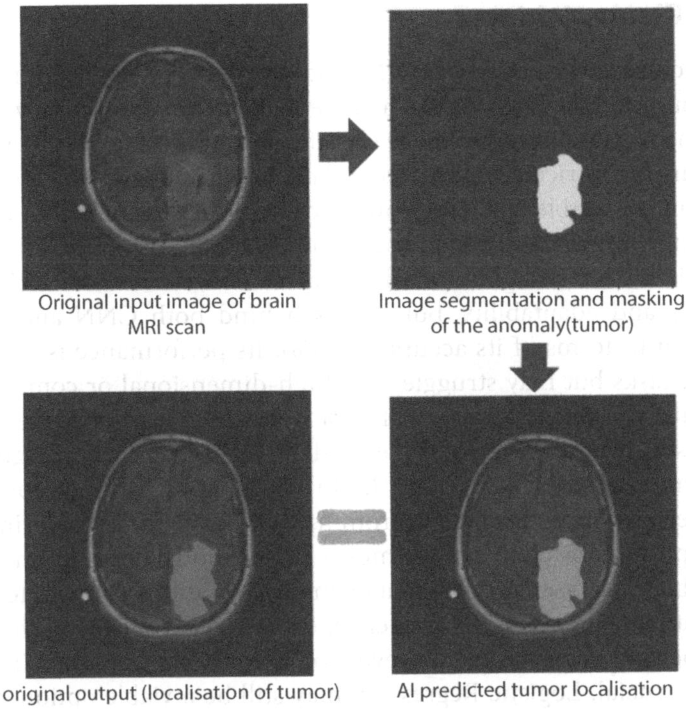

Figure 8.2 Working overview of tumor detection and localization.

controlled by α_1, and similarly, the magnitude of penalties for false negatives (FNs) is controlled by β_1 (see Figure 8.2).

8.4 Experimentation

8.4.1 Dataset

The dataset used in this paper is available at https://www.kaggle.com/datasets/mateuszbuda/lgg-mrisegmentation. This dataset comprises magnetic resonance (MR) brain images and the accompanying manual segmentation masks for FLAIR abnormalities. These image data were sourced from The Cancer Imaging Archive (TCIA). The archive contains data from 110 patients who were part of The Cancer Genome Atlas (TCGA) collection for lower-grade gliomas. To be included in this dataset, patients were required to have available fluid-attenuated inversion recovery (FLAIR) sequence data as well as genomic cluster information. Additional information about the tumor genomic clusters and the data collected from the patients can be found in the data.csv file.

8.4.2 Results Achieved

The structure and working of CNN model have been described in Figures 8.3, 8.4 and 8.5. The CNN model had the highest average accuracy (98.1%), indicating its suitability for image classification tasks. It excels in automatically learning intricate features from data. Logistic Regression, while simple and interpretable, achieved lower accuracy (85%) compared to CNN, suggesting limitations in capturing complex patterns. Thus, it may be more suitable for straightforward binary-classification tasks. KNN offers simplicity and adaptability, but it falls behind both CNN and Logistic Regression in terms of its accuracy (80%). Its performance is reasonable for some tasks but may struggle with high-dimensional or complex data. SVM, with an average accuracy of 71%, performed least effectively in this comparison. The accuracy of these models has been shown in Figures 8.6, 8.7, 8.8 and 8.9. SVM's strengths lie in handling high-dimensional data, but its performance may benefit from further tuning or considering other model options. The choice of the most suitable model depends on the specific problem, dataset size, and data complexity. In this context, for image classification tasks, the CNN model appears to be the preferred choice due to its superior performance. However, for simpler tasks, or when interpretability is crucial, Logistic Regression may still be a viable option. Careful consideration of the problem's requirements and data characteristics is essential when selecting a machine learning model and collaborating with such esteemed professionals.

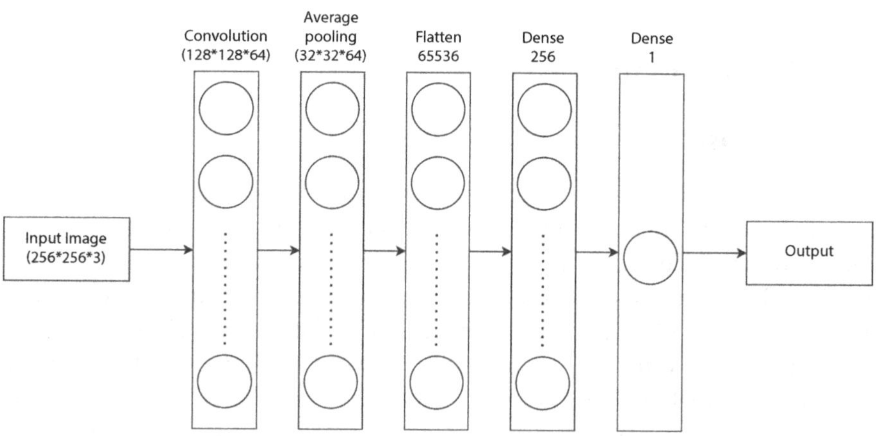

Figure 8.3 CNN model for tumor detection.

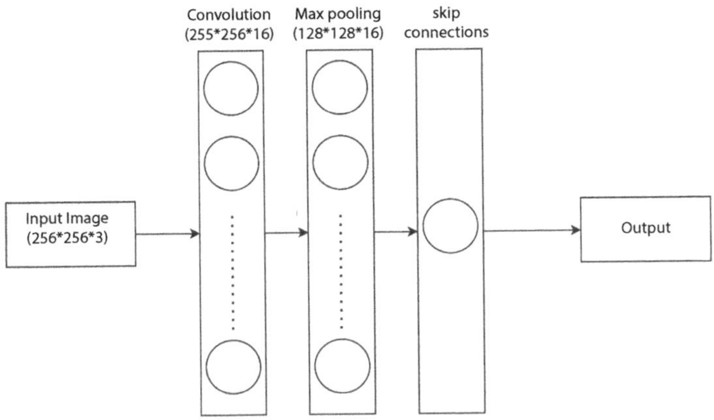

Figure 8.4 CNN model for tumor localization.

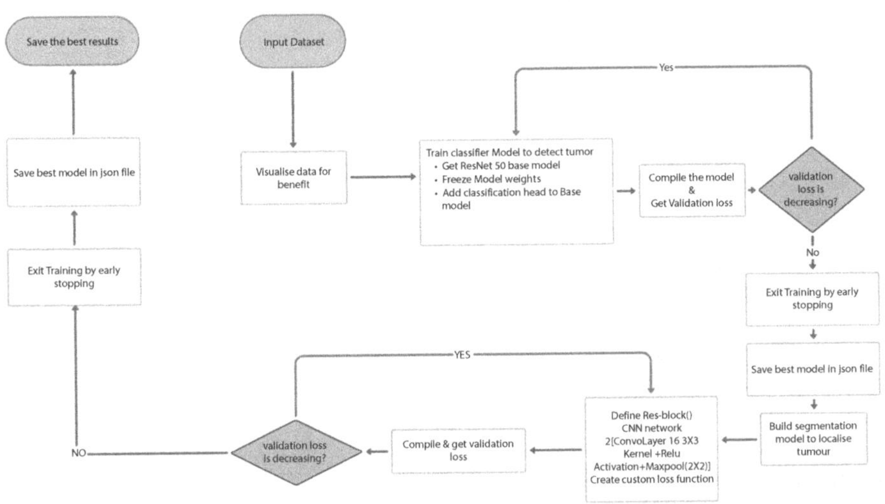

Figure 8.5 Flowchart on the overview for the tumor detection and localization using CNN.

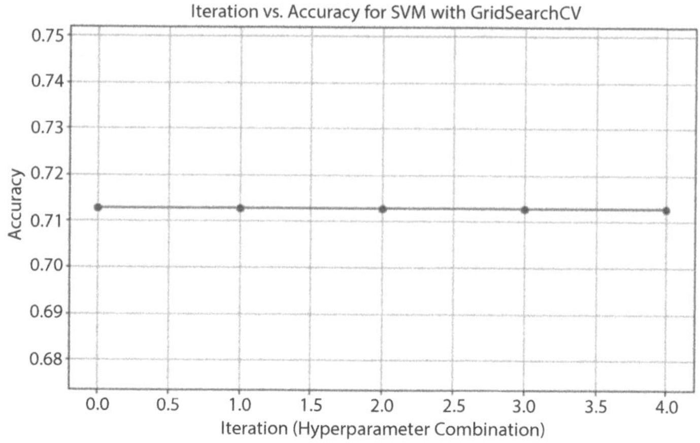

Figure 8.6 Accuracy through GridSearchCV.

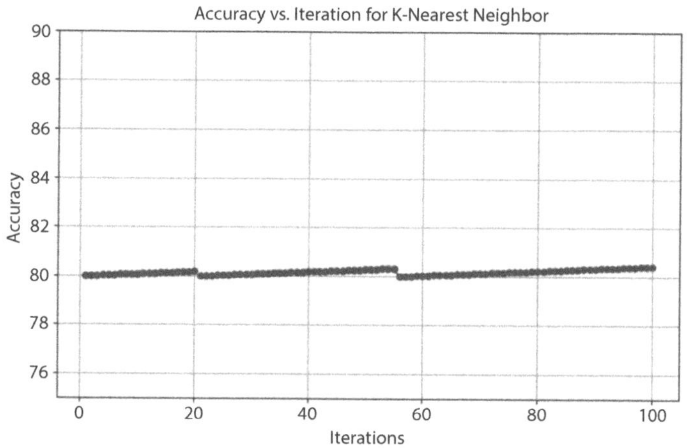

Figure 8.7 Accuracy through K-nearest neighbor.

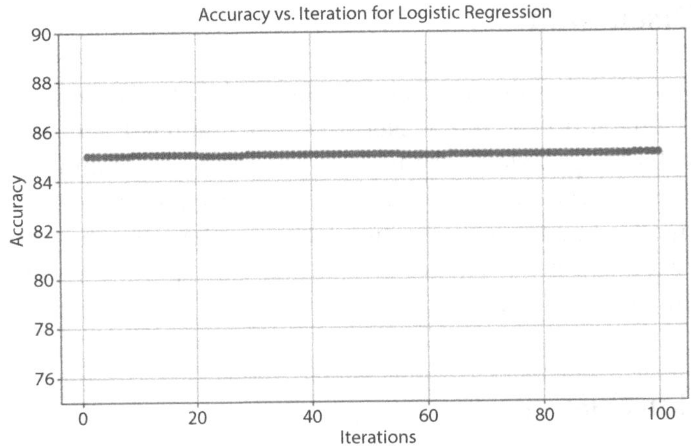

Figure 8.8 Accuracy through logistic regression.

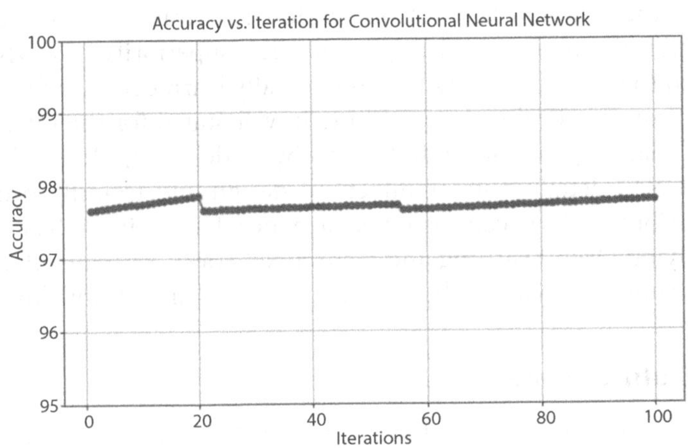

Figure 8.9 Accuracy through CNN.

Table 8.2 Comparison of evaluation metrics.

Algorithm	*Algorithm*	*Precision*	*Recall*	*F1-score*
SVM	*71.28*	*0.67*	*0.67*	*0.66*
KNN	*80.32*	*0.6*	*0.66*	*0.63*
Logistic Regression	*85.19*	*0.7*	*0.63*	*0.61*
CNN	*98.09*	*0.97*	*0.99*	*0.98*

8.5 Discussion

From the table of evaluation metrics, i.e., Table 8.2, it can be observed that the Convolutional Neural Network, when applied with the Transfer Learning Technique, yields the highest precision and accuracy for tumor detection and localization. These findings underscore the significance of CNN in medical image segmentation tasks, emphasizing their potential to enhance accuracy and efficiency and ultimately improve patient diagnosis and treatment planning.

8.6 Conclusion

Image segmentation is a crucial component of medical image processing, particularly in the context of MRI. In this study, we explored and compared several classification methods such as SVM, KNN, and Logistic Regression. However, the spotlight lies in Convolutional Neural Networks (CNN) as they exhibit the most promising results. The superiority of CNN can be attributed to its innate ability to automatically learn complex features and patterns from medical images, making it well-suited for the intricacies of medical image segmentation. In this study, we delve into the methodology behind CNN, detailing its architectural design and training procedures that contribute to its exceptional performance. Hence, it can be concluded that applying Deep Learning and Neural Networks is highly efficient and accurate compared with traditional Machine Learning Algorithms.

8.6.1 Future Scope

Continuous improvement and expansion of the dataset can lead to better model performance. Collecting more diverse MRI images, including different tumor types, stages, and patient demographics, can help improve the model generalization. Advanced data augmentation techniques can artificially increase the size and diversity of datasets. Moreover, it can improve the robustness and generalization of the model. In addition, fine-tuning the hyperparameters, such as the learning rate, batch size, and optimizer choice, will optimize the performance of the model. Exploring different pre-trained models and architectures for transfer learning, such as EfficientNet, Inception, and NASNet, may capture different features and improve performance.

References

1. Fernando, T., Gammulle, H., Denman, S., Sridharan, S., Fookes, C., Deep learning for medical anomaly detection—A survey. *ACM Comput. Surv.*, 54, 7, 1–37, Sep. 2022, doi: 10.1145/3464423.
2. Clerk Maxwell, J., *A Treatise on Electricity and Magnetism*, 3rd ed., vol. 2, pp. 68–73, Clarendon, Oxford, 1892.
3. Lakshmi, M.J. and Rao, S.N., Brain tumor magnetic resonance image classification: A deep learning approach. *Soft Comput.*, 26, 13, 6245–6253, Jul. 2022, doi: 10.1007/s00500-022-07163-z.
4. Jun, W. and Liyuan, Z., Brain tumor classification based on attention guided deep learning model. *Int. J. Comput. Intell. Syst.*, 15, 1, 35, Dec. 2022, doi: 10.1007/s44196-022-00090-9.
5. Rehman, A., Naz, S., Razzak, M., II, Akram, F., Imran, M., A deep learning-based framework for automatic brain tumors classification using transfer learning. *Circuits, Syst., Signal Process.*, 39, 2, 757–775, Feb. 2020, doi: 10.1007/s00034-019-01246-3.
6. Alam, M.S. *et al.*, Automatic Human Brain Tumor Detection in MRI Image Using Template-Based K Means and Improved Fuzzy C Means Clustering Algorithm. *Big Data Cogn. Comput.*, 3, 2, 27, May 2019, doi: 10.3390/bdcc3020027.
7. Patil, P.G., Karande, K.J., Surwase, S.V., Detection of brain tumor using optimized fuzzy C-means and SVM classifier. *AIP Conf. Proc.*, (Vol. 2494, No. 1), AIP Publishing, October 2022.
8. G.R., S.S., N.M., P.S., A.R., V.M., An Investication Report on Spoting and Diagnosing Diseases from the Images of Brain by Convolutional Neural Method Using Fusion Support Vector Machine. *2022 International Conference on Power, Energy, Control and Transmission Systems (ICPECTS)*, Chennai, India, pp. 1–4, 2022, doi: 10.1109/ICPECTS56089.2022.10046672.
9. Gurusamy, R. and Subramaniam, V., A machine learning approach for MRI brain tumor classification. *Comput. Mater. Contin.*, 53, 91–108, 2017.
10. Nagabushanam, M. *et al.*, Detection and localization of brain tumors using Fractional Hartley Transform and adaptive neuro-fuzzy inference system classification methods. *J. Ambient Intell. Hum. Comput.*, 14, 7, 8851–8858, 2023.
11. Li, M., Kuang, L., Xu, S., Sha, Z., Brain Tumor Detection Based on Multimodal Information Fusion and Convolutional Neural Network. *IEEE Access*, 7, 180134–180146, 2019, doi: 10.1109/ACCESS.2019.2958370.
12. Juan-Albarracín, J. *et al.*, Automated glioblastoma segmentation based on a multiparametric structured unsupervised classification. *PloS One*, 10, 5, e0125143, 2015.
13. Ahmadi, M. *et al.*, Detection of brain lesion location in MRI images using convolutional neural network and robust PCA. *Int. J. Neurosci.*, 133, 1, 55–66, 2023.

14. Abd-Ellah, M., Awad, A., Khalaf, A. *et al.*, Two-phase multi-model automatic brain tumour diagnosis system from magnetic resonance images using convolutional neural networks. *J. Image Video Proc.*, 2018, 97, 2018, https://doi.org/10.1186/s13640-018-0332-4.
15. Pereira, S., Pinto, A., Alves, V., Silva, C.A., Brain Tumor Segmentation Using Convolutional Neural Networks in MRI Images. *IEEE Trans. Med. Imaging*, 35, 5, 1240–1251, May 2016, doi: 10.1109/TMI.2016.2538465.
16. Xu, Y., Jia, Z., Ai, Y., Zhang, F., Lai, M., Chang, E., II, Deep convolutional activation features for large scale Brain Tumor histopathology image classification and segmentation. *2015 IEEE International Conference on Acoustics, Speech and Signal Processing (ICASSP)*, South Brisbane, QLD, Australia, pp. 947–951, 2015, doi: 10.1109/ICASSP.2015.7178109.
17. Solanki, S., Singh, U.P., Chouhan, S.S., Jain, S., Brain Tumor Detection and Classification Using Intelligence Techniques: An Overview. *IEEE Access*, 11, 12870–12886, 2023, doi: 10.1109/ACCESS.2023.3242666.
18. Fahmy, S.A., Dawoud, A., Zeinelabdeen, Y.A., Kiriacos, C.J., Daniel, K.A., Eltahtawy, O., Abdelhalim, M.M., Braoudaki, M., Youness, R.A., Molecular Engines, Therapeutic Targets, and Challenges in Pediatric Brain Tumors: A Special Emphasis on Hydrogen Sulfide and RNABased Nano-Delivery. *Cancers*, 14, 21, 5244, 2022.
19. https://www.cancer.org/cancer/types/brain-spinal-cord-tumorsadults/about/keystatistics.html#:˜:text=The%20American%20Cancer%20Society's%20estimates,in%20females
20. Rasool, M., Ismail, N.A., Al-Dhaqm, A., Yafooz, W.M.S., Alsaeedi, A., A Novel Approach for Classifying Brain Tumours Combining a SqueezeNet Model with SVM and Fine-Tuning. *Electronics*, 12, 1, 149, Dec. 2022, doi: 10.3390/electronics12010149.
21. Aiwale, P. and Ansari, S., Brain tumor detection using KNN. *Int. J. Sci. Eng. Res.*, 10, 12, 187–193, 2019.
22. Nankani, H. *et al.*, Detection analysis of various types of cancer by logistic regression using machine learning. *Int. J. Eng. Adv. Technol. (IJEAT)*, 9, 1, 99–104, 2019.
23. Saeedi, S., Rezayi, S., Keshavarz, H. *et al.*, MRI-based brain tumor detection using convolutional deep learning methods and chosen machine learning techniques. *BMC Med. Inf. Decis. Making*, 23, 16, 2023, https://doi.org/10.1186/s12911-023-02114-6.
24. Deisenroth, M.P., Faisal, A.A., Ong, C.S., *Mathematics for machine learning*, Cambridge University Press, Cambridge, New York, 2020.

9

Integrating Apriori Algorithm with Data Mining Classification Techniques for Enhanced Primary Tumor Prediction

Khalid Mahboob[1]*, Nida Khalil[2], Fatima Waseem[3] and Abeer Javed Syed[2]

[1]*College of Computer Science & Information Systems, Institute of Business Management, Karachi, Pakistan*

[2]*Software Engineering Department, Sir Syed University of Engineering & Technology, Karachi, Pakistan*

[3]*Software Engineering Department, Capital University of Science and Technology, Islamabad, Pakistan*

Abstract

In the realm of data mining and medical diagnostics, the integration of the Apriori algorithm with data mining classification techniques is a promising approach aimed at improving the accuracy and efficacy of primary tumor prediction. The Apriori algorithm, which is renowned for its association rule mining capabilities, is merged with classification techniques to enhance the prediction accuracy of primary tumors based on relevant medical attributes. The Apriori algorithm excels in mining frequent itemsets and establishing associations within large datasets. By integrating this algorithm with data mining classification methods, a synergistic effect was achieved. The Apriori algorithm effectively identified significant patterns and associations, providing valuable insights into the relationships between medical attributes and primary tumor occurrence. These patterns, when combined with classification techniques, contribute to a refined predictive model. Classification techniques within data mining offer a robust framework for constructing predictive models. By leveraging these techniques in conjunction with the knowledge gleaned from the Apriori algorithm, a more accurate and precise primary tumor prediction model was developed. This hybrid approach utilizes the discovered association rules to enrich the feature set for classification, resulting in an improved predictive performance. Thus, the integration of the Apriori

**Corresponding author*: khalid.mahboob@iobm.edu.pk

Neha Sharma, Korhan Cengiz and Prasenjit Chatterjee (eds.) Intelligent Data Analytics for Bioinformatics and Biomedical Systems, (213–234) © 2024 Scrivener Publishing LLC

algorithm with data mining classification techniques holds immense promise for enhancing the primary tumor prediction accuracy.

***Keywords*:** Data mining, cancer, classification, prediction, tumors, malignant, gene, bioinformatics

9.1 Overview

The history of tumors is an anecdote of intrigues, exploration, and advancement. Humanity has struggled with the mystery of these abnormal growths over time, progressively solving their puzzles and creating cutting-edge technologies to identify and cure them. Although they are frequently linked to cancer, tumors are not always cancerous. Tumors can be benign or malignant, and can appear anywhere in the body. Efficient medical management and patient education are needed to have a thorough understanding of the many tumor types, their causes, and available treatments. There are two categories of tumors: benign and malignant.

Benign tumors are non-cancerous growths that do not spread to other parts of the body or invade neighboring tissues. They have often clearly defined borders and moderate growth rates. Benign tumors are often not life-threatening, but depending on their size and location, they might result in health issues. Fibroids that develop in the uterus, lipomas that develop in fat tissue, and moles are typical examples of benign tumors. However, malignant tumors are cancerous. They are harmful because they can spread (metastasize) to other areas of the body and infect the surrounding tissues. Malignant tumors can be divided into different groups based on the tissue from which they originate.

Some common types of malignant tumors include the following:

i. Carcinomas: These cancers develop from epithelial cells that coat organs and cover the body's surfaces. Lung, breast, prostate, and colon cancer are common carcinomas.
ii. Sarcomas: Sarcomas grow in connective tissues including muscles, cartilage, and bones. Sarcomas are cancers of bones and muscles, such as osteosarcoma and leiomyosarcoma.
iii. Lymphomas: Lymphomas affect lymphatic tissues, including lymph nodes, in the body. Two common types of lymphoma are Hodgkin and non-Hodgkin.
iv. Leukemia: Leukemia begins in the bone marrow and other blood-forming tissues. They cause aberrant white blood

cell production. Leukemia includes acute myeloid leukemia (AML) and chronic lymphocytic leukemia (CLL).

v. Gliomas: In the brain or spinal cord, gliomas can form as tumors. A particularly dangerous type of glioma is called glioblastoma multiforme.

Although the precise cause of tumors is not always clear, several factors, such as genetics, age, hormones, deficiency of the immune system, and environmental factors, can increase the risk of their development:

i. Hormones: Unbalanced hormone levels or exposure to hormone analogs can affect the growth of specific malignancies, including breast and prostate cancer.
ii. Factors in the environment: Exposure to environmental pollutants, such as radiation, tobacco smoke, and certain chemicals, can increase the risk of tumor development.
iii. Age: As cells acquire genetic alterations over time, the risk of developing cancer generally increases with age.
iv. Immune System Deficiency: The body may be less able to fight off tumor cells if the immune system is compromised, whether as a result of illness or immunosuppressive drugs.
v. Genetics: Some individuals may be born with genetic mutations that predispose them to develop particular tumor types. For instance, individuals with particular gene mutations, such as BRCA1 and BRCA2, are more likely to develop breast and ovarian cancers.

Depending on the type, location, size, and malignancy of the tumor, several treatment methods are available. Some of the typical methods for treating tumors are as follows:

i. Radiation therapy: Cancer cells are targeted and eliminated by high-energy X-rays or other radiation sources. This approach is frequently used to treat cancerous tumors.
ii. Surgery: Surgical excision of benign tumors is the first-line treatment and is sometimes curative. Malignant tumors may undergo surgery to remove as much of the tumor as possible and then undergo other therapies.
iii. Targeted Therapy: Targeted therapies concentrate on specific molecules involved in the development and spread of cancer. They are frequently used in conjunction with other therapies.

iv. Chemotherapy: Chemotherapy uses medications to either destroy or inhibit cancer cell growth. When malignant tumors spread, they are frequently utilized as systemic treatment.
v. Immunotherapy: Immunotherapy uses the immune system to combat cancer. It has demonstrated potential in the treatment of several malignant cancers.

Therefore, because of the above scenario, data mining techniques, and machine learning algorithms have been applied to predict primary tumors in various medical fields. These methods have been employed, notably in the context of liver tumors, to identify patterns and connections between blood test features and tumors [1]. Early tumor detection is crucial for effective treatment, and classification models using data mining predictive algorithms have been employed to classify tumors based on blood test values [2]. Data-mining techniques have also been used to forecast various tumor forms and improve prognosis and treatment [3]. A variety of classification techniques, including decision trees, naive Bayes, and K-nearest neighbors, have been used to create prediction models for tumor prognosis [4]. Furthermore, data mining methods have been used to predict non-small cell lung carcinoma (NSCLC) using algorithms such as logistic regression, random forest, k-nearest neighbors, decision trees, and support vector machines [5].

By enhancing early identification and treatment planning, the application of data mining classification algorithms for the prediction of primary cancers has transformed healthcare. Data-mining algorithms can find patterns and links in big databases of medical data that might not be obvious to human observers. Here, classification approaches for data mining are used to improve the prediction of primary tumors.

9.1.1 Feature Selection

The dataset contains a variety of features (attributes); however, not all are equally useful for predicting tumors. The most useful qualities that aid in precise classification are found using feature selection strategies. This improves the performance of the model and decreases the complexity of the data.

9.1.2 Hyperparameter Tuning

Hyperparameter tuning involves maximizing the parameters of the algorithm to produce the best prediction results. Grid search and random searches are popular methods for this purpose.

9.1.3 Enhanced Primary Tumor Prediction

The classification model can be applied to primary tumor prediction on new, unexplored patient data after training and assessment. Based on the input features, the model assigns a probability or class label to reflect the possibility of a primary tumor being present.

9.1.4 Continuous Improvement

Data mining for tumor prediction is a procedure that is constantly being improved. To increase the precision and adjust to shifting patterns in the occurrence and diagnosis of tumors, models can be updated using fresh data. Its continued efficacy in predicting primary tumors is ensured by regular monitoring of model performance and upgrading the most recent medical knowledge.

9.1.5 Clinical Integration

By incorporating the predictions made by data mining models into the clinical workflow, healthcare workers can make better-informed decisions regarding patient care and treatment design. Healthcare professionals can improve primary tumor prediction by utilizing data mining classification algorithms, resulting in earlier diagnosis and more efficient treatment plans. This strategy may enhance patient outcomes while easing the financial and personal toll that cancer has on society.

The Apriori approach can improve primary tumor prediction by exposing hidden correlations in clinical data, increasing feature representation, enhancing model performance, and offering insightful information for medical practitioners. This method optimizes tumor prediction in healthcare applications by combining the benefits of classification and association-rule mining.

The Apriori algorithm can improve primary tumor prediction when combined with data mining categorization methods. A common method for finding patterns in data mining is association rule mining, which uses algorithms such as the Apriori algorithm [6]. It has been used in many fields, including medicine [7]. Additionally, connections between blood test characteristics and blood tumors have been found using data mining approaches, such as rule induction and deep learning, which have enabled early prognosis and improved healing ability [8]. Another study suggested applying the AdaBoost algorithm to CT lung scans to detect lung cancer with high accuracy [9]. Additionally, cancer prediction, dataset categorization using FUZZY classification methods, and feature selection have both been applied. Therefore, by utilizing association rule mining and other cutting-edge techniques, merging the Apriori algorithm with data mining classification techniques can improve primary tumor prediction.

9.2 Previous Studies on Tumor Prediction Using Data Mining and Apriori Algorithm

The study in [10] used data mining techniques to evaluate various survival indicators for cancer prognosis. A dataset encompassing data from several data profiles, such as clinical, therapeutic, and overall life quality from 140 advanced ovarian cancer patients was collected and utilized to predict cancer patient survival. The combined dataset was categorized using relevant machine learning methods after adequate preprocessing. Using an ensemble technique with sequential pattern mining and time intervals of two months between treatments, the proposed integrated model approach achieved the best accuracy of 76.4%.

Predicting a person's tumor (normal, benign, or malignant) based on tumor properties such as fractal dimension, concavity, compactness, texture, perimeter, radius, etc. is estimated in the study [11]. Machine learning and data mining classification techniques have been applied to these issues. Decision Tree (DT), Random Forest (RF), Random Tree (RT), and Artificial Neural Network (ANN) with 10-fold cross-validation were used in this study, and accuracy is calculated using error rates. The Correlation Coefficient (CC), Mean Absolute Error (MAE), Root Mean Squared Error (RMSE), and Root Relative Squared Error (RRSE) were used to assess model performance. The ANN outperformed the other proposed models in terms of error rate and accuracy.

The study [12] addressed cervical cancer prediction using data mining techniques, such as boosted decision tree, decision forest, and decision jungle algorithms, along with performance evaluation based on the Area under Receiver operating characteristic curve (AUROC), accuracy, specificity, and sensitivity. A 10-fold cross-validation approach was used to validate the results, and the boosted decision tree produced the best results. When the Hinslemann screening approach was applied, the boosted decision tree generated an extremely high prediction of 0.978 on the AUROC curve. The other classifiers produced substantially worse results than the boosted decision tree.

The goal of this study [13] is to offer a report on breast cancer to construct prediction models for breast cancer survivability. The prediction models were developed utilizing a large dataset of (683 breast cancer occurrences) using three common data mining methods: Naive Bayes, Radial Basis Function (RBF) Network, and J48 DT. The results based on the average accuracy breast cancer dataset showed that the Nave Bayes was the best predictor with 97.36% accuracy on the holdout sample, the RBF Network was second with 96.77% accuracy, and J48 DT was third with 93.41% accuracy.

The study in [14] employed 32 classification methods from six categories, including Bayes, function-based, lazy, meta-, rule-based, and tree-based, to locate the best and most commonly used categories and methods in healthcare data mining. In the performance evaluation of the classification algorithms, 17 healthcare datasets relating to thyroid, cancer, skin disease, heart disease, hepatitis, lymphography, audiology, diabetes, surgery, arrhythmia, post-survival, liver, and tumor were employed. The tree-based classification methods outperformed the other approaches, with an average classification accuracy of 79.92%, and a maximum accuracy of 99.50%, and an analysis time of 3.91 s for the logistic model tree classifier.

Based on gene expression profiles gathered using DNA microarrays, the research in [15] provided an intelligent decision support system (IDSS) for early cancer diagnosis. The proposed methodology selects the most essential characteristics from the input patterns using information gain (IG). The chosen characteristics (genes) were then decreased using the gray wolf optimization (GWO) technique. For cancer type classification, the system employs a support vector machine (SVM) classifier. The proposed methodology was tested on two datasets (Breast and Colon) and its classification accuracy, which is the most important performance indicator in illness diagnosis, was examined.

The study in [16] examined gene expression data from 1,157 kidney cancer patients to identify specific genes associated with prognosis. The experimental findings show that the proposed methodology can improve the stability of classification accuracy and feature selection. The proposed approach combines the empirical wavelet transform (EWT) to reconstruct the loss in nonlinear Feature Extraction, and a neutral network to recover the loss in neutral categorization. Medical information and genetic data were used to establish the best classification algorithm and assess classification accuracy using sample category, primary detection, tumor level, and vital stage as risk variables. The results of this study revealed that DAGAN outperforms traditional machine learning and data mining methodologies in predicting kidney cancer prognosis using gene expression data.

Data mining is an important aspect of the learning disclosure process in which intelligent agents are used to extract patterns. Therefore, the study in [17], which depicts numerous data mining approaches, will be useful for medical practitioners and analysts to accurately identify illnesses. Data-mining applications in medical services have enormous potential and utility. Nevertheless, the effectiveness of data-mining techniques in the healthcare domain is contingent on the availability of detailed healthcare data. In this study, the authors presented a few classifiers utilized in medical data analysis. Several disease prediction analyses have also been considered, including breast cancer prediction, heart disease diagnosis, thyroid prediction, and diabetic prediction. The results suggest that the DT method is ideally suited for disease prediction because it yields outcomes with higher accuracy.

9.3 Data Mining Process

Data mining is a way of extracting useful information from enormous volumes of data. To find patterns, correlations, and trends in the data, multiple procedures and methods must be used [20]. Making the data useful, helping those who work in healthcare and education, and providing reliable information are all made possible through data mining. Numerous industries, including health, business, market research, banking, finance, exchange, risk analysis, resource utilization for corporations, trade, consumer analysis, shopping, banking, medical, science, engineering, insurance, and education, can benefit from data mining [18].

The steps that make up the process of data mining are typically outlined in subsequent subsections: Section 9.3.1, which covers data collection and pre-processing; Section 9.3.2, which covers model(s) selection and how to

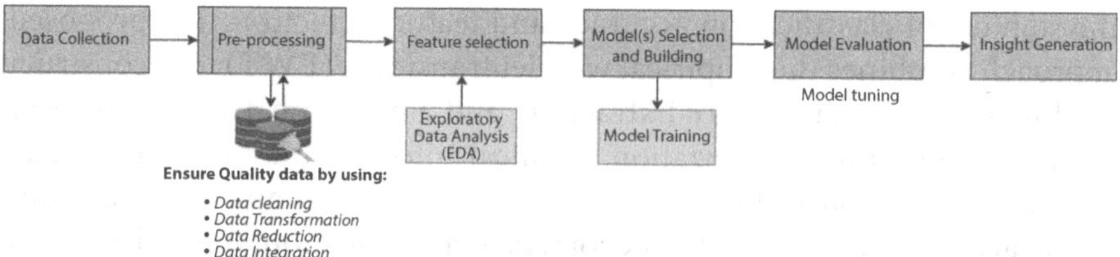

Figure 9.1 Representation of data mining process.

construct the chosen model; and Section 9.3.3, which covers evaluation and exploratory data analysis.

The data mining procedure is appropriate for every project, as shown in Figure 9.1, and includes the following process details:

9.3.1 Data Collection and Pre-Processing

The process of data mining begins with collecting data. This entails compiling reliable and pertinent data from a variety of sources. The validity and dependability of future analyses and insights directly depend on the quality and reliability of the data that were obtained [18, 19]. This subsection examines the value of precise data collection and highlights the requirements of extensive and varied data sources. Several methods are used to collect data, including surveys, interviews, observations, and experiments.

Once the data is gathered, it endures preprocessing, which is the procedure of cleaning, modifying, decreasing, and combining raw data before analysis [18]. This section examines the various data preprocessing stages and emphasizes their importance in guaranteeing data quality and eliminating noise and inconsistencies.

9.3.1.1 Data Cleaning

Data cleaning entails identifying and correcting errors, conflicts, and missing values in collected data. To guarantee the accuracy and dependability of the data, it uses methods such as outlier identification, addressing missing data, and reconciling inconsistencies [21].

9.3.1.2 Data Transformation

The process of data transformation involves converting the data into a format suitable for analysis. In this stage, the categorical variables are scaled, normalized, and encoded. Researchers can make the results more comprehensible and comparable by changing the data [21].

9.3.1.3 Data Reduction

Data reduction techniques seek to reduce the dataset's dimensionality by removing duplicate or irrelevant elements. Feature selection and feature extraction techniques aid in lowering dataset complexity, enhancing computational performance, and preventing overfitting [21].

9.3.1.4 *Data Integration*

Data integration is the process of merging information from various sources to produce a single dataset for analysis [21]. To create a comprehensive view, this stage requires fixing data format errors, correcting semantic discrepancies, and integrating datasets.

9.3.1.5 *Data Discretization*

In data mining and machine learning, the process of "data discretization" transforms continuous data into discrete values or intervals. Because many data mining approaches, such as association rule mining and decision trees, are designed to work with discrete or categorical data, it is frequently necessary to perform this procedure. Discretization can also aid in cleaning the data's noise and improving its readability.

9.3.2 Model(s) Selection and Building

Model selection and building in the context of data mining refer to the phase in which suitable models or algorithms are selected to derive conclusions and make predictions from the data. This step is fundamental to achieving precise and significant results. The selection of models is influenced by the nature of the issue, data offered, and desired result [22].

In data mining, various strategies and procedures are available for model selection and building. Several typical strategies include the following:

9.3.2.1 *Supervised Learning*

A type of machine learning called supervised learning uses input features to guide the algorithm while learning from labeled data to make predictions or to analyze data. Supervised learning can be applied to the following problems in bioinformatics:

i. Amino acid sequences were used to predict protein structure and function.
ii. Partitioning genes as disease-connected or non-disease-connected.

iii. Based on information about gene expression, classifying, or defining disease subgroups.
iv. Drug-target interaction prediction.

In bioinformatics, algorithms that are frequently used for supervised learning include decision trees, support vector machines, and deep learning techniques such as neural networks.

9.3.2.2 *Unsupervised Learning*

By contrast, unsupervised learning works with unlabeled data. In the absence of predetermined classes or labels, the objective is to find hidden patterns or structures in data [22]. Algorithms used in unsupervised learning discover patterns and structures in unlabeled data. Unsupervised learning can be applied to bioinformatics tasks as follows:

i. Based on information regarding their expression or sequence, we grouped related genes or proteins.
ii. Identifying obscure patterns or subcategories in biological data, such as cancer subtypes.
iii. Visualization of highly-dimensional data using dimensionality reduction.

In bioinformatics, dimensionality reduction methods, such as principal component analysis (PCA) and t-distributed stochastic neighbor embedding (t-SNE), as well as clustering algorithms, such as k-means and hierarchical clustering, are frequently used. Clustering has several purposes, such as medical diagnosis, text mining, web analytics, and biological computation [23].

9.3.2.3 *Reinforcement Learning*

Reinforcement learning is a machine learning technique that allows an agent to acquire knowledge in an interactive environment through experimentation and failure while using feedback from its actions and experiences [24]. Through reinforcement learning, an agent can be taught to act in a way that maximizes the reward signal. Reinforcement learning is still used, although it is less popular in bioinformatics than in other sciences [23]. Examples include:

i. Drug optimization and discovery, where the agent looks for the best possible drug candidates.
ii. 3D structure prediction using protein-folding simulations.

Policy gradient approaches or deep Q-networks (DQN) for reinforcement learning can be applied to bioinformatics issues when necessary [23, 24].

9.3.2.4 Ensemble Method

Several machine learning models have been combined using ensemble methods to increase the reliability and accuracy of the predictions. In bioinformatics, ensemble approaches are important for increasing prediction accuracy and managing complex biological data [23]. Examples comprise:

i. Random forests for classifying and analyzing gene expression.
ii. Several models have been used to combine and forecast protein–protein interactions.
iii. Various docking techniques have been used to predict drug–protein binding.

Ensemble techniques can capture several facets of complicated biological data, while reducing overfitting. To analyze and understand biological data successfully, bioinformatics pipelines frequently use a combination of these techniques. The best methodologies must be chosen, and the results must be interpreted in a physiologically meaningful manner, which requires domain competence.

9.3.3 Evaluation and Exploratory Data Analysis

To determine the quality of the data, comprehend its properties, and assess the effectiveness of data-mining models, evaluation and exploratory data analysis are crucial steps in the data-mining process.

Exploratory data analysis is a crucial stage of the data-mining process that entails the initial examination and analysis of the dataset to learn more about its organization, trends, and potential correlations. It aids in the detection of irregularities, missing values, outliers, and data distributions. Data transformation, data visualization, and summary statistics are examples of EDA approaches [25].

Data mining evaluation entails the evaluation of the efficacy and effectiveness of data mining models or algorithms. It seeks to establish whether a model achieves the goals of the analysis and how effectively it generalizes to fresh, untested data. The accuracy, precision, recall, F1-score, ROC curves, and confusion matrices are examples of typical evaluation measures. To evaluate the model performance, cross-validation and hold-out validation were used [25, 26].

9.3.3.1 *Evaluation Techniques in Data Mining*

i. Cross-validation: K-fold cross-validation is a method for evaluating the performance of a model that involves repeatedly dividing the data into training and testing sets and averaging the outcome.
ii. Hold-Out Validation: The data must be split into a training set and a distinct testing set to assess the performance of the model on untested data.
iii. Confusion Matrix: A confusion matrix that includes true positives, true negatives, false positives, and false negatives is used to comprehensively breakdown a model's classification performance.
iv. ROC Curve: Particularly in binary classification situations, the Receiver Operating Characteristic (ROC) curve is used to visualize a model's performance over various thresholds.
v. Precision-Recall Curve: This curve emphasizes the trade-off between recall and precision and is particularly helpful when working with unbalanced datasets [27].

For data preparation, feature selection, model selection, and model tuning decisions to be well-informed, effective EDA, and evaluation are essential. These procedures aid in ensuring that the data mining findings are trustworthy and offer useful information on the particular issue at hand.

9.4 Data Mining in Bioinformatics

Bioinformatics is an interdisciplinary field that involves the collection, storage, and analysis of biological data. To comprehend and interpret biological data, biology is combined with computer science, mathematics, and statistics. Bioinformatic applications include discovering the 3D structures of proteins and DNA, designing new drugs, and researching therapeutic activity [28].

Data mining techniques have been extensively employed in bioinformatics research and development. These methods are used to draw conclusions and discover patterns in biological data such as DNA, RNA, and protein. These include tasks such as pattern recognition, association, outlier detection, prediction, classification, and prediction. Bioinformatic applications such as gene and protein structure categorization, gene expression analysis, co-disease association, outlier detection, protein structure prediction, and drug development have all demonstrated the effectiveness of data mining [29–31]. This enables researchers to better understand gene expression, medication strategies, and other genomics- and proteomics-related issues by providing insightful connections from huge and complicated bioinformatics datasets [32].

However, processing a massive volume of data and extracting knowledge may be difficult because of issues such as dealing with incomplete and handwritten data. Overall, data mining is essential for bioinformatics because it makes it easier to analyze and interpret biological data for a variety of applications.

Applications of data mining in bioinformatics include gene discovery, protein function inference, domain detection, function motif detection, disease diagnosis and prognosis, disease treatment optimization, protein and gene interaction network reconstruction, data cleansing, and protein subcellular location prediction.

9.5 Cancer and Tumor Biology

The Latin version of the Greek word for crab is where the word cancer first originated. In the beginning, Hippocrates described cancer as having a central body with a propensity to spread outward like "the arms of a crab." Neoplasia is a more technical name for cancer, in addition to the widely used, general term "cancer" that is used by most people. Neoplasia, often known as neoplasm, literally translates to "new tissue" in Greek (neo = new, plasia = tissue or cells). This phrase implies that malignancies are new cellular growths within the body, and "malignant tumor" is another phrase for cancer. In this context, it alludes to a collection of unorganized, brand-new cells that serve no discernible function in the body's physiological processes [34].

Our knowledge of cancer biology has advanced enormously over the last century. Technological and conceptual advancements in several areas, including massive next-generation sequencing, the inclusion of "omic" sciences, high-resolution microscopy, molecular immunology, flow cytometry, analysis and sequencing of individual cells, new cell culture techniques, and the creation of animal models, have been particularly responsible for this progress over the past few decades. However, there are still many unanswered questions and issues with this condition that need to be resolved [33].

Contrary to popular beliefs, cancer is a collection of more than 100 distinct diseases. Unchecked proliferation and spread of aberrant cells is a feature of many disorders. Genetic mutations that result in unregulated cell proliferation cause cancer. DNA damage that interferes with normal cell cycle regulation can be induced by both internal (inherited mutations, hormones, immunological disorders) and external (tobacco, chemicals, radiation exposure) factors. Although benign tumors may not metastasize like malignant malignancies, they both involve dysregulated cell proliferation caused by genetic abnormalities [33]. In the process of metastasis, cancer cells move from one area of the body to another through the lymphatic or circulatory system. This enables cancer cells to develop new tumors in different organs after leaving the initial site [35].

There are two ways to categorize cancers: by the primary site, which is the area of the body where the cancer initially appears, and by the type of tissue in which the cancer originates, also known as the cancer's histological type. Hundreds of distinct malignancies are classified histologically into five core groups: carcinoma, sarcoma, myeloma, leukemia, and lymphoma. In addition, there are few mixed-type malignancies. Cancers are usually described by their histological type by medical professionals. However, depending on their primary sites, the general public is more familiar with cancer names as the skin, lungs, female breasts, prostate, colon, rectum, cervix, and uterus are the most prevalent places where cancer arises. Depending on the organ from which it originates, cancer can develop in several locations and exhibit various behaviors. For example, breast cancer differs from lung cancer in its characteristics. It is critical to recognize that when cancer spreads to another area of the body from one organ, it retains its characteristics. For instance, when examined under a microscope, metastatic breast cancer in the lungs continues to act and appears as breast cancer that first appears in the breast [34].

Mutations in apoptosis-related genes can cause the cells to develop malignancies. Less than usual suppression of cell cycle progression is provided by altered genes (tumor-suppressor genes), while increased cell cycle progression is provided by oncogenes. Increased anti-apoptotic signals, decreased pro-apoptotic signals, or both. Methods that utilize apoptosis for clinical purposes might be created as we learn more about cell death. These techniques may entail the selective activation of apoptosis in tumor cells while deactivating it in normal tissue, correction of apoptotic defects in cancer cells by reactivating the concerned gene, or prevention of apoptosis in normal tissues using substances that shield normal tissues from radiation and chemotherapy damage to deliver higher radiation doses to tumor cells without harming normal tissues [36].

9.6 Data Mining Classification Techniques

Classification, a prevalent technique in data mining, involves the creation of a model using pre-classified records to categorize a large volume of data. For instance, researchers may use classification algorithms, such as decision trees or neural networks, to analyze pre-classified genomic data for cancer research. By training the model on known genomic variations associated with different types of cancers, the algorithm can later classify new genetic mutations to identify potential cancer-linked variations. Decision tree- and neural network-based categorization algorithms frequently utilize this method. Both learning and classification are integral parts of the data-classification process. During this process, a classification algorithm analyzes the training data to establish classification rules. The accuracy of these rules is evaluated using classification tests. If the accuracy meets these criteria, rules can be applied to new data entries. Bioinformatics researchers may use classification techniques to categorize gene expression data based on specific experimental conditions. This allows them to understand how genes respond to different treatments or environmental factors, aiding drug discovery and personalized medicine. The classifier training method utilizes pre-classified samples to determine the essential

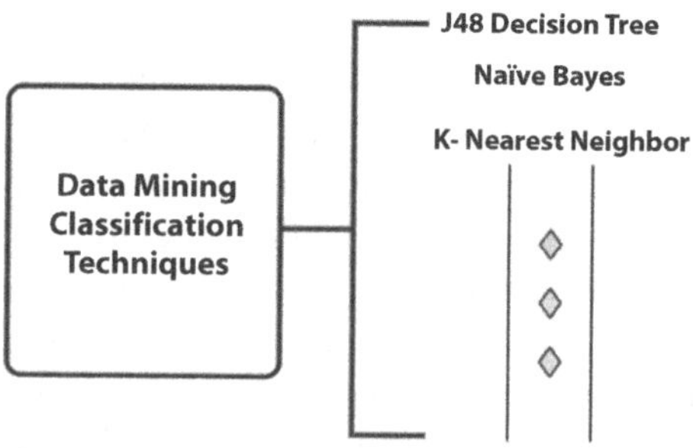

Figure 9.2 List of classifiers.

discrimination parameters, which are then encoded into a model known as a classifier [37].

Figure 9.2 shows the list of classifiers that are used in data mining.

9.6.1 J48 Decision Tree

A decision tree (DT) functions as a machine learning or data-mining model that utilizes multiple attribute values from the provided data to determine the target value (dependent variables) for a new sample. The inner nodes of the tree represent various quality attributes, whereas the branches connecting the nodes indicate the likely values of these attributes based on the observed samples. Ultimately, terminal nodes signify the definitive value (classification) of the dependent variable. The dependent variable refers to an attribute whose value is influenced by the criteria set by the other features. The additional features present in the dataset that aid in predicting the value of the dependent variable are referred to as independent variables [38].

9.6.2 Naïve Bayes

The Naive Bayesian model allows rapid construction and analysis of extensive datasets. Simple Bayesian classification approaches often outperform more complex methods. It calculates the posterior probability (P(c)), assessing the predictor (x) impact on class (c) independently of other predictors [39].

9.6.3 K-Nearest Neighbor

K-Nearest Neighbor (IBK) is a supervised learning approach that partitions a dataset into multiple groups. During the training phase, the classifier retains the features and class labels from the training sets. To classify new instances, it utilizes a voting mechanism that returns the highest probability estimate for each class. Euclidean distance metrics were applied to assign the items to the most frequently identified classes. For each test object, the distances were computed using appropriate K values. This process involves constructing a decision tree based on insights obtained from a labeled dataset. The attribute selection for data partitioning is determined by the feature with the highest normalized information gain. This iterative process is performed on smaller subsets, and splitting occurs if all the instances within a subset belong to the same class. The resulting leaf node is added to the decision tree to guide the user in selecting the class [40].

9.7 Apriori Algorithm and Association Rule Mining

The widely used algorithm for extracting several frequently occurring collections of items from transaction data stored in databases is the Apriori Algorithm, which is based on association rule mining. The Boolean association rule is used in an apriori manner to determine the itemsets that appear in a dataset the most frequently. The method's name comes from the fact that it utilizes prior information on typical itemset qualities. To do this, k-frequent itemsets are used to find k + 1 itemsets using an iterative method known as the level-wise approach [41].

Association rules are expressed as "IF–THEN" statements, aiding interpretation. Typically, rules are filtered using support, confidence, and lift ratio metrics, with only those exceeding predefined thresholds considered for further analysis. The support reflects rule frequency, confidence indicates reliability and lift ratio measures rule dependence strength [41, 42].

The Apriori algorithm is a commonly employed technique for uncovering association rules, particularly in domains such as hypothesis testing, numerical analysis, and large-scale data processing. Although it demonstrates proficiency in diverse applications, its classical iterative method may not match the efficiency of more advanced depth-first approaches. Nevertheless, the core concept of detecting frequent items within a database remains versatile and applicable to association-rule mining, albeit with a focus on depth-first strategies. The Apriori algorithm is a well-liked method, locating frequently occurring itemsets in a dataset and deriving association rules from them are its intended uses. To uncover intriguing connections or correlations between objects or variables in huge datasets, association-rule mining is a technique. Market basket analysis, recommendation systems, and other fields are among the many most frequently used areas [43].

The Apriori algorithm comprises two pivotal stages: first, the identification of frequently occurring item sets within the dataset and second, the generation of association rules derived from these frequent item sets. The initial step presents a greater challenge and exerts a substantial impact on the overall performance of association rule mining, garnering the majority of research emphasis [42].

9.8 Conclusion and Future Work

In conclusion, integrating the Apriori algorithm with data mining classification techniques has shown significant promise in enhancing primary tumor prediction. The Apriori algorithm, originally designed for association rule mining, has been successfully adapted to identify meaningful patterns and relationships within medical datasets related to primary tumor prediction. By integrating Apriori with classification techniques such as decision trees, support vector machines, or neural networks, we can exploit the discovered patterns to improve the accuracy and efficiency of primary tumor prediction. This fusion of Apriori's association rule mining capabilities with classification models enables a more comprehensive understanding of the underlying features and their impact on tumor prediction, leading to more informed and precise predictions.

There are several avenues for future work to explore and enhance the integration of the Apriori algorithm with data-mining classification techniques for primary tumor prediction. First, research should focus on refining and optimizing the integration process to achieve better efficiency and scalability, particularly with large and complex medical datasets. Additionally, investigating the potential of incorporating other advanced association rule mining algorithms beyond Apriori could further improve the pattern discovery and prediction accuracy. Furthermore, exploring the integration of ensemble learning approaches with association-rule mining may provide a more robust and accurate prediction model. Finally, considering real-world deployment and validation of the integrated approach on diverse medical datasets can validate its effectiveness and practical applicability, ultimately benefiting healthcare professionals in the domain of tumor prediction and diagnosis.

References

1. El-Halees, A.M. and Shurrab, A.H., Blood Tumor Prediction Using Data Mining Techniques. *Health Informatics - An International Journal (HIIJ)*, 6, 2, 23–30, 2017, doi: 10.5121/HIIJ.2017.6202.
2. Geetha, C. and Arunachalam, A., Liver tumor prediction by data mining and machine learning techniques in health care environment. *Int. J. Health Sci. (IJHS)*, 6, S4, 6722–6729, 2022, doi: 10.53730/ijhs.v6ns4.10398.
3. Mohana Lakshmi, G. and Mythili, K., Survey of gene-expression-based cancer subtypes prediction. *International Journal of Advances in Computer Science and Technology (IJACST)*, 3, 3, 207–211, 2014.
4. Saleema, J.S., Deepa Shenoy, P., Venugopal, K.R., Patnaik., L.M., Cancer Prognosis Prediction Model using Data Mining Techniques. *Data Min. Knowl. Eng.*, 6, 1, 21–29, 2014.
5. Uma, R., Ramkumar, P., Anith Ruth, J., Valarmathi, R., Devi., M.S., Prediction of Lung Cancer using Data Mining Techniques. *In 2022 3rd International*

Conference on Smart Electronics and Communication (ICOSEC), IEEE. pp. 975–977, , 2022, doi: 10.1109/ICOSEC54921.2022.9952118.

6. Thamilselvan, P., Lung Cancer Prediction and Classification Using Adaboost Data Mining Algorithm. *Int. J. Comput. Theory Eng.*, 14, 4, 149–154, 2022, doi: 10.7763/ijcte.2022.v14.1322.
7. Padmapriya, A. and Maragatham, K.S.C., Priority Based Apriori Algorithm For Cancer Prediction Using Fuzzy Classification. *Int. J. Eng. Res. Technol.*, 2, 4, 2259–2266, 2013.
8. Jadhav, M.S., Gondhale, P.R., Kharya, M.R., Sharma., A.R., Classification of Brain Tumor Based On Data Mining Techniques. *Int. J. Adv. Res. Innov. Ideas Educ.*, 4, 3, 243–250, 2018.
9. Hemanth, G., Janardhan, M., Sujihelen, L., Design and Implementing Brain Tumor Detection Using Machine Learning Approach. *2019 3rd International Conference on Trends in Electronics and Informatics (ICOEI),* Tirunelveli, India, pp. 1289–1294, 2019, doi: 10.1109/ICOEI.2019.8862553.
10. Kaur, I., Doja, M.N., Ahmad, T., Ahmad, M., Hussain, A., Nadeem, A., Ahmed, A., An integrated approach for cancer survival prediction using data mining techniques. *Comput. Intell. Neurosci.*, 2021, 1, 6342226, 2021.
11. Krishnaveni, A. and Ahmed, M., II, Fractal dimension feature based breast tumor classification using data mining. *J. Data Acquis. Process.*, 38, 2, 1208, 2023.
12. Alam, T.M., Khan, M.M.A., Iqbal, M.A., Abdul, W., Mushtaq, M., Cervical cancer prediction through different screening methods using data mining. *Int. J. Adv. Comput. Sci. Appl. (IJACSA),* 10, 2, 2019. Available at SSRN: https://ssrn.com/abstract=3474371
13. Chaurasia, V., Pal, S., Tiwari, B.B., Prediction of benign and malignant breast cancer using data mining techniques. *J. Algorithms Comput. Technol.*, 12, 2, 119–126, 2018.
14. Jha, S.K., Pan, Z., Elahi, E., Patel, N., A comprehensive search for expert classification methods in disease diagnosis and prediction. *Expert Syst.*, 36, 1, e12343, 2019.
15. AbdElNabi, M.L.R., Wajeeh Jasim, M., El-Bakry, H.M., Hamed N. Taha, M., Khalifa, N.E.M., Breast and colon cancer classification from gene expression profiles using data mining techniques. *Symmetry*, 12, 3, 408, 2020.
16. Sakthivel, N., Subasree, S., Sivakumar, S., Mohan, M.M., Classification of kidney cancer data using depth aware generative adversarial networks approach. *The Seybold Report,* 18, 557–564, 2023.
17. Deepika, M. and Kalaiselvi, K., A empirical study on disease diagnosis using data mining techniques, in: *2018 second international conference on inventive communication and computational technologies (ICICCT),* IEEE, pp. 615–620, 2018.
18. Bilici, Z. and Özdemir, D., Data mining studies in education: Literature review for the years 2014-2020. *Bayburt Eğitim Fakültesi Dergisi*, 17, 33, 342–376, 2022.

19. Sikibi, M., Use data mining cleansing to prepare data for strategic decisions, in: *Data Mining-Concepts and Applications*, Ciza Thomas (Ed.), IntechOpen, 2022.
20. Chhabra, P. and Madaan, R., Data mining concepts in healthcare with discussion on prediction of diseases, in: *2022 International Conference on Machine Learning, Big Data, Cloud and Parallel Computing (COM-IT-CON)*, vol. 1, IEEE, pp. 71–77, 2022, May.
21. Durugkar, S.R., Raja, R., Nagwanshi, K.K., Kumar, S., Introduction to data mining, in: *Data Mining and Machine Learning Applications*, pp. 1–19, 2022.
22. Witten, I.H., Frank, E., Hall, M.A., Chapter 4: Data Preprocessing, Chapter 5: Algorithms: The Basic Methods, in: *Data Mining: Practical Machine Learning Tools and Techniques*, 4th ed., Morgan Kaufmann, Elsevier, 2016.
23. Mughal, M.J.H., Data mining: Web data mining techniques, tools and algorithms: An overview. *Int. J. Adv. Comput. Sci. Appl. (IJACSA)*, 9, 6, 2018.
24. François-Lavet, V., Henderson, P., Islam, R., Bellemare, M.G., Pineau, J., An introduction to deep reinforcement learning. *Found. Trends Mach. Learn.*, 11, 3–4, 219–354, 2018.
25. Witten, I.H., Frank, E., Hall, M.A., Pal, C.J., Chapter 5, in: *Data Mining: Practical Machine Learning Tools and Techniques*, Morgan Kaufmann, Elsevier, 2016.
26. Provost, F. and Fawcett, T., *Data Science for Business: What You Need to Know about Data Mining and Data-Analytic Thinking*, O'Reilly Media Inc., 2013.
27. Hossin, M. and Sulaiman, M.N., A review on evaluation metrics for data classification evaluations. *Int. J. Data Min. Knowl. Manag. Process (IJDKP)*, 5, 2, 1, 2015.
28. Branco, I. and Choupina, A., Bioinformatics: new tools and applications in life science and personalized medicine. *Appl. Microbiol. Biotechnol.*, 105, 937–951, 2021.
29. Thareja, P. and Chhillar, R.S., A detailed survey on data mining based optimization schemes for bioinformatics applications. *ECS Trans.*, 107, 1, 4689, 2022.
30. Nasser, F.K. and Behadili, S.F., A Review of Data Mining and Knowledge Discovery Approaches for Bioinformatics. *Iraqi J. Sci.*, 63, 9, 3169–3188, 2022.
31. Khan, M.N.R., Bala, S., Yesmin, S., Abedin, M.Z., Bioinformatics: The importance of data mining techniques, in: *Sentimental Analysis and Deep Learning: Proceedings of ICSADL 2021*, Springer Singapore, pp. 411–422, 2022.
32. Singh, P. and Singh, N., Role of data mining techniques in bioinformatics. *Int. J. Appl. Res. Bioinf. (IJARB)*, 11, 1, 51–60, 2021.
33. Piña-Sánchez, P. *et al.*, Cancer Biology, Epidemiology, and Treatment in the 21st Century: Current Status and Future Challenges From a Biomedical Perspective. *Cancer Control*, 28, 107327482110387, Jan. 2021, doi: 10.1177/10732748211038735.
34. Ruddon, R.W., *Cancer biology*. Oxford University Press, 2007.

35. Siegel, R.L., Miller, K.D., Fuchs, H.E., Jemal, A., Cancer statistics, 2022. *CA Cancer J. Clin.*, 72, 1, 7–33, 2022 Jan, doi: 10.3322/caac.21708, Epub 2022 Jan 12, PMID: 35020204.
36. Weinberg, R.A. and Weinberg, R.A., *The biology of cancer.* WW Norton & Company, 2006.
37. Mia, M.R., Akhter Hossain, S., Chhoton, A.C., Ranjan Chakraborty, N., A Comprehensive Study of Data Mining Techniques in Health-care, Medical, and Bioinformatics. *2018 International Conference on Computer, Communication, Chemical, Material and Electronic Engineering (IC4ME2)*, Rajshahi, Bangladesh, pp. 1–4, 2018, doi: 10.1109/IC4ME2.2018.8465626.
38. Posonia, A.M., Vigneshwari, S., Rani, D.J., Machine Learning based Diabetes Prediction using Decision Tree J48. *2020 3rd International Conference on Intelligent Sustainable Systems (ICISS)*, Thoothukudi, India, pp. 498–502, 2020, doi: 10.1109/ICISS49785.2020.9316001.
39. Rahmi, N.S., Wardhani, N.W.S., Mitakda, M.B., Fauztina, R.S., Salsabila, I., SMOTE Classification and Random Oversampling Naive Bayes in Imbalanced Data : (Case Study of Early Detection of Cervical Cancer in Indonesia). *2022 IEEE 7th International Conference on Information Technology and Digital Applications (ICITDA)*, Yogyakarta, Indonesia, pp. 1–6, 2022, doi: 10.1109/ICITDA55840.2022.9971421.
40. Firdaus Abdullah, M., Noraini Sulaiman, S., Khusairi Osman, M., Karim, N.K.A., Lutfi Shuaib, I., Danial Irfan Alhamdu, M., Classification of Lung Cancer Stages from CT Scan Images Using Image Processing and k-Nearest Neighbours. *2020 11th IEEE Control and System Graduate Research Colloquium (ICSGRC)*, Shah Alam, Malaysia, pp. 68–72, 2020, doi: 10.1109/ICSGRC49013.2020.9232492.
41. Cong, Y., Research on Data Association Rules Mining Method Based on Improved Apriori Algorithm. *2020 International Conference on Big Data & Artificial Intelligence & Software Engineering (ICBASE)*, Bangkok, Thailand, pp. 373–376, 2020, doi: 10.1109/ICBASE51474.2020.00085.
42. Wang, P.-J., Shi, L., Bai, J.-N., Zhao, Y.-L., Mining Association Rules Based on Apriori Algorithm and Application. *2009 International Forum on Computer Science-Technology and Applications*, Chongqing, China, pp. 141–143, 2009, doi: 10.1109/IFCSTA.2009.41.
43. Dash, S.R., Dehuri, S., Rayaguru, S., Discovering interesting rules from biological data using parallel genetic algorithm. *2013 3rd IEEE International Advance Computing Conference (IACC)*, Ghaziabad, India, pp. 631–636, 2013, doi: 10.1109/IAdCC.2013.6514300.

10

Deep Learning in Genomics, Personalized Medicine, and Neurodevelopmental Disorders

Ajay Sharma[1,2*], Shashi Kala[3], Aman Kumar[1], Shamneesh Sharma[1], Gaurav Gupta[2] and Varun Jaiswal[2]

[1]upGrad Campus, upGrad Education Private Limited India, Bangalore, Karnataka, India
[2]Yoga Nanda School of Artificial Intelligence and Machine Learning, Shoolini University of Life Science and Business Management, Solan, HP, India
[3]Jaypee Institute of Information Technology, Greater Noida, UP, India

Abstract
The combination of computer science (artificial intelligence) and healthcare in medication can change medical services. Prevision medication techniques distinguish patient aggregates with uncommon treatment reactions or exceptional medical service needs for the curation of the disease. Artificial intelligence creates a source of knowledge by utilizing modern computation and surmising, permitting the framework to learn and engage clinician work through expanded insight. The current study examines the combination of medications that will support the goal of addressing the most difficult standing-up problems in personalized medication. Personalized medicine analysis and prognosis will be facilitated by a combination of genomic and non-genomic determinants, along with patient-side effects, clinical history, and lifestyle data. This comprehensive approach will help to identify individualized treatment plans for patients. Precision medication is another way to deal with clinical examination, and patient consideration that spotlights the understanding and treatment of illness through the coordination of multi-modular or multi-omics information from a person to pursue patient-custom fitted choices. Novel procedures for processing and comprehendong the huge and complex datasets produced by personalized medication require analytical methodologies. Simultaneously, software engineering has progressed quickly to foster

**Corresponding author*: ajaysharmadharmani@gmail.com

Neha Sharma, Korhan Cengiz and Prasenjit Chatterjee (eds.) Intelligent Data Analytics for Bioinformatics and Biomedical Systems, (235–264) © 2024 Scrivener Publishing LLC

procedures for putting away, handling, and investigating these complex datasets, an accomplishment that conventional insights and early registration innovations could not accomplish. AI is a part of the computerized perception that recognizes a complex pattern in the information that can be utilized to make expectations or characterizations of beforehand concealed information or for cutting-edge exploratory information examination. AI investigation of multi-model precision medication information empowers the expansive examination of enormous datasets and, finally, a superior comprehension of human well-being and infection. This book chapter on the utilization of AI for precision medication's "big data" in hereditary qualities, genomics, and other fields of data.

Keywords: Genomics, healthcare, personalized medicine, machine learning, neurodegenerative disorder, machine learning, neuroscience

10.1 Introduction

Precision medicine, also known as personalized healthcare, is an innovative method for understanding health and illnesses based on personalized patient data. This approach involves assortment and examination of various types of patient data, including medical diagnoses, clinical phenotypes, biological investigations, and environmental, demographic, and lifestyle factors. The combination of these datasets, referred to as multimodal data, provides a comprehensive picture of a patient's health status. The growth of personalized medicine has been deeply influenced by advancements in technology in fields such as medicine, genetics, multi-omics, metabolic neuroscience, and imaging. These technological advancements are permissible for the collection of huge amounts of biological data for each patient, which can help the healthcare caregiver make different diagnosis plans for a person based on their definite needs. However, the extensive number and range of diagnostic tests available can generate complex data that can be challenging to understand and analyze, especially in datasets containing information from multiple patients. Therefore, new tools and techniques are continually being developed to help healthcare professionals better understand and interpret these data to provide personalized treatment plans that optimize patient outcomes [1]. Precision medicine holds the promise of revolutionizing healthcare by enabling more targeted treatment and improving patient outcomes. With continued advancements in technology and research, precision medicine will remain critical in the future of healthcare. The field of precision medicine has greatly benefited from the evolution of computer science, which has enabled efficient storage and analysis of vast volumes of data. This development has played a crucial role in advancing precision medicine diagnostics and therapeutics because computer science methodologies can be used to interpret data collected in healthcare systems [1, 11].

Computer science methodologies, such as Artificial Intelligence (AI), Machine Learning (ML), and Deep Learning (DL), are particularly useful for processing complex and diverse datasets such as multimodal data in precision medicine. Computer science can recognize patterns, behaviors, and relationships from a large dataset produced by healthcare companies through human analysis [29, 33]. As is the case for specific patients, physicians diagnose more accurately and can design a personalized treatment plan with definite medication requirements. The integration of computer science technology and personalized medicine has revolutionized the healthcare industry by allowing efficient treatment to improve patient health. Furthermore, ongoing research and technological advancements in both fields will continue to enhance the capabilities of precision medicine and ultimately benefit patients by providing more personalized and targeted healthcare solutions [5, 34, 38].

The term "precision medicine" has evolved, making it difficult to pinpoint its exact origin. One of the earliest grounds to adopt a precision medicine method was transfusion medicine, which emerged in the early 1900s as we have grown in information technology. This approach resulted from the discovery of blood types that transformed blood transfusions. Difficulties associated with unmatched blood types can be avoided by using identical donor and recipient blood types. Since then, precision medicine has come a long way away, with innovative methods of prevention, diagnosis, intervention, and treatment that alter the medicinal scene. Today, precision medicine seeks to personalize medical care based on a person's exclusive genetic, environmental, and lifestyle factors, providing targeted interventions that are more effective and efficient. With advancements in technologies such as genomics, proteomics, metabolomics, immunology, cheminformatics, and artificial intelligence, precision medicine is poised to continue evolving and revolutionizing healthcare in the years to come [33].

Precision medicine has made remarkable growth in the treatment of formerly fatal illnesses, with precision medicine therapies extending patients' lives and refining their superiority of life. For instance, gene therapy has revolutionized the treatment of spinal muscular atrophy (SMA) type-I in infants, a condition that was after inevitably lethal formerly the age of two. Gene therapy has revolutionized the medical world by extending the lives of children with SMA type I. This ground-breaking treatment improves health and reduces the number of severe respiratory complications requiring invasive respiratory support. As a result, the lives of both patients and their families have transformed, offering a newfound sense of hope and happiness. Precision medicine has now become a well-established field that is receiving substantial funding from research and scientific funding agencies, governments, politicians, private supporters, and other government officials. This assistance is due to its past successes, which demonstrates its potential to change the future of medicine. In this context, this study aims to explore how machine learning can become an invaluable tool for precision medicine in the future. Research has been conducted in the fields of genetics and genomics using big data technology and the latest ML algorithms, their applications, and neuroscience [30]. Additionally, ethical and legal considerations were examined to ensure responsible use of machine learning. Personalized medicine and machine learning (ML) play a vital role in deciphering complex data and identifying individualized treatment plans. The vast amount of data generated through genomic sequencing, electronic medical records, and wearable devices can be analyzed using machine learning algorithms, paving the way for personalized medicine. However, it is essential to take ethical and legal considerations into account, including data privacy and ownership, algorithm bias, and the potential for discrimination [30]. Overall, this study provides a summary of how machine learning can be leveraged in precision medicine and neuroscience and explores related ethical and legal thoughts. By embracing the full potential of machine learning, we can accelerate progress in the area of personalized medicine and offer hope to millions of patients worldwide.

10.1.1 Genomics, Genetics, and Personalized-Medicine Genetics

The branch of genetics and genomics has progressed at an unprecedented rate since Friedrich Miescher's discovery of DNA in 1869, and Watson, Crick, and Franklin's first descriptions of DNA in the late 1950s and 1980s. Both the branches of biological genetics and genomics are instrumental in the introduction of the personalized medicine revolution, as they study genes, their parts in inheritance, and the interactions between a human-specific genome and the larger environment [14, 15]. Genetics and genomics are the main focuses of personalized medicine. This focus has been facilitated by the significant reduction in the cost and time required for genetic testing. In the early days of genomics, the sequencing of the first complete human genome was a massive project that took over a decade to complete and incurred a monstrous cost of $3 billion. However, with rapid advancements in technology, this process has become much more efficient and cost-effective. Currently, the human genome can be sequenced in just 24 h and at a fraction of the cost of approximately $1,000. This remarkable progress in genomics has propelled the field of precision medicine and is anticipated to become increasingly important in the future. The ability to decode an individual's genome can provide valuable insights into their unique genetic makeup and potential health risks, thereby enabling personalized medical care and targeted interventions. Genomics can change and transform our understanding of disease and develop new treatments for specific patients. With continued advancements in genomics and related fields, the potential of precision medicine to improve health outcomes and revolutionize healthcare is enormous [18].

10.1.2 The "Omics" Revolution a Bioinformatics Perspective

Precision medicine has grown to incorporate data from numerous fields, beyond genetics and genomics. Omic sources such as epigenetics, proteomics, metabolomics, radiomics, pharmaceutical comics, macrobiotics, and environmental omics have been combined into personalized medicine through refinement techniques. The integration of data from numerous domains such as proteomics, genomics, metabolomics, transcriptomics, and other "omics" fields has given rise to the term "multi-omics." The analysis of extensive and deep phenotyping datasets in precision medicine is a demanding endeavor that necessitates the application of data science approaches and accumulated processing capacity. Newly created data science approaches are essential for decision-making and are required to successfully preprocess, comprehend, develop, and use this information. In recent years, there has been an increasing desire to integrate data from many areas to obtain thorough understanding of complex biological systems. This method, informally known as "multi-omics," incorporates data from many sources, including genomes, transcriptomics, and metabolomics, to provide a broader understanding of how a biological system functions. Interpreting these enormous and heterogeneous multi-omics datasets without the assistance of information science and collective computing capacity is a challenging task. Machine learning(ML), a subset of AI, has emerged as a viable data-science technique. ML approaches entail teaching computer models to process and analyze data, recognize complicated patterns, and forecast future situations. These methods have proven indispensable in evaluating multi-omics datasets, which are vital for the advancement of precision medicine. Machine learning algorithms can identify biomarkers, categorize patients into subgroups, and forecast treatment results, all of which are critical for customized medicine [18]. Machine learning models can provide more thorough knowledge of a patient's health state by utilizing several sources of information, such as clinical and environmental data. In summary, the incorporation of machine learning and data science into precision medicine has the potential to transform the discipline and improve patient outcomes by allowing us to quickly process, analyze, comprehend, and give results on a large volume of complicated data [18].

Novel data-science approaches are required to address the challenges involved in processing, analyzing, and exploiting complex data in precision medicine. Machine learning has emerged as a key tool for evaluating these datasets among these methodologies. Machine learning methods, as a subset of artificial intelligence, enable the training of AI/ML models to absorb and grasp massive volumes of data, discover complicated patterns, and forecast new situations. ML algorithms can handle enormous amounts of information faster than traditional statistical approaches, allowing researchers to discover new insights and reveal previously undiscovered associations. The use of machine learning (ML) has a wide range of potential applications in precision medicine, including forecasting disease risk and discovering novel therapeutic targets for designing tailored treatment strategies. Machine learning algorithms, for instance, may evaluate enormous amounts of genomic data to identify genetic variants that relate to illness risk or treatment resistance, thereby assisting in the creation of tailored therapeutics. Many elements of our daily lives, such as speech recognition, image search, and natural language processing (NLP), have already been altered by machine learning. Machine learning may be used in healthcare to forecast disease susceptibility, identify patient subgroups, and customize therapies. Machine learning, with its capacity to evaluate complex and diverse data, can aid in the discovery of novel biological discoveries that are difficult or impossible to discover using previous approaches. To fully realize the potential of machine learning, certain obstacles must be overcome. Algorithm biases, the requirement for large and diverse datasets, the interpretation of machine learning outcomes, and ethical issues related to data privacy and security are all examples of these in data handling. To address these issues, researchers must work across disciplines to combine data from multiple areas and to create novel analytical approaches. Moreover, machine learning algorithms can analyze data from electronic medical records and wearable devices to identify illness patterns, forecast disease progression, and evaluate therapy efficacy [18, 31, 32]. Machine learning algorithms may provide a comprehensive perspective on an individual's health by merging data from numerous sources, allowing the development of individualized treatment regimens.

In summary, machine learning has altered many aspects of our daily lives and has played a vital role in the future of precision medicine. Data science technologies such as machine learning will become increasingly significant in the field of customized medicine as datasets become more sophisticated and vaster. In conclusion, machine learning has emerged as a vital tool in the future of personalized medicine, assisting in the analysis of massive and heterogeneous multi-omics datasets to identify new perspectives and allow for personalized treatment and medication. Although several challenges need to be addressed, the potential of machine learning to transform healthcare is immense. As technology advances, we expect to see even more significant breakthroughs in precision medicine, improving patient outcomes and quality of life.

10.2 Machine Learning in Personalized Medicine and Neurogenerative Disorder

Once considered an invention of the imagination by artists, philosophers, and science fiction writers, the advent of artificial intelligence (AI) has revolutionized medicine and research by introducing "smart" machines and technology [6]. Machine learning, a subset of AI, involves creating computer models that can detect and analyze patterns in complex datasets to develop classification and prediction based on the training data set. Arthur Samuel, a former IBM employee, popularized the term "machine learning" in the 1950s, and it has come a long way since then. Machine learning can be divided into supervised, unsupervised, and reinforcement learning methods. The positive (+ve) input data point in the dataset trains the ML model to replicate the process of decision in the future, whereas negative (−ve) data points train the model to avoid making the decision. Reinforcement learning is less significant in personalized medicine than other ML approaches, such as supervised or unsupervised ML methods, where we do not need to directly input data [22, 23, 28].

Unsupervised ML approaches are strong strategies in which patterns in unlabeled data are recognized and groupings of similar cases in a dataset are detected. This approach is most effective when solving queries that require understanding of the underlying structure of a dataset, such as identifying illness subgroups or spotting disparities between patients and healthy people. Once identified, these clusters can be further studied or displayed using typical statistical methods. This allows researchers to discover important links between variables, gain insight into the characteristics of certain subgroups, and forecast future trends based on these patterns. Principal component analysis (PCA), k-nearest neighbors, and autoencoders are among the most extensively used techniques in unsupervised ML models. The principal component analysis (PCA) is a method for recognizing shapes and patterns in massive datasets by lowering the dimensionality of the data while maintaining the majority of its variability. The k-nearest neighbor algorithm is a clustering technique that is used to locate and group comparable data points. Variational autoencoders (VAEs) are a form of neural networks that can learn the underlying distribution of data and generate new data points depending on the provided information [4]. In general, unsupervised machine learning is critical for discovering significant patterns in unstructured information, which can lead to greater comprehension of complex biological systems and disorders. It has evolved into a crucial tool in precision medicine, allowing researchers to identify patient subgroups, design individualized therapies, and enhance patient outcomes [8, 22, 33].

In recent years, supervised machine learning methods have grown in popularity due to their ability to accurately predict outcomes based on input data. In contrast, supervised machine learning approaches use labeled data to detect patterns in complicated datasets, such as differentiating between healthy and unhealthy samples, for predicting the result scores. This approach involves training a model on a dataset with known labels to maximize its performance for a specified goal. The obtained ML algorithm patterns can subsequently be used to categorize fresh datasets or create data-driven predictions tailored to particular patients. Classification-based ML models were employed to categorize the data, whereas regression models were used to anticipate continuous result scores. SVM, RF, linear models, and DNN are prominent supervised machine learning algorithms. These strategies are applicable to both classification and regression issues, where classification entails predicting various categorical variables and regression entails predicting continuous variables from a given dataset [4, 22]. Support vector machines are examples that are often used to solve classification issues by identifying the most optimal hyperplane that divides multiple classes of data points. Similarly, support vector regression is used to solve regression issues by identifying the best-fitting line that captures the relationship between I/O input and output variables. Random forests, on the other hand, increase the model's stability and accuracy using a collective technique that integrates several decision trees, resulting in improved accuracy and prediction. Linear models, such as logistic regression, are basic yet effective strategies that can be used for both classification and regression-based issues.

Deep neural networks are another type of AI-based model that can learn from complex representations/patterns of data through multiple layers of nonlinear transformations. Overall, supervised statistical and machine learning methods have an extensive range of applications in fields such as healthcare, finance, and manufacturing [4]. They are valuable tools for making predictions and providing insights into complex systems, and their popularity is expected to grow continuously in the future [4, 8, 33, 36].

For machine learning methods to be effective, numerous critical factors must be considered. First, the quality of the input data must be ensured with minimal noise and artifacts. The accuracy of the ground-truth labels is crucial because incorrect labeling can significantly impact the presentation and outcome of the ML model. Thus, the precision of the actual labels during the data pre-processing process must be ensured using proper diagnostic labels and diagnoses. Machine learning models typically require complete training sets deprived of missing input data features to produce more accurate results. Methods such as random attribution of data can fill in missing data, which is a requirement for completing a dataset for an ML model. Larger datasets remain preferred as they allow the ML model to study the accurate difference in the data while minimizing the risk of outliers negatively distressing the model. Collecting large datasets can be challenging, particularly for rare diseases. Precision and accuracy are both critical in classification algorithms, and machine learning models need to be optimized. Finally, before using machine learning models for clinical decision making or computer-aided diagnosis, it is essential to validate the model. One way to validate the model is to train it using datasets comprising cases identified by a physician, and then independently analyze new cases by both the doctor and the ML model and compare the consequences to authenticate the model. ML models can be deployed for both classification and regression-based problems. However, selecting an appropriate model for a specific clinical problem requires consideration of each model's strengths and weaknesses. Researchers and engineers can consult textbooks such as Applied Predictive Modeling or available research articles and review papers, such as a newly available tutorial for clinicians to understand the details of each machine learning process [4, 8, 22, 35].

10.2.1 Machine Learning Using Artificial Deep Neural Networks (DNN)

Artificial neural networks (ANN) remain modeled after the interconnectivity of neurons, in addition to interconnections in the human brain.

They typically comprise an input layer, one or more hidden layers, and output layer. Each layer in the model contains many artificial nodes that are linked to the nodes in the next layer via weights, which simulate the connections between brain cells. This is called the feed-forward network (FFN). In a classification problem, such as identifying patients with or without a disease, the number of neurons in the input layer is frequently the same as the number of input characteristic features; however, the number of neurons in the output layer is the same as the number of classes required for classification. The network's ability to handle complex nonlinear problems increases with the number of hidden layers and neurons in each layer. Figure 10.1 describes the working of the neural network, hidden layer (FC) layers, and output layers. However, as the number of hidden layers increased, the network became more difficult to optimize and train. Deep neural networks are artificial neural networks with multiple hidden layers, as shown in Figure 10.1 [34, 35].

The background of artificial neural networks (ANN) dates to World War II 1943 when Walter Pitts and Warren McCulloch introduced the first computer model of a neuron [13]. However, due to the limited hardware and algorithms at the time, training these networks was computationally exclusive, making them less accessible for widespread use. It was not until the 1980s that the first recurrent neural network was introduced by James Hopfield, and backpropagation was popularized by Geoffrey Hinton and colleagues for neural network training [12]. This allows for the additional efficient training of complex neural networks. In the early 20th century and early 2000s, new hardware, such as specialized graphical processing units (GPUs), especially NVIDIA, and even more efficient algorithms were developed. These advancements have allowed for the development and training of neural networks through composite architectures and multiple

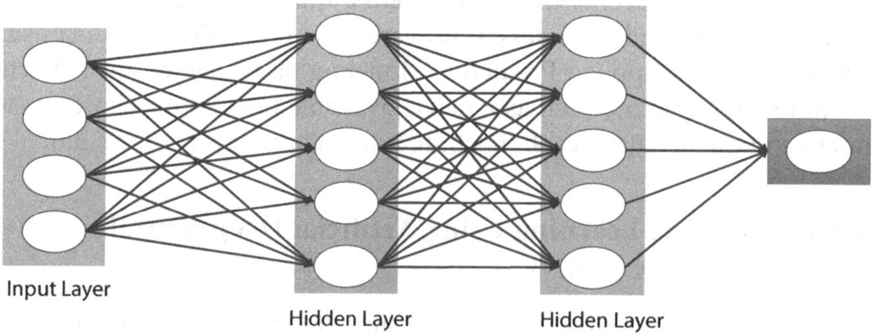

Figure 10.1 Conception of a fully connected feed-forward (FC-FW) artificial neural network with hidden layers.

hidden layers, outperforming many classical ML techniques, such as support vector machines (SVM) and random forests (RF). Artificial neural networks are extensively used in numerous domains, including computer vision, natural language processing, autonomous vehicles, and biomedical image processing [12, 32, 35, 36]. Their flexibility, scalability, and ability to learn complex relationships from large datasets make them powerful tools for data-driven decision making [30].

In recent years, deep learning models have emerged as powerful tools that surpass out-of-date machine learning models in numerous tasks and, in some cases, smoothly outperforming humans. Dedicated or specialized neural network architectures have been established for different applications, such as recurrent neural networks for processing sequential time-series data and convolutional neural networks (CNN) [34, 35, 36, 38] for solving complex signal processing and image processing tasks. For instance, convolutional neural networks are highly effective in automating image-based tumor staging owing to the use of convolutional filters in the initial layers. These filters identify significant sequential or spatial features in datasets, such as whole-genome sequence (WGS) data or 3D-imaging data, without requiring handcrafted feature extraction filters [39]. The filters are optimized alongside the network weights, and the raw dataset is fed directly into the deep convolutional neural network (CNN), which automatically identifies the optimum features aimed at the given machine-learning problem. Considering their effectiveness and potential, deep learning methods, including CNN and recurrent neural networks (RNNs) are likely to play an increasingly significant role in personalized medicine applications in the future.

10.2.2 Limitations and Advantages of ML Over Traditional Approaches

With the advent of precision medicine, ML, particularly artificial neural networks (ANNs), provide a range of benefits for data analysis. Machine learning models do not have any strict assumptions regarding data distribution, such as a normal distribution. Consequently, they can effortlessly associate multi-omics information, which includes binary, categorical, discrete, and continuous variables, deprived of the essential for widespread data pre-processing. ML models can effectively manage noisy data and a large variance within the dataset due to one functionality called regularization, which is employed in many ML algorithms. Reducing noise is preferable. Machine learning models have specific categories and architectures that can be trained on small datasets, particularly those with many features relative to observations. Multifaceted machine learning models can detect complex calculations and nonlinear patterns in training data that a human being cannot observe and may overlook [42, 43].

Although machine learning offers significant benefits, it has some limitations. One such limitation is the difficulty of interpreting complex, non-linear patterns associated with simpler linear models, which leads to ML models being viewed as a "black box." Therefore, it is crucial to guarantee that machine learning models do not overfit the training data, which can negatively impact their generalizability. Overfitting occurs when the machine learning model significantly improves the training datasets compared to the testing data, which means that the model is not intelligent enough to specify the data well. Overfitting is more frequent in increasingly complicated machine learning models such as DNN with millions of input parameters. Underfitting the training dataset using ML models may result in decreased accuracy for both the training and testing data. A self-governing test set must be used to ensure that the model is not overfitting or underfitting in the data when evaluating machine learning models [42, 43].

10.3 Machine Learning in Genomics

Machine learning algorithms have been shown to be quite successful in dealing with huge and complicated genomics datasets, which are frequently difficult to evaluate using antiquated statistical or linear ML models. Artificial intelligence (AIML) has a significant impact on genomics. There are several exclusive and Nobel examples where machine learning models have successfully tackled the difficulties presented by such data, leading to clinically significant outcomes. This study discusses selected examples to demonstrate the wide applicability of machine learning across various domains [19].

Genome-wide association studies have employed machine learning to recognize variants related to specific traits or phenotypes. For instance, Type I diabetes patients have been identified using SVM models based on GWAS data, indicating that genotype-based sickness risk valuation may be possible for diseases where SNP capture a significant risk quantity. Researchers have compared various conventional ML models to classify persons with Crohn's disease using the method called genotyping of data and genome-wide notation. Their study, which involved 18,227 Crohn's disease patients' persons and 34,050 healthy persons, used non-linear classification methods such as the boosted tree algorithm, and an NN with more than one hidden layer outperformed linear models such as logistic regression [19]. Figure 10.2 highlights the prediction of disease in genomics with the help of heatmaps. The use of machine learning models for patient treatment and early diagnosis has several advantages.

- These models can analyze data obtained from previous patients to identify those who would benefit from detailed treatment.
- ML models can analyze data from various sources, including electronic medical records, to identify patients who could benefit from early conduct or contribute to clinical trials of new interventions. The potential of machine learning in cancer treatment is demonstrated by developing and testing an SVM model for predicting drug specificity and sensitivity using genomic data.
- Machine learning approaches and deep learning techniques have proven useful in pharmacogenomics to predict drug response and aid in personalized drug design. By identifying non-responders to specific treatments, clinicians can avoid administering unnecessary treatments and select the most active treatment based on the patient's genome.

Machine learning has been instrumental in discovering new biomarkers for various diseases and facilitating early disease detection, treatment response prediction, and disease outcome prediction.

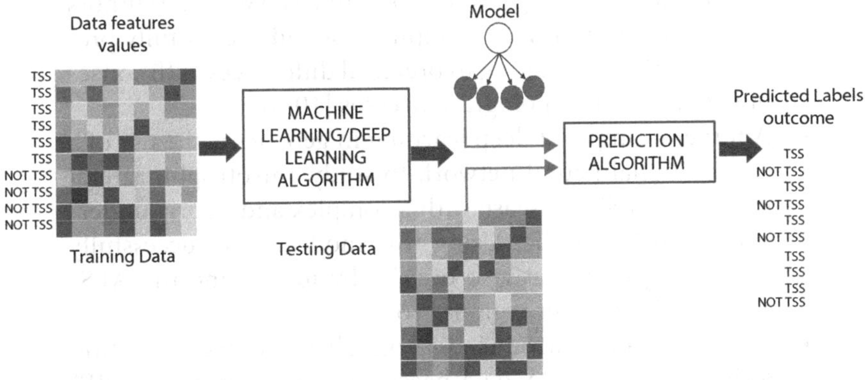

Figure 10.2 Deep learning in genomics heatmaps shows the prediction of a disease.

- The availability of large freely accessible datasets, such as the UK Biobank and the Alzheimer's Disease Neuroimaging Initiative (ADNI), has aided many such studies. For instance, one study utilized unsupervised machine learning on data from more than over 10,000 tumor datasets across ~32 types of cancer to comprehend their similarities and differences. The objective of this study was to discover potential cancer therapeutic targets by investigating how cancer develops from the original cells and the factors that affect tumor growth, with immunological aspects and related issues [22, 23].
- Other approaches are being explored, such as using genetic data in a DL model to determine cancerous cell genome biomarkers linked to improved survival rates in bladder cancer patients and categorizing them into survival subtypes [27].
- Researchers have successfully used novel deep learning models to study heritable conditions beyond cancer. The author has created a deep learning model that uses statistically important SNPs associated with the obesity phenotype to classify obese patients, which effectively identifies applicable SNPs and connections for precise tasks [27].
- A Deep Learning model named DeepVariant was developed to assist, in categorizing genetic variants in Whole-Genome Sequence (WGS) data. DeepVariant is particularly useful in distinguishing true variants from sequencing errors, outperforming other methods [10, 15].
- DeepSEA was designed to identify the practical belongings of non-coding variations, which comprise most disease-associated SNPs in the genome. To train DeepSEA, the authors used chromatin profiles as input data and successfully predicted the SNPs resulting in practical differences with consequences for anthropological diseases [10, 16].
- Another example of deep learning in genetics is the use of a convolutional neural network to study amyotrophic lateral sclerosis (ALS), a disease with a complex and poorly understood genetic profile. Using this model, they successfully identified patients at risk of ALS by identifying the ALS-associated promoter regions [16].
- The researcher introduced a mutable variable collection technique for GWAS data based on a random forest (RF) technique that ranks SNPs based on their prognostic control.

This is because of its high performance on datasets with numerous variables and significantly rarer observations. The ML model can be applied to various genomic data analysis study, including pathway analysis, classification, regression, feature selection, genetic association, and epistasis recognition from the dataset obtained in the laboratory *in vivo* [9].

- A new ML-based model was established to address the limitations of GWAS, which can only account for a minor proportion of common diseases. These models are particularly useful in understanding epigenetics and epigenomics, which alter gene expression without altering DNA sequences [9, 21].
- DeepBind, a CNN-based network, aids in the cutting-edge discovery of genetic variants linked to human disease by predicting the arrangement of document-binding proteins present in DNAs and RNAs. DeepChrome and DeepHistone are used to determine whether histone protein modifications have combinatorial effects on gene expression and may serve as biomarkers for epigenetic changes that have the potential to adapt and modify health and disease in patients [2, 7, 22].
- Epigenetics and epigenomics enhance additional layers of complications in previously complex genetic and genomic datasets, making this novel machine-learning model invaluable in advancing biological models and understanding the molecular basis of human diseases, which is especially crucial because it is essential to deliberate epigenetic mechanisms [26].

10.3.1 Multi-Model Data Integration Using Machine Learning

The combination of multiple omics data sources with machine learning aims to enhance our understanding of the genotype–phenotype relationship. Medical imaging provides a vast amount of data for analysis and has become an important tool in the diagnosis and administration of many diseases. However, integrating medical imaging with genetic data can be challenging, as it requires identifying the links between deep genetic and high-dimensional imagination topographies to better understand how hereditary variations influence organ anatomy and function to comprehend disease phenotypes. To address this challenge, the field of imaging genetics has emerged, which seeks to identify the genetic underpinnings of imaging features and to use them to better understand disease mechanisms.

Recently, Jonsson *et al.* developed a CNN model to estimate brain age using high-resolution T1-weighted MRI data. The researchers then used this information to examine its relationship with genome-wide association study (GWAS) data. This approach can potentially reveal genetic variants associated with structural and functional brain changes that may underlie cognitive decline and other neurological disorders. By integrating deep genetic information with high-dimensional imaging features, imaging genetics can pave the way for the development of personalized medicine and targeted treatment for various diseases. They identified two sequence variants associated with atypical brain aging. Researchers have presented a method that utilizes genetic and imaging data to automatically diagnose craniofacial syndromes using 3D facial images. Their approach had a well-adjusted accuracy of 73% for classifying genetically established craniofacial conditions. Several global initiatives, such as the IMAGEN study, employ brain imaging and genetics to explore the psychological, biological, and ecological factors that affect brain development and mental health. With these efforts, the future of precision medicine is promising [37, 41].

Advanced ML methods can be utilized to associate multi-omics data to diagnose, predict, and treat diseases, as well as to investigate the relationship between genotype and phenotype. This approach allows the incorporation of important information across different disciplines of medicine, such as genetics and metabolomics. The field of medical imaging has been a focus of attention in recent years owing to the vast amount of data gathered in the healthcare sector. However, it is often challenging to establish a link between high-dimensional tomographic features and genetic variations that can influence organ anatomy and function to better understand various disease phenotypes. To address this challenge, researchers have focused on imaging genetics. Researchers conducted a study that demonstrated a significant improvement in the classification accuracy of patients with schizophrenia by combining functional MRI and SNP data, compared to using either imaging or SNP data alone. A boosted tree machine learning model was used to predict the period until Alzheimer's disease diagnosis in normal participants and patients with moderate cognitive impairment using genetic information, neuroimaging, and clinical data. Bayesian networks have also been used to discover relationships among neuropsychological testing scores, single genetic variations, pathways, and imaging characteristics. Machine learning has been used to predict therapeutic responses, in addition to illness categorization and diagnosis. Lin *et al.*, for example, developed a DL model that used SNP, demographic, and clinical data to predict antidepressant treatment response in patients with severe depressive disorders, achieving a model sensitivity of 75% and specificity of 69%.

These findings show that machine learning has the potential to improve the comprehension of the complicated interactions between genetic variants, imaging characteristics, and disease phenotypes in the field of medical imaging. This demonstrates the potential of modern ML model algorithms to integrate multi-omics data for precision medicine. Despite machine learning algorithms having the capability to evaluate complicated multi-omics data, many studies in this field continue to concentrate on single-data modalities. This might be caused by a lack of collaboration among specialists in many domains, which makes gathering and integrating actual multi-omics data challenging. Consequently, machine learning models in personalized medicine have immense potential to fully exploit the abundance of information accessible from multi-omics data for research and patient treatment.

10.4 Machine Learning and the Future of Medicine in Healthcare

The growth of medical science and technology has resulted in increasingly complex medical practices. Advancements in the fields of sciences, such as genetics, metabolomics, and immunology, have brought new insights into and caused numerous diseases, while genetic testing and imaging technologies have allowed for more accurate diagnoses and individualized therapies. These new technologies and fields have created new research opportunities, leading to the development of innovative treatments and therapies. However, they have introduced new obstacles, such as the requirement to analyze large and complicated datasets and interpret the results in a clinically meaningful manner. Despite these obstacles, the merging of various professions and technologies has the potential to significantly improve patient outcomes and change medical practices. Doctors are today more specialized than ever; however, despite the arrival of technology that was supposed to replace physicians, the clinician's role in the practice of medicine remains critical. Machine learning algorithms can evaluate complicated findings, interpret and explain of those results, and consider persistence in the backdrop of their lives, which are crucial tasks that require the special talent of a physician. Although precision medicine offers immense potential, it will not replace physicians in the near future.

However, it can help therapists with analysis, prediction, and behavior by analyzing patient-specific data using machine learning approaches.

10.4.1 Ethical and Legal Considerations of Precision Medicine

The application of machine learning in precision medicine is a promising discovery with the potential to significantly enhance patient outcomes. However, this creates serious ethical, legal, and moral issues that must be addressed. Thus, data privacy is a serious issue. Because machine learning models require large datasets to train and enhance their accuracy, it is vital to share medical data from many places. Maintaining patient privacy in the data is critical, and care must be taken to ensure that any shared dataset does not include patient identification information. Distributed machine learning, which utilizes a traveling model that learns locally from available data before moving it to another location, might be an answer to this problem. Patient privacy is better safeguarded by avoiding transferring data from its source, and the model is less likely to include identifying patient information. This strategy is interesting because it solves privacy, ethical, and legal problems while also benefiting from local training, which is more efficient than centralized training. However, more research is needed to verify that distributed ML models are as effective and exact as centralized models. Another ethical concern is that machine learning has the potential to aggravate current health inequities. Machine learning algorithms trained on datasets that do not appropriately reflect certain groups may be less accurate when applied to those communities, resulting in uneven treatment and outcomes. To avoid unintentional biases and harmful repercussions, machine learning models must be trained on various datasets and verified across different populations. Figure 10.3 demonstrates the many features of customized medicine in omics. Machine learning has enormous potential in precision medicine, and it is critical to evaluate the ethical, legal, and moral aspects to ensure that these technologies are used equally and responsibly.

The implementation of machine learning in precision healthcare poses several ethical, legal, and moral issues. Data security is one of the most pressing challenges, as model performance often increases with more datasets acquired from numerous sites. To protect patient privacy, the datasets must not contain identifiable information. Distributed machine learning models that train locally before moving to the next center can resolve privacy concerns associated with data transfer; however, more research is needed to achieve the same level of effectiveness and accuracy as centralized models. Figure 10.3 highlights the aspects of machine learning

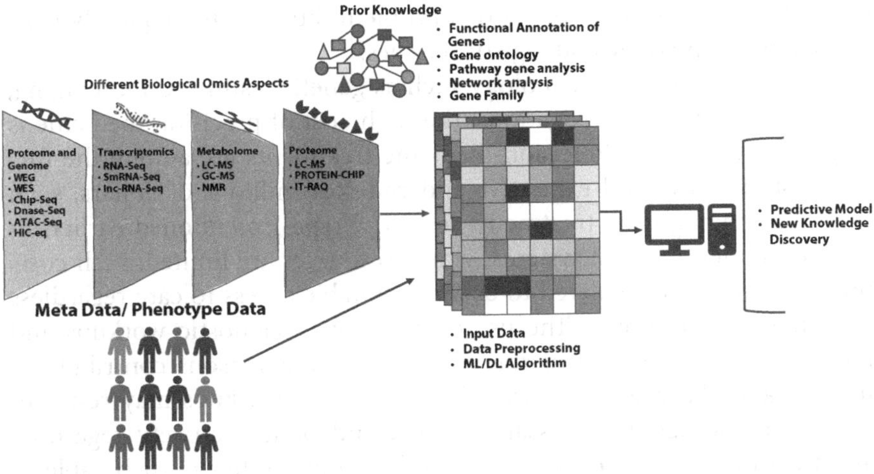

Figure 10.3 Machine learning in different aspects of omics and personalized medicine.

in personalized medicine. Interpreting machine learning models poses a major challenge, particularly as the complexity of input data and models increases. This lack of transparency poses ethical and legal issues as clinicians may not fully comprehend how the model arrives at a specific decision. Researchers are exploring ways to develop more interpretable models that are vital for clinical decision-making. Such models will enable clinicians to understand how the model arrives at its decision, allowing them to appropriately adjust patient care. Another ethical consideration is the accountability of errors caused by machine learning models. It is not clear who should be held accountable when a model chooses poorly. Regulatory agencies for medical devices and AI software are evaluating the safety and effectiveness of AI-powered devices. Currently, these tools are marketed as diagnostic aids instead of as autonomous diagnostic tools because they are meant to assist clinicians in making decisions. These concerns highlight the need for responsible and transparent development and use of machine learning models in precision medicine [22, 34, 35].

In addition to the ethical and legal concerns discussed earlier, machine learning has some technical limitations that raise moral, permissible, ethical, and honest concerns. Typically, machine learning models are developed based on the quality of the datasets with which they are trained. The training datasets are often incomplete, noisy, and biased; as a result, the models built using such datasets may not be applicable after implication to datasets from other healthcare centers or topographical locations, interpreting them as useless for general use. Increasing the amount of training data is the simplest solution to this problem, but this is frequently constrained by permissible and logistical issues.

Despite advances in technology such as genetic testing (GT), imaging, and other scientific investigations, the high cost of precision medicine is a significant concern. Precision medicine treatments are among the furthermost exclusive and expensive and can cost millions of dollars, such as life-prolonging gene treatments for SMA type I mentioned earlier. In publicly funded medical systems, where resources are limited, such costs must be carefully considered to ensure equitable access to care regardless of socioeconomic status. The use of expensive diagnostic workups and interferences that are out of spread for numerous reasons contribute to unacceptable disparities in care. These extensive workups may result in incidental findings, unnecessary testing, and patient anxiety regarding analytical uncertainty. Future machine learning models must be able to identify the most important features of a specific clinical question to avoid unnecessary assessments and reduce harm to patients. While the cost of gaining data is a concern, reducing unhelpful treatment side effects, improving diagnosis, and enhancing patient management can offset this cost [22, 23].

Patient selection can lead to biases that compromise the validity and generalizability of ML models, while exacerbating disparities based on socioeconomic position, race, gender, aptitude, and class. Furthermore, precision medicine is generally restricted to the developed world, with populations in emerging and third-world countries excluded from tests and treatments due to practical and economic constraints. To increase empathy and treatment of health and illness for all humankind, we must make active efforts to incorporate these communities into precision medicine research and development. Such efforts might involve establishing plans for increasing access to funding and resources for precision medicine in underserved communities, addressing cultural sensitivity and inclusivity issues, and promoting collaborations and partnerships between researchers and healthcare providers worldwide.

Precision medicine's potential influence on individual behavior raises serious ethical concerns. Will patients be motivated to change their behavior if they are aware of the genetic or epigenetic risk factors for illnesses such as heart disease or obesity? A new group of "patients-in-waiting" who are not yet sick but have been recognized as high-risk may be created, causing severe psychological suffering for these individuals and their families. As a result, before introducing precision medicine, physicians must examine individuals and their surroundings. It is critical that patients understand the possible hazards and advantages of genetic testing and individualized therapies as well as the psychological impact of knowing one's hereditary risk. Healthcare practitioners and providers must provide sufficient counseling and assistance to people designated as high-risk to ease their worry and guide them in making educated health decisions.

10.5 Genomics Technology and Application

As genomic sequencing has increased since the human genome project was completed in 2003, certain technologies, methods, and tools are needed to interpret and decipher genomic data. There is a certain application that uses genomic applications worldwide. Some of these applications are discussed in the succeeding sections.

10.5.1 High-Throughput DNA Sequencing Technology

Advancements in the next-generation sequencing (NGS) have revolutionized the field of genomics by enabling faster and more precise sequencing. With continuous improvements in technology, the cost of DNA sequencing has been steadily decreasing. It is now possible to sequence a human genome in just a few thousand dollars ($3–5K), and this cost is expected to decrease even further. Consequently, NGS has rapidly become a common tool in clinical practice. Recent reviews have highlighted various genomic technologies and the cost of studies per genome. Due to the increased demand for specialized sequencing, greater read lengths, cheaper prices, and the capacity to perform quick sequencing on current platforms, NGS has emerged as a leading transcriptomic tool [17].

A comprehensive review of several high-volume DNA sequencing approaches and their applications highlighted numerous major features. These tools have transformed genomics, providing researchers with a better knowledge of the genome, its activities, and its role in numerous disorders. Whole-genome sequencing (WGS) has emerged as a potent technique in clinical genomics, enabling the discovery of genetic variations linked to illness susceptibility, prognosis, and therapy response. WGS technology has progressed dramatically over the years and its use has shifted from a research tool to a clinical tool capable of guiding therapeutic therapies. Clinical exome sequencing (CES), also referred to as whole-exome sequencing (WES), is a powerful diagnostic technique for the study of uncommon genetic disorders and composite diseases. It includes whole sequencing of the protein-coding sections of the genome, which constitute only approximately 2% of the genome but includes approximately 85%

of known disease-causing variations. CES has become an essential tool in clinical practice, allowing for the discovery of pathogenic variations that cause hereditary illnesses. Whole-transcriptome sequencing (WTS) is a powerful method for analyzing genome functional components and gene expression variations over time. RNA sequencing (RNA-Seq) is a commonly used technology that allows researchers to examine gene expression patterns in different cells, organs, or network pathways. RNA-Seq offers vital insights into gene regulation and alternative splicing, allowing the identification of novel therapeutic targets. Single-cell sequencing is a relatively new technique that has attracted considerable interest in recent years. Because of its efficacy in many genomics' investigations and research issues, single-cell sequencing was named the technique of 2013. Individual cells can be analyzed using this method, revealing insights into cellular heterogeneity, clonal development, and disease progression. Recent breakthroughs in droplet microfluidics technologies have enabled unrivalled single-cell DNA research and output, enabling the identification and detection of the human genome and genetic variation across and within a population, a concept known as precision genomics. In theory, high-throughput DNA sequencing tools have changed genomics to a field of study, allowing researchers to investigate the genome's complexity and its role in many disorders. These technologies have opened new pathways for hereditary disease detection, prognosis, and therapy, and their implementation has progressed from research to clinical practice. Advances in these technologies hold enormous promise for near-term perception of precision medicine [18, 30].

10.5.2 Pharmacogenomics (PGx)

Genetic factors can contribute to pharmacological treatment failure and cause adverse responses in individuals. Pharmacogenomics (PGx) involves the study of genetic differences that affect the pharmacological effects of medications, including therapeutic responses and antagonistic reactions. PGx is intended to create safe and effective pharmaceuticals and doses tailored to an individual's genetic composition by merging pharmacology and genomics. Enzymatic inhibition and induction caused by drug–gene interactions may affect drug metabolism, resulting in individual differences in medication responses. Individual differences in drug response can be explained by genetic polymorphisms, such as single polynucleotide polymorphisms (SNPs) in metabolic and action pathways of commonly prescribed medications, such as selective serotonin reuptake inhibitors (SSRI), tricyclic antidepressants (TCA), opioid pain medications, beta-blockers, and anti-arrhythmic drugs [40]. Examples of such polymorphisms include CYO450 2C19+, CYP450 2C9−, VKORC1, CYP2D6, CYP450 3A4/3A5, Factor II, Factor V Leiden, MTHFR, OPRM1, UGT1A1, and UGT2B7c.

10.5.3 The Study of Drug Action is Divided into Different Categories: Pharmacokinetics and Pharmacodynamics

Pharmacokinetics is the process of establishing how much medication is needed to circulate and act on each target in the human body, and it includes ADMET aspects such as absorption, distribution, metabolism, and excretion. Pharmacodynamics, on the other hand, focuses on how target cells respond to medications via numerous components such as receptors, ion channels, enzymes, and the immune system. One major benefit of PGx is its ability to offer personalized therapeutic approaches by providing actionable information about which treatments may be most effective and which drugs to avoid due to potentially adverse effects. To achieve this, PGx can classify patients' specific absorbing gene variations as slow, intermediate, normal, or ultrafast metabolizers of each drug, categorizing them as poor, intermediate, extensive, or ultrarapid metabolizers.

10.5.4 Circulating Cell-Free Nucleic Acids

Cell-free nucleic acids are a diverse group of small DNA fragments that can circulate freely in the blood. These include cfDNAs, messenger RNAs (mRNAs), and microRNAs. The presence of cell-free nucleic acids in the bloodstream results from normal biological processes, such as cellular turnover and apoptosis, as well as numerous clinical conditions, such as cancer, metabolic disorders, cardiovascular diseases, and embryonic abnormalities. cfDNA, in particular, has been the focus of much research in recent years due to its potential applications in non-invasive prenatal testing, cancer diagnosis, and monitoring of treatment response. When cells die by apoptosis or necrosis, their contents, including cfDNA, are released into circulation, where they may be identified and examined. Fetal-derived cfDNA can be identified in the maternal plasma of pregnant women, allowing for noninvasive prenatal testing for fetal genetic disorders. Other forms of cfNA that have received interest for their potential diagnostic and therapeutic uses are mRNA and microRNA. mRNAs can represent variations in gene expression in different cells, tissues, or circumstances, providing information about disease development and therapeutic responses. MicroRNAs can influence gene expression by binding to messenger RNA, making them potential therapeutic targets. The detection and analysis of cfNA in blood samples has grown in popularity in clinical practice because it provides a noninvasive and cost-effective alternative that involves invasive procedures such as tissue biopsy. Advances in sequencing technology have enabled the high sensitivity and specificity of cfNA analysis, allowing its transition from research to clinical practice. Finally, cell-free nucleic acids such as cfDNA, mRNA, and microRNA circulate freely in the blood and provide important insights into a variety of clinical diseases and biological processes. The detection and analysis of cfDNA in blood samples has enormous potential for non-invasive diagnosis, illness progression monitoring, and individualized therapy methods [25].

10.5.5 Circulating Tumor Cells (CTCs)

CTCs are malignant cells that break away from the original abnormal cell growth and enter circulation, potentially causing new tumors to form in distant critical tissues (metastasis). CTCs have become increasingly significant in current malignancy research since the mid-1990s, when it was revealed that even at an early stage of the disease, tumors shedding cells at less than 1.0% per day may be identified in the blood. This was demonstrated by the application of highly sensitive magnetic separation technologies based on ferrofluids such as colloidal magnetic nanoparticles and high-gradient magnetic separators. Subsequently, various other methods have been used to enumerate and identify CTCs [24].

CTCs have been termed a "liquid biopsy" because they provide insights into the metastatic process by using information on the patient's illness position. CTC examination is preferred over tissue biopsies, which are not effective in assessing metastatic risk, disease development, and behavioral efficacy due to their invasiveness, poor accuracy, and inability to be repeated. Numerous research techniques for isolating and counting CTCs have been developed, and the CellSearch System is the only FDA-approved technique for CTC enumeration in whole blood. Clinical studies have shown that the presence of CTC has been demonstrated to be a powerful predictive predictor for inclusive existence in patients with metastatic breast, colorectal, or prostate cancer [3, 24].

10.5.6 Mitochondrial DNA (mtDNA)

Mitochondria are distinct cellular organelles with mitochondrial DNA (mtDNA) as their genetic material. Unlike nuclear DNA, which is packed and forms chromosomes, mtDNA in humans is a circular molecule of approximately 16,500 base pairs that encodes a small proportion of the total DNA present in cells. Mutations in mtDNA have been linked to several illnesses and disorders, including malignancies of the breast, colon, stomach, liver, and kidneys. These mutations can develop spontaneously or as a result of environmental factors such as exposure to chemicals or radiation. Mutations in mtDNA can have far-reaching implications on cellular metabolism and general health because mitochondria play a critical role in energy generation and other key cellular activities. Because of its unique characteristics, mtDNA is being used in a variety of scientific studies, including human evolution and population genetics. mtDNA analysis has been used in forensic investigations to identify human remains and trace maternal lineages in criminal cases. Advances in DNA sequencing technology have permitted accurate and sensitive examination of mtDNA, aiding the identification of disease-causing mutations and the creation of personalized treatment strategies. Overall, mtDNA research has produced useful insights into human health and evolution, with potential applications in various domains of research and clinical practice [20].

The discovery of mitochondrial DNA alterations has been effective in the diagnosis of unsolved cases of cancer, such as prostate, ovarian, lung, and pancreatic malignancies, as well as endometriosis. Even earlier outdated histological means can detect disease, and mitochondrial genomic deletions can occur. By identifying biochemical signatures associated with these genomic deletions, the onset of the disease can be predicted with greater accuracy and at an earlier stage than can be observed by a pathologist, providing more time for treatment and intervention. To improve diagnostic accuracy, researchers are working on combining analysis of CTCs and cfDNA in a single system to confirm the presence of a reported mutation and rule out false positives [20].

10.6 Artificial Intelligence and Neurodegenerative Disorders

Deep learning has made extraordinary developments in the field of neuroimaging, and this progress has increased from mature to medical images. In recent years, there has been a systematic evaluation of the latest research in this area, which aims to shed light on the common deep learning approaches and architectures used in neuroimaging, including convolutional neural networks (CNN), autoencoders, and generative adversarial networks (GAN). A non-exhaustive tilt of widely accessible neuroimaging datasets and repositories was also included in the study, surveyed by a definite study of new efforts in MRI-based deep learning studies. Over the last few decades, traditional MLs, such as SVM and logistic regression, have been regularly implemented for pattern detection and image analysis identification. However, the advancement of DL techniques, such as CNN, has propelled machine learning to new heights [35, 36]. The deep architecture of neural networks and the nonlinear function units of these techniques allow them to deal with large amounts of data. Traditional ML and DL applications for medical imaging have been thoroughly reported, notably in the field of MRI neuroimaging research. MRI is an essential diagnostic imaging method for researching the brain due to its non-ionic and high-contrast resolution. This approach is based on the nuclear magnetic resonance process, which occurs when atomic nuclei in a magnetic field are stimulated by oscillating radio waves. The human body contains a high concentration of hydrogen nuclei, which may be used in magnetic resonance imaging (MRI) examinations [36]. The hydrogen nuclei were aligned using a magnetic field scanning device. When an oscillating radio frequency was delivered, the nucleus's magnetic momentum was briefly displaced away from the field. When the radio pulse is withdrawn, the realignment of the hydrogen nuclei produces signals that the receiver coil can detect. This is the foundation of MRI, a neuroimaging technology used to visualize brain anatomy and function. Functional MRI is a subset of MRI that monitors changes in blood flow and oxygenation around brain cells to reveal information regarding brain activity. This technique relies on the blood oxygenation level-dependent (BOLD) signal and is typically used in two ways. Resting-state MRI is performed after the patient is in a resting state, whereas task fMRI monitors the brain's response throughout an allocated task. Diffusion tensor imaging (DTI) is another technique that uses MRI to estimate the signs of water molecules in the brain. This information can be used to study the connectivity between different brain regions and white matter tracts [36].

In recent years, deep learning approaches have become increasingly useful in neuroimaging training in adults for neuropsychiatric disorder recognition, brain tissue and structure segmentation, and scientific outcome prediction. However, comparatively few deep learning trainings have been led in MRI. This knowledge gap is significant because neuroimaging is essential for understanding the developing brain and identifying potential neurological disorders in early life. This chapter seeks to fill this void gap by providing a thorough evaluation of recent efforts in MRI-based deep learning experiments. The author is interested in anticipating prospective applications of deep learning in neuroimaging and inspiring more research in this field.

10.7 Conclusion

The author has highlighted the following outcomes while writing the manuscript:

- Precision medicine is a paradigm that strives to enhance human illness diagnosis, treatment, and prevention by combining data from various sources. Machine learning approaches, particularly sophisticated deep learning models, are becoming increasingly important for evaluating and processing large-scale multi-omics data to achieve this aim. These data-driven methodologies allow for categorization and prediction of illness outcomes for both individuals and residents, supporting the creation of tailored and accurate treatments.
- Genetics and genomics have played crucial roles in the evolution of precision medicine, and are especially complementary to machine learning technology. When the data are combined with additional clinical, lifestyle, and environmental assessments, they can provide more comprehensive knowledge of illness causes and inform more effective preventive and treatment efforts.
- The integration of precision medicine and machine learning has led to significant advancements in the understanding of anthropological health and disease, and their potential impact on the future of healthcare is enormous. By leveraging large-scale multi-omics data, machine learning technologies can help identify novel therapeutic targets, accelerate drug development, and improve patient outcomes. Therefore, the continued development and application of precision medicine and machine learning methodologies holds great potential for the future of medicine and human health.

Conflict of Interest

The authors declare no conflicts of interest, financial or otherwise.

Acknowledgments

The authors would like to thank all anonymous peer reviewers for their valuable comments and suggestions for further improving the quality of this book chapter. The authors also extend their gratitude to the Shoolini University Department of Computer Science and the upGrad campus (Banglore, Karnataka), Department of Computer Science and Engineering (AI/ML Data Science), and Lovely Professional University Jalandhar Punjab India, for their collaborative effort, which inspired the writing of this book chapter. Special thanks are given to Dr. Neha Sharma from Chitkara University for providing the opportunity to contribute a manuscript to her book.

References

1. Agusti, A., The path to personalised medicine in COPD. *Thorax*, 69, 9, 857–864, 2014.
2. Alipanahi, B., Delong, A., Weirauch, M.T., Frey, B.J., Predicting the sequence specificities of DNA-and RNA-binding proteins by deep learning. *Nat. Biotechnol.*, 33, 8, 831–838, 2015.
3. Alix-Panabières, C. and Pantel, K., Challenges in circulating tumour cell research. *Nat. Rev. Cancer*, 14, 9, 623–631, 2014.
4. Bell, J., What is machine learning?, in: *Machine Learning and the City: Applications in Architecture and Urban Design*, pp. 207–216, 2022.
5. Bhattacharyya, S., Snasel, V., Hassanien, A.E., Saha, S., Tripathy, B., *Deep Learning: Research and Applications*, Walter de Gruyter GmbH & Co KG, India, 2020.
6. Cheng, L. and Yu, T., A new generation of AI: A review and perspective on machine learning technologies applied to smart energy and electric power systems. *Int. J. Energy Res.*, 43, 6, 1928–1973, 2019.
7. Divyananda, J., McKenna, S., Prathiba, V., Mohan, V., Trucco, E., Deep Learning in Genomics. https://www.researchgate.net/publication/328343467_Deep_Learning_in_Genomics
8. El Naqa, I. and Murphy, M.J., What is machine learning?, in: *Machine Learning in Radiation Oncology*, vol. 1 (1st edn), Springer, pp. 3–11, 2015.. https://link.springer.com/book/10.1007/978-3-319-18305-3
9. Enoma, D.O., Bishung, J., Abiodun, T., Ogunlana, O., Osamor, V.C., Machine learning approaches to genome-wide association studies. *J. King Saud Univ. - Sci.*, 34, 4, 101847, 2022.

10. Eraslan, G., Avsec, Ž., Gagneur, J., Theis, F.J., Deep learning: new computational modelling techniques for genomics. *Nat. Rev. Genet.*, 20, 7, 389–403, 2019.
11. Harvey, A., Brand, A., Holgate, S.T., Kristiansen, L.V., Lehrach, H., Palotie, A., Prainsack, B., The future of technologies for personalised medicine. *New Biotechnol.*, 29, 6, 625–633, 2012.
12. Hinton, G.E., How neural networks learn from experience, in: *Scientific American Magazine*, 267, 3, p. 144, 1992.
13. Ivakhnenko, A.G., Savchenko, E.A., Ivakhnenko, G.A., GMDH algorithm for optimal model choice by the external error criterion with the extension of definition by model BIAS and ITS applications to committees and neural networks. *Pattern Recognit. Image Anal. C/C Of Raspoznavaniye Obrazov I Analiz Izobrazhenii*, 12, 4, 347–353, 2002.
14. Jarroux, J., Morillon, A., Pinskaya, M., History, discovery, and classification of lncRNAs, in: *Long non coding RNA biology*, pp. 1–46, 2017.
15. Jones, W., Alasoo, K., Fishman, D., L. Parts, Computational biology: deep learning. *Emerg. Top. Life Sci.*, 1, 3, 257–274, 2017.
16. Karim, A., Su, Z., West, P.K., Keon, M., Shamsani, J., Brennan, S., Wong, T., Milicevic, O., Teunisse, G., Rad, H.N., Molecular classification and interpretation of amyotrophic lateral sclerosis using deep convolution neural networks and Shapley values. *Genes*, 12, 11, 1754, 2021.
17. Kircher, M. and Kelso, J., High-throughput DNA sequencing concepts and limitations. *Bioessays*, 32, 6, 524–536, 2010.
18. Kumar, R. and Sharma, A., Computational strategies and tools for protein tertiary structure prediction, in: *Basic Biotechniques for Bioprocess and Bioentrepreneurship*, pp. 225–242, Elsevier, India, 2023.
19. Libbrecht, M.W. and Noble, W.S., Machine learning applications in genetics and genomics. *Nat. Rev. Genet.*, 16, 6, 321–332, 2015.
20. Lin, Y.-H., Lim, S.-N., Chen, C.-Y., Chi, H.-C., Yeh, C.-T., Lin, W.-R., Functional role of mitochondrial DNA in cancer progression. *Int. J. Mol. Sci.*, 23, 3, 1659, 2022.
21. MacEachern, S.J. and Forkert, N.D., Machine learning for precision medicine. *Genome*, 64, 4, 416–425, 2021.
22. Park, C., Took, C.C., Seong, J.-K., Machine learning in biomedical engineering. *Biomed. Eng. Lett.*, 8, 1–3, 2018.
23. Park, Y. and Kellis, M., Deep learning for regulatory genomics. *Nat. Biotechnol.*, 33, 8, 825–826, 2015.
24. Paterlini-Brechot, P. and Benali, N.L., Circulating tumor cells (CTC) detection: clinical impact and future directions. *Cancer Lett.*, 253, 2, 180–204, 2007.
25. Pös, O., Biró, O., Szemes, T., Nagy, B., Circulating cell-free nucleic acids: characteristics and applications. *Eur. J. Hum. Genet.*, 26, 7, 937–945, 2018.
26. Qureshi, I.A. and Mehler, M.F., Advances in epigenetics and epigenomics for neurodegenerative diseases. *Curr. Neurol. Neurosci. Rep.*, 11, 464–473, 2011.

27. Rusk, N., Deep learning. *Nat. Methods*, 13, 1, 35–35, 2016.
28. Samuel, A.L., Machine learning. *Technol. Rev.*, 62, 1, 42–45, 1959.
29. Sarker, I.H., Deep learning: a comprehensive overview on techniques, taxonomy, applications and research directions. *SN Comput. Sci.*, 2, 6, 420, 2021.
30. Savard, J., Personalised medicine: a critique on the future of health care. *J. Bioeth. Inq.*, 10, 197–203, 2013.
31. Sharma, A. and Guleria, V., Biosensors In Bioinformatics, Biotechnology, And Healthcare, in: *Blockchain and Deep Learning: Future Trends and Enabling Technologies*, pp. 329–349, Springer, India, 2022.
32. Sharma, A., Guleria, V., Jaiswal, V., The Future of Blockchain Technology, Recent Advancement and Challenges, in: *Blockchain and Deep Learning: Future Trends and Enabling Technologies*, pp. 329–349, Springer, India, 2022.
33. Sharma, A., Gupta, A., Jaiswal, V., Solving image processing critical problems using machine learning, in: *Machine Learning for Intelligent Multimedia Analytics: Techniques and Applications*, pp. 213–248, 2021.
34. Sharma, A. and Kumar, R., Recent Advancement and Challenges in Deep Learning, Big Data in Bioinformatics, in: *Blockchain and Deep Learning: Future Trends and Enabling Technologies*, pp. 251–284, Springer, India, 2022.
35. Sharma, A., Kumar, R., Jaiswal, V., Classification of heart disease from MRI images using convolutional neural network. *2021 6th international conference on signal processing, computing and control (ISPCC)*, IEEE.
36. Sharma, A., Pal, T., Jaiswal, V., Heart disease prediction using convolutional neural network, in: *Cardiovascular and Coronary Artery Imaging*, pp. 245–272, Elsevier, India, 2022.
37. Singh, A.P., Singh, R., Verma, S.S., Rai, V., Kaschula, C.H., Maiti, P., Gupta, S.C., Health benefits of resveratrol: Evidence from clinical studies. *Med. Res. Rev.*, 39, 5, 1851–1891, 2019.
38. Stewart, J., Sprivulis, P., Dwivedi, G., Artificial intelligence and machine learning in emergency medicine. *Emerg. Med. Australas.*, 30, 6, 870–874, 2018.
39. Uelze, L., Grützke, J., Borowiak, M., Hammerl, J.A., Juraschek, K., Deneke, C., Tausch, S.H., Malorny, B., Typing methods based on whole genome sequencing data. *One Health Outlook*, 2, 1–19, 2020.
40. Van der Lee, M., Kriek, M., Guchelaar, H.-J., Swen, J.J., Technologies for pharmacogenomics: a review. *Genes*, 11, 12, 1456, 2020.
41. Wadhwa, A., Bhardwaj, A., Verma, V.S., A review on brain tumor segmentation of MRI images. *Magn. Reson. Imaging*, 61, 247–259, 2019.
42. Wuest, T., Weimer, D., Irgens, C., Thoben, K.-D., Machine learning in manufacturing: advantages, challenges, and applications. *Prod. Manuf. Res.*, 4, 1, 23–45, 2016.
43. Xu, C., Fu, L., Lin, T., Li, W., Ma, S., Machine learning in petrophysics: Advantages and limitations. *Artif. Intell. Geosci.*, 3, 157–161, 2022.

11

Emerging Trends of Big Data in Bioinformatics and Challenges

Ajay Sharma[1,2*], Tarun Pal[3], Utkarsha Naithani[3], Gaurav Gupta[1] and Varun Jaiswal[1]

[1]*School of Electrical and Computer Science Engineering, Shoolini University Solan, Himachal Pradesh, India*

[2]*upGradCampus, upGrad Education Private Limited India, Bangalore, Karnataka, India*

[3]*School of Bioengineering and Food Technology, Faculty of Applied Sciences & Biotechnology, Shoolini University, Himachal Pradesh, India*

Abstract

Current technologies are much more advanced, and they greatly outpace storage, organizing, analyzing, and extracting capabilities. The rapid and cost-effective generation of biological data has led to a heap of "big biological data." A variety of bioinformatics fields, including drug omics, proteomics, immunological informatics, cheminformatics, and structural bioinformatics, are covered in the current repertoire. We are discussing sophisticated ways to effectively handle data from biological experiments, including big data approaches, software, computational tools, and biological databases. Big data, or very large volumes of data generated by a variety of biological experiments, are produced using NGS technology and are crucial for genomic and biomedical research. In NGS experiments, there is a need for the creation of novel computer algorithms that satisfy the analysis requirements of high-performance computing. The authors have reviewed current techniques for processing large datasets in PDB (Public Domain Database), NCBI (IEDB), DDBJ (Document-Based Database), and other databases using technologies such as Apache Pig (No SQL), H-base (Hibernication), and Hive (Map-Reduce Programming Framework). Using a new database management system (DBMS) is an approach to deal with the problem of storing big data files for efficient search queries in a reasonable amount of time. The healthcare industry generates a large amount of data for various purposes, such as the research and

**Corresponding author*: ajaysharmadharmani@gmail.com

Neha Sharma, Korhan Cengiz and Prasenjit Chatterjee (eds.) Intelligent Data Analytics for Bioinformatics and Biomedical Systems, (265–290) © 2024 Scrivener Publishing LLC

development of medications, clinical operations, and care and analysis of patient profiles. A report claimed that in 2011, the amount of data related to healthcare in the United States exceeded 150 exabytes. Therefore, it is critical that researchers comprehend the significance of big data technologies. Personalized healthcare is being developed as a result of the rapid development of applications for mobile healthcare and additional monitoring tools, which aid the analysis of analytics data generated by these tools regarding patient profiles.

Keywords: Bioinformatics, big data, NGS, health, structural biology, immunology, HPC

11.1 Introduction

Imagine in 2050 Venter met Biden and Biden asked, "Venter how is your Research going on?" Venter answers, "Now we have access to 1,000 Petabytes of data storage, a 10 million-node GPU cluster with more than 1,000 Terabytes of RAM" and a new data integration engine that collects and maps all databases across the globe. Finally, we prioritized and generated the hypothesis regarding big data's significance in bioinformatics.

The availability of a large amount of data in molecular biology and the objective of using this information to understand the molecular mechanisms behind the living world, with the help of information technology resources, has emerged as a new field called bioinformatics. Bioinformatics provides computational tools, software, packages, databases, and web servers to analyze and understand the biological molecular mechanisms of life on Earth. An enormous amount of biological data has been produced as a result of the completion of the human genome project. Scientists took a long time to analyze, correlate, and store information, which has led to the development and rapid growth of biological databases. As time passed, biological experimental data became big data, which can be used to check everything from the regulation of genes that resulted in the evolution of genomes to questions such as why coastal algae bloom. What kinds of microorganisms reside in the human body, which cavities exist, how the human brain works, what kinds of genes are responsible for different cancers, and which medicines influence cancer treatment? The European Bioinformatics Institute (EBI) in the UK, which is part of the European Molecular Biology Laboratory, is one of the largest biological data repositories. EBI currently has ~21 petabytes (1 petabyte is 1,024 terabytes) of data and backups of regulatory genes, amino acids, protein structures, and small molecules. This data is growing at an exponential rate, in the last year, EBI handled 9 million queries per day to mine the data from the biological dataset, which is growing by 60% each year [42, 63].

Genomic data (gene expression), including both overexpressed and under-expressed genes, have become available in a more efficient manner, providing sensitive and specific analyses of data that account for ~2 petabytes. This number doubles every three years. Big data has become an essential part of biological experiments, providing a scheme for organizing, decision-making (Decision Support System), representing (labeling), pattern finding, pattern matching, and making it possible to access data for humans and computers in biological and biomedical research worldwide. The human genome project, which was completed two decades ago, still requires big data and other high-end technologies to be decoded comprehensively with the fusion of other information present in heterogeneous sources.

11.2 Human Genome

After more than 200 gigabytes of data were collected, the "Human Genome" Project produced a single sequence comprising over three billion nucleotides in the haploid human genome. For scientists, managing such massive datasets in terms of storage, analysis, and comparison is challenging. However, all people have similar genomic sequences, and for the ability to decipher sequences to start delivering real benefits, it is necessary to create and develop methods that allow reading a certain number of copies of the same genome simultaneously. There are currently a number of approaches available, each with its own pros, cons, and limitations. However, all of them are sufficiently inexpensive and quick to be used in medical clinics, in addition to specialized laboratories. With their introduction, it has become possible to quickly determine the extended genomic sequences of specific patients; for example, to identify mutations in genes that may lead to the development of various diseases and physical and mental disorders in the human body. Modern high-performance sequencing technologies enable *de novo* sequencing and resequencing of genomes (DNA-Seq), the investigation of single-cell transcriptomes (cRNA-Seq) and whole-body transcriptomes (RNA-Seq), the study of epigenomes and metagenomes, and the nature of DNA–protein interactions (ChIP-Seq), among other topics [10, 11]. All omics can obtain vastly different datasets from the same sequencer; the only things that vary are the sample preparation techniques (protocols) used to create sequencing libraries. Next-generation sequencing (NGS) has evolved significantly since its discovery over a decade ago.

The capacity of NGS has increased more than a hundred times, transforming its ability to tackle and decode huge amounts of information present in the genomes of almost all types of life forms.

11.3 Next-Generation Sequencing

The last 10 years have seen a massive increase in the amount of data generated in biomedical science and genomics, primarily due to advancements in NGS technology [59]. Since the first human genome sequence was completed in 2002, it has taken 10 years and approximately $3 billion to complete. However, owing to advances in computing power and high-throughput experimentation methods such as NGS, we can now complete the same task in a few hours for less than $1,000. Reduced expenses resulted in increased data generation, potentially reaching exabytes (1,024 PB). Within the next 10 years, it is anticipated that approximately 2 billion human genomes will be sequenced [59]. Several businesses, such as Roche and Illumina, produce approximately 2 PB of data annually.

Sequencing machines (sequencers) permit the parallel preparation of billions of sections of nucleic acids. These nucleic acids are repeated several times in the same type of operation, every one of which brings about the acquisition of vast information indexes for analysis. Each DNA sequencer has computer server hardware to handle, which takes care of issues of appropriate reading of billion nucleotides every hour, obtaining a fragment of a given length (reads), which are then aligned and commented on to produce a genomic sequence. There are distinctive stages and diverse markers for sequencing machines [36]. The principal stages of second-generation NGS are the products of Roche and Pacific Bioscience, Illumina Inc., and Thermo-Fisher Scientific [9, 15]. They are largely identified with the use of polymerase chain reaction, mechanization of the primary phases of DNA reuse and depend on parallelizing the way toward reading DNA fragments. To continue running the sequencer in one run, it is conceivable to determine the essential primary structures of several fragments of the genome. Each of these techniques has its limitations, such as the number of reads in sequence, its cost, the accessibility of programming software, and other different parameters; however, every one of these is large and effectively created with a specific end goal to provide quick and shabby sequencing of any genomic information. The volume of this information is colossal; it should first be stored, dissected, and exhibited in a frame helpful to the researcher. A wide range of techniques, individual computer programs developed internally and through community improvement by network individuals, as well as a variety of data formats, databases, and information, must be understood by scientists in light of the variety of sequencing machines, each with its own application domain [63, 64].

Next-generation sequencing (NGS) experiments generate a large amount of data that require high-throughput analysis to extract meaningful information, and other available information can be incorporated for interpretation. This information requires huge computational resources and can be considered big data. The NGS sequencer generates massive datasets, which present a challenging computational task for biologists [53]. For instance, according to the NCBI GenBank database, the data from various NGS experiments alone are estimated to have required two trillion CPU hours by 2025 [59]. Since 1982, the bank doubled its base every 18 months. Refer to Figure 11.1. Third-generation sequencing technology (TGS), which is based on sequencing by synthesis (SBS) and produces more than 90% of biological sequence data worldwide, is currently in the developmental stage. TGS technology can sequence 1,000 bp (base pairs) of input-length reads. TGS technology can also be used to directly sequence cDNA and RNA sequences [58]. Currently, accuracy-related challenges persist with TGS, and the error rate is very high compared with NGS. However, next-generation sequencing is a widely used technology that generates a high volume of data, which poses a challenge and requires

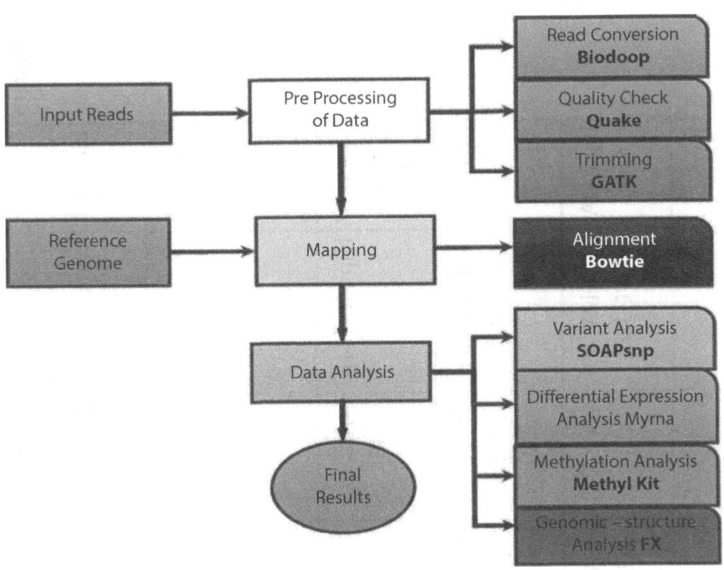

Figure 11.1 Flow chart of NGS working tool and pipeline.

Table 11.1 Table showing big data algorithm in next-generation sequencing, parallel and distributed computing for processing large scale biological experimental data sets.

Meta	Kraken [73]	Mash [51]	SBT [66]	Compareds [39]	**HPC System**	CLOSET [74]	Sigma [46]	MEGAHT [36]	-
Count	BF Counter [45]	KMC2 [17]	Kmer Stream [44]	Jally fish [40]		BioPig [49]	Dec GPU [37]	Gerbil [19]	-
EC	Fiona [62]	Karect [2]	Musket [38]	Fiona [62]		Cloud RS [12]	BLESS2 [28]	Dec GPU [37]	FADE
Assembly	Light assembler [18]	MHAP [4]	Minia [56]	Hip Mer [24]		Cloud Brush [11]	Hip Mer [24]	F-Assem [40]	
RNA	HISAT [31]	KALLISTO [8]	RNA-Skim [75]	HPG Aligner [43]		Myrna [33]	HPG Aligner BW [41]	HPG Aligner [69]	Dragen [72]
Align	Bowtie2 [34]	Balaur [54]	Bio Bloom [14]	Bit Mapper [13]		Big BWA [1]	CUSHAWA3-UPC [26]	Arioc [72]	FHAST [21]
Big Data Algorithm	**1**	**2**	**3**	**4**		**1**	**2**	**3**	**4**

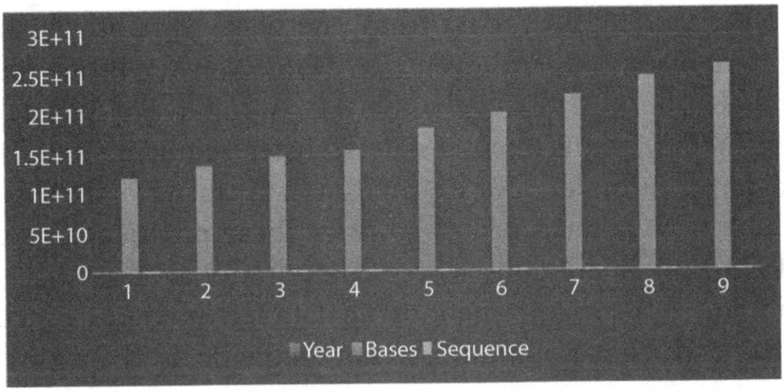

Figure 11.2 Ten-year growth of NCBI database deposited growth nucleotide sequence submission rapid growth of nucleotide where data size is doubled in every 18 months data rep in $e^x * 10$.

high-end computational technology. According to the research requirements and data, the complete next-generation sequencing pipeline algorithm (Table 11.1) can be used and designed (Figure 11.1). Similarly, based on the requirement that various big data algorithms are available for NGS data analysis (Figure 11.1), Figure 11.2 shows growth in the nucleotide dataset. There are different operations on NGS dataset that are computationally challenging and require special treatment, which is currently provided through big data technology and is discussed further [59].

11.3.1 Challenges of NGS in Big Data

Data Flooding: The first problem in NGS is the very large size of NGS FASTAQ files—the "data deluge" problem. NGS experiments can be exceeded from microplate readings or digitized gel photos. For example, a compressed FASTAQ NGS file with a 60× human genome of approximately ~200 GB. Now imagine that a small project of 10–20 genome sequencing (WGS) can generate ~4 TB of raw data, more disk space will be required for downstream sampling of the data analysis.

Storing of NGS data:

- High-end enterprise cluster and SAN (Storage Area Network)
- At least two mirrored server or cloud
- Hard drives/NAS or RAID -5/6 configuration

Moving Data: Moving NGS data from one place to another is challenging and time-consuming, and even FTP (File Transfer Protocol Port No: 20 (Control channel), 21 (Data channel)) may suffer. For Whole Genome Sequencing (WGS), experimental data transfer requiring external drives may be the only option left. For example, a data cluster of 200 Tb can take 56 h with a data transfer speed of 1 GB/s. These practical challenges are associated with other domains where computational assistance was considered and due to the requirement of big data technologies, especially in a data-rich field, which is not limited to any single field.

11.4 Bioinformatics Big Data Architecture

a. Hadoop Distributed File System-Hadoop framework on commodity Linux cluster accommodates voluminous data in Distributed File System (DFS). HDFS follows a master/slave architecture system consisting of a solitary Name Node and a master server and manages access to files by clients. In structural bioinformatics, Hadoop offers a framework for working with the Protein Data Bank, which aids in structural alignment, protein–ligand docking, and protein–ligand complex clustering [3].
b. Map Reduce Framework-MapReduce is a framework introduced by Google plays an important role in programming model and processing paradigm for handling huge data in distributed computing environments. This framework divides the task into two fundamental operations: mapping and reduction. These tasks are then efficiently distributed across nodes within a Hadoop cluster, fostering parallelism and scalability [70].
c. Bioinformatics Data Sources-In the age of big data, the comprehensiveness and heterogeneity of bioinformatics data contribute to the richness of research work. GenBank, ENSEMBL, and the UCSC Genome Browser house extensive genomic data [20, 30]. The Protein Data Bank (PDB) archives experimentally determined protein structures, while databases such as Uni-Prot and Inter-Pro offer comprehensive protein information. MG-RAST, QIIME, and Meta-Phi provide platforms for analyzing metagenomic data, enabling studies on microbial diversity and function. Illumina, PacBio, and Oxford Nanopore are major players

in generating vast amounts of raw sequencing data used in genomic and transcriptomic studies [10, 35, 67].

11.5 Big Data in Immunology

The innate and adaptive immune systems, which are further subdivided into humoral and cell-mediated immunity, comprise an extremely complex human immune system. In humoral immunity, B-cell produce antibodies to prevent the spread of infection by extracellular pathogens and help neutralize, although T cells can also activate B cells [75]. Human cellular immunity includes phagocytes, cytotoxic T-lymphocytes (CTLs), and the release of cytokines in response to pathogens with T-cell receptor (TCR). T cell identify pathogens that interact with the Major Histocompatibility Complex (MHC) with CD4 or CD8 receptors. The Immune Epitope Database (IEDB) hosts nearly 451,990 cell epitopes which include 449,341 peptide epitopes and 2,649 non-peptide epitopes as of July 2018 [71]. The Immunogenetic Database (IMGT) contains MHC, T-cell receptors, and immunoglobulin molecules in all vertebrates. The ease of data distribution and high-quality IGMT has important implications in medical research, such as autoimmune diseases, lymphomas, AIDS, antibody engineering, therapeutic approaches, and genetic evolution engineering. IGMT is further divided into two databases, IMGT/LIGM-DB (~355 species,~196,471 entries) translation of fully interpreted nucleotide sequences of I_g and TcR of all vertebrates, and the second one is IMGT/HLA-DB (~29,417 allele, ~55,268 entries (HLA Class-I Allele: ~21,040, HLA Class-II: ~7,898, HLA Alleles: ~28,983, Other Non-HLA ~479)), which includes human leukocyte antigens of all species of humans [57]. Peptides present on the surface of MHC induce an immune response by T cells called T-cell epitopes. The diversity of B cell epitopes is huge. This diversity is due to mutations, selection, and affinity maturation. High polymorphisms present in immune-associated proteins are found; furthermore, the frequency of the different types of MHC is different in various types of human population indices. This polymorphism contributes to the genetic basis of the immune response. Polymorphism in species is also responsible for the proactive and revived nature of individuals towards disease. This polymorphism also affects the structure of these biological proteins; this associated data is massive in volume, which can be used to design vaccine drugs and to understand the complex biology behind it. However, the associated amount of data is variable and not homogenous (string, 3D structures, clinical data, and image data). Dynamism is also associated with biomolecules; therefore, the storage and processing of these data is a challenge in the digital world. Databases such as FLUDB [29] and Epicombflu [29] can store such different types of data for pathogens. The Influenza Research Database (IRD) uses cloud and high-performance computing to store data for the research and development of vaccines, theoretic, and diagnostic against influenza viruses from various resources, along with data mining and visualization tools. In contrast, Epicombflu provides information on influenza proteins, epitopes, and their associated information for vaccine design. Figure 11.3 shows the complete life cycle of the data flow in biological experiments related to the immune system in living cells.

The dynamics of the immune system can be studied through analysis of specific B or T cells, single-cell manipulation, mass spectrometry, cytometry, and high-throughput sequencing of B and T cell receptors (BCR and TCR). When BCR and TCR are combined with technology to identify the epitope recognized by the receptors, big data immunology can be used to develop vaccines, antibody-drug combinations, and clinical diagnoses.

Transcriptomes are an important starting point for the regulatory network in the activation of immune cells in bioinformatics. A network such as this can be helpful for a particular gene class (transcriptional factor) that the transcriptome data computational model can analyze [53]. The main factors influencing big data in life sciences (immunology) are "omics," which refers to the growth in next-generation sequencing data, sequencing capacity, different methods for sequencing DNA, structure or methylation,

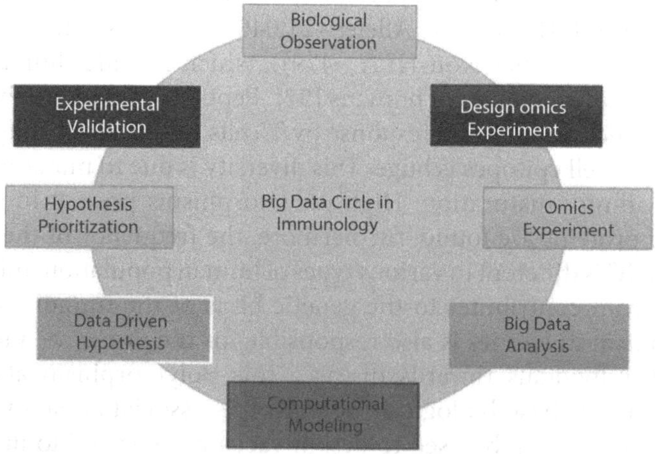

Figure 11.3 The big data strategy circle showing data flow in immunological data experiments generated a hypothesis for experimental validation in functional exp in *vivo/vitro/silico* disease modeling, and observational approaches in living cell images.

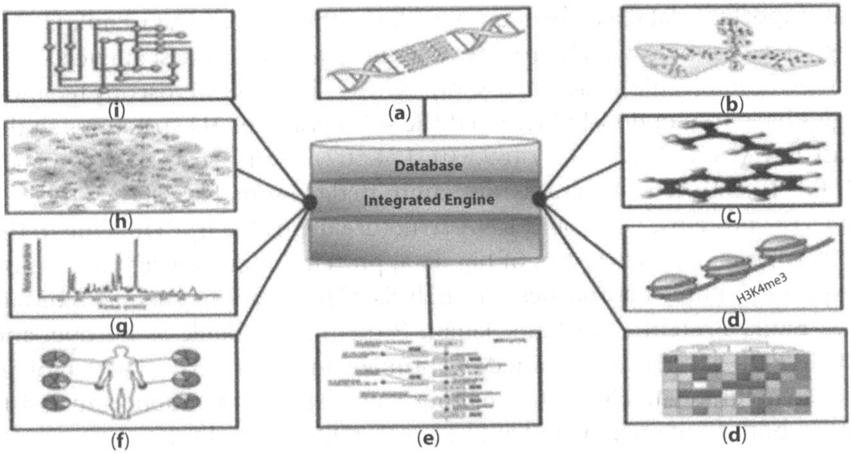

Figure 11.4 Figure shows some of the fields that produce tremendous amounts of data in biological and biomedical experiments (a). Genome, (b). Cytome, (c). Drug omics, (d). Transcriptome, (e). Lipidome, (f). Microbiome, (g). Proteome, (h). Interactome, and (i). Metabolome.

DNA protein interaction, and distinct RNA protein interactions. The experiment's data quality improved even more with the introduction of big data in omics technology. For instance, a significant undertaking was the Cancer Genome Atlas (TCGA). In this project, the genomes of more than 20,000 cancer patients were sequenced. New genetic variations linked to cancer have been identified [52, 61].

There are different areas of research that greatly overlap with immunology and benefit from big data analysis, including Genomics, Glycosmis, Transcriptome, Metabolome, Lipidome, Epigenome, Proteome, Cytome, Interactome, Drug omics, and some microbiome data (see Figure 11.4). Biological experiments in these research areas also produced data, which could be considered as big data.

11.6 Structural Biology

The amount of data has increased dramatically in recent years due to advances in structural biology and bioinformatics. An X-Ray Free-Electron Laser (XFEL) gathers data on individual crystal proteins from all angles. It is estimated that ~150–200 petabytes of data are generated within 48 h from ~10 million X-ray images [68]. Thus, structural biology, such as new technologies, could be a matter of research for big data engineers.

An important database for biomolecules is the Protein Data Bank (PDB) digital data source, which provides a single gateway for the sequenced conserved biomolecule structures. X-ray, NMR, Electron microscopy technologies have tremendously increased the submission of 3D structures in the past few years (2012–2021) (69,510–174,507). Every year, approximately 8,000–10,000 new structures are submitted. Figure 11.5 shows the last ten-year proteins, DNA, and RNA structure deposited in PDB. Due to the fundamental characteristics of big data, protein 3D structure information requires multiple approaches for analysis. Organizations such as BioMag, Res-Bank, Protein Data Bank Japan, Protein Data Bank or Europe, and RCSB PDB have been combined to optimize our ability to deal with biological structural data efficiently, making it available to the public and assisting in both fundamental and applied research globally [32].

Structural bioinformatics assists in the analysis, prediction, and manipulation of generated data in biological projects funded by various agencies. A better outcome could be achieved by bridging the large knowledge gap in the structure using structural bioinformatics tools and algorithms. Currently, the Protein Data Bank (PDB) contains over 174,507 structures, 46,620 distinct protein structures, 42,159 human sequence structures, and 10,890 structures containing nucleic acids. Nevertheless, approximately 810 times larger protein-sequencing data can be accessed through UniProt and NCBI (National Centre for Biotechnology Institute). Protein sequences also have complex, varied, and volumetric one-dimensional information, and as sequencing techniques have advanced recently, more sequences (from approximately 7 ∗ 106 to 19 ∗ 106) are being deposited [32].

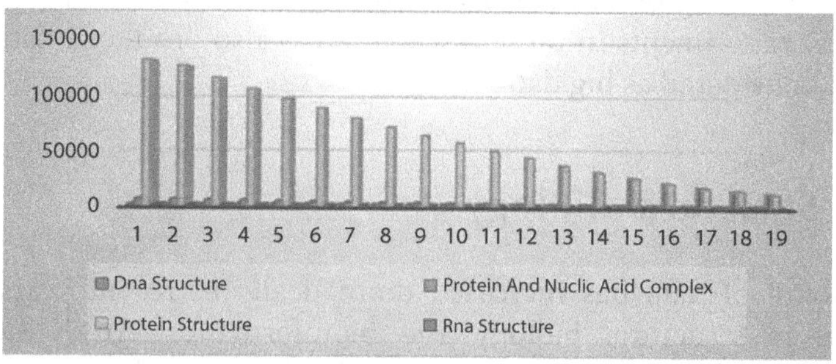

Figure 11.5 Twenty years of cumulative growth of the structure deposited in the PDB. The plot indicates rapid growth in the deposition of protein structure, DNA, RNA, and Protein nucleic acid complexes.

11.7 Computer Science

The field of computer science is used in bioinformatics to analyze and comprehend biological data, thereby facilitating research on genomes, proteomics, and drug development. In healthcare, computer science engineering has driven advances in clinical informatics, allowing the creation of electronic health records, medical imaging systems, and predictive analytics for personalized therapy. In biotechnology, computer science plays an important role in modeling biological systems, generating innovative therapies, optimizing bioprocesses, and improving the effectiveness and efficacy in the development of drugs and industrial biotechnology. The ability to analyze genomes of varying complexity, ranging from microorganisms to humans, on a large scale has become feasible in modern bioinformatics, owing to its high computing power. A wealth of new information about the mechanisms by which these biological codes operate, which is currently unknown, has been discovered through accumulated data. The problem is not only in the storage or transmission of the data, but also in the processing of this biological experimental data because of the sheer volume of generated data (storing a single genomic sequence on a computer storage medium will require hundreds of gigabytes).

It is challenging to piece together the genome from billions of sequenced reads. It is necessary to apply recent advancements in bioinformatics to address problems involving genomic sequences. Thus, as far as gathering large dimensions (volume, variety, velocity, veracity, variability) of genomic information is concerned, more effective, accurate, and specific methods for analyzing this heterogeneous information based on modern methods, available tools, and software for evaluating large amounts of experimental data have become critical [27, 48, 64].

IT solutions developed in fields such as networked artificial intelligence (AI), business information, and analytics to analyze biological data can be used to create them. First, we must create statistical and mathematical techniques for data processing, analysis, and information retrieval algorithms that can be used with large biological datasets. Statistical analysis algorithms (such as A/B testing and time-series analysis), machine learning algorithms (GA Genetic Algorithm, ACO Ant Colony Optimization), predictive analytics, natural language processing (NLP) techniques, exploratory data analysis (EDA), and advanced data mining tools (such as clustering and regression analysis with the aid of Weka and Rapid Miner) are a few examples of these techniques. In addition, information technologies provide software and instrumental tools that enable the processing and storage of extraordinarily large volumes of data. Organizing distributed computing using a large number of computational nodes, most often integrated into a parallel computing system, is the primary method for resolving these issues [63, 64].

The MapReduce (Figure 11.6) programming platform from Google and the freely distributed Hadoop framework from the Apache Software Foundation are the most well-known examples of distributed computing models implemented in large parallel clusters of computing nodes. Hadoop is designed to develop and support the execution of distributed computing programs [50].

The MapReduce model for the distributed file system (HDFS), which is designed to store large files dispersed among the computational cluster's nodes, is the foundation of Hadoop. Moreover, Hadoop has large-scale data processing programs such as Apache Spark, Hive, and Pig. A high-level language for data analysis, which is included in Apache Pig, is a platform for analyzing sizable experimental datasets. The infrastructure is included with Apache Pig so that these computer-coded programs can be assessed for data analysis. It enhances the overall efficiency of data processing by optimizing the script's execution of operations and performing different optimizations, such as combining several MapReduce jobs [25]. The extensible nature of Apace Pig enables users to create user-defined functions in Python, Java, and other languages. This facilitates the integration of customized logic into user data-processing workflows [25].

One of the key features of Pig programs, a high-level scripting language created at Yahoo, is its structure, which allows for significant data parallelization. This allows the Pig program to process very large datasets easily. Reading, writing, and managing massive datasets stored in distributed storage via SQL relational databases is made easier by Facebook's development and maintenance of Apache Hive data warehouse software.

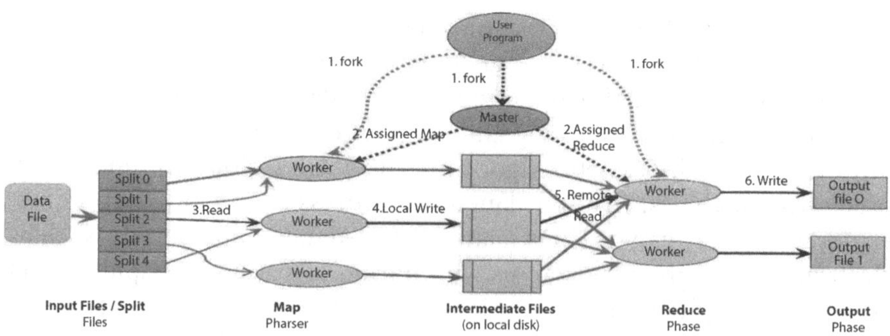

Figure 11.6 An applied conceptual big data analysis architecture.

The large-scale distributed processing of unstructured and weakly structured data contained in files can be accomplished using the Apache Spark software framework [15]. Furthermore, an excess of commercial software systems employing a variety of technology classes, capabilities, and destinations is available from relatively small businesses such as Cloudera, Coursera Hortonworks, Map-R, and others, as well as from larger vendors such as IBM and Microsoft [48].

Specialized high-performance hardware/software complexes represent the next technological component of this tool for processing large amounts of biological data. The technology used in these products is based on the paradigm of in-memory analytics, which maximizes the use of RAM for processing systems, such as the IBM supercomputer at Oak Ridge National Laboratory, which was recently announced. The primary purpose of this supercomputer is to solve big-data problems. It is equipped with up to 9,216 (approximately 20 two-core), 4.0 GHz dedicated processors based on POWER9 architecture, 27,648 NVIDIA Tesla V100 GPU, high bandwidth DDR4 SDRAM, super-fast memory with a capacity of up to ~250 TB of storage, and the ability to support up to ~9,000 virtual servers. Its design maximum performance is more than 111,000 million of operations per second (MIPS), and it can handle 200 GB/s of communication traffic between nodes and intercommutes [60]. Additional providers of solutions, including Teradata, Oracle, SAP, and SAS, also provide specialized supercomputers.

Example: Consider the problem of storing and mapping the value in the database. Pseudocode for mapping the values in the database

```
// map(StringKey, String Value)
   _id: ObjectId("90z8245b67sdfd845r9fgt3c"),
   cust_id: "10xbigdata",
   ord_date: new Date("25, 07, 2018"),
   status: 'p',
   price: 250,
   items: big: "mmm", qty: 20, price: 25.5 ,
          big: "nnn", qty: 15, price: 30.5
//mapfunction custid&place
Total Price Per Customer:
var mapFunction1 = function() {
                 emit(this.cust_id, this.price);
             }
```

Big Data Analysis on traditional platforms is facilitated by HPC clusters because they have access to grid computing. One of the key drawbacks of grid computing, which has led to the creation of cloud computing to conduct large-scale analysis, is the inability to customize computations according to user requirements. To manage the enormous volume of data produced by throughput technologies, the primary applications are cluster computing, Xeon Phi, GPU, and cloud computing. GPU computing offers a powerful, reasonably priced, and highly performant solution with high floating performance. The GPU and Xeon Phi demonstrated a 30% increase in performance when comparing the two devices. Cluster computing is highly scalable for many types of big data analysis because it leverages the parallel data approach for data analysis.

As a result, we currently possess a sophisticated set of techniques for examining vast amounts of data, enabling the extraction of the required knowledge. But as previously noted, the vast majority of big data technologies and techniques are successfully applied and utilized almost solely in business sectors due to the steadily expanding volumes of biological data [63, 64, 67].

11.8 Healthcare

The healthcare sector has produced a significant amount of data. Big data is overwhelming the healthcare industry due to its volume, diversity of data types, and speed of generation (Figure 11.7). A big data scientist can use this enormous amount and collection of data to analyze it and convert it into complete, meaningful information. Big data analytics has the potential to enhance healthcare, save lives, and reduce the cost of drug discovery and clinical trials by identifying correlation and Knowledge Data Discovery (KDD) patterns and trends within the data. Big data plays a vital role in drug discovery pipelines. Among *in vivo*, *in vitro*, and *in silico* approaches, *in silico* is a very common approach that gives rise to molecular docking simulations in which one target screens millions or drugs, leading to the development of new drug molecules [6, 7, 47]. Pharmacogenomic approaches for drug development require the integration of multiple resources like (genomics, proteomics, and other omics) [61] (see Figure 11.5). The FDA has approved more than 138 drugs, including pharmacogenomic biomarkers with their functional labels.

Large numbers of gene expression samples collected *in silico* for drug development can be handled as big data and effectively arranged and managed in a Hadoop cluster along with their co-related expressions. The

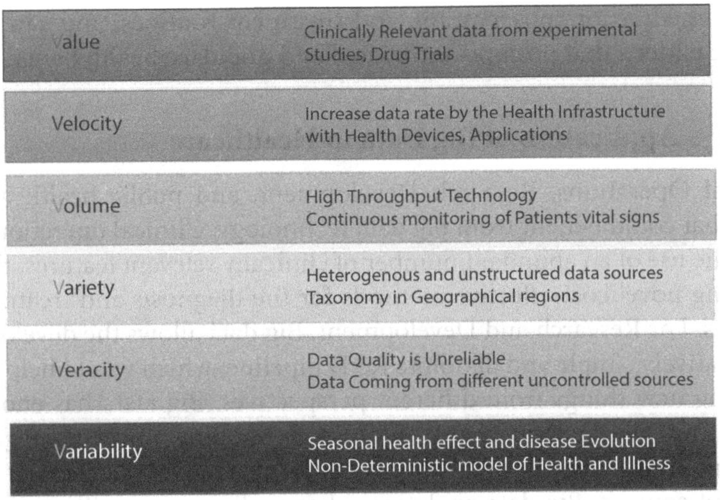

Figure 11.7 Six Vs of big data used in the healthcare (value, velocity, volume, variety, veracity, variability).

development of personalized medicine is sped up by combining the same set of genes with pre-existing gene expression with other related data. In the near future, creating a new technique and boosting computer power for *in silico* drug development will take only a few hours. For instance, Yabuuchi sought to characterize and illustrate the intricacy among 1,060 chemical compounds for the compound-protein structure.

While analyzing and visualizing possible lead chemical molecules for drug development requires the effective use of big data in the creation of new techniques, additional resources should also be considered. Tools use the explosion of data to discover hidden knowledge in data (KDD) with less investment in healthcare big data analytics software [23]. Big data analytics in healthcare has the potential to produce better outcomes in a variety of scenarios. For instance, the creation of mobile applications and other devices, aids in the analysis of patient health characteristics and care outcomes to identify the most clinically and financially advantageous disease treatments. This influences provider behavior by applying advanced analytics to patient profiles, such as monitoring vital signs (heartbeat, blood pressure, etc.). Many software companies, hospitals, and research institutes are developing and deploying mobile health apps that help patients manage and maintain a record of their daily routines, care, locate providers, and improve their health. Through examination, pharmaceutical organizations, inquire about offices and specialists, allowing them to screen for proper medication, observation, and treatment routines, and can distinguish a pattern that prompts individual and populace health benefits [65].

11.8.1 Application of Big Data in Healthcare

Clinical Operations, Research Development, and public health are key areas that could benefit from big data technology. Clinical operations promote the use of an abundant number of clinically relevant features, thereby reducing novel cost-effective methods for the diagnosis and treatment of patients. For Research and Development, Big data allows the development of a relatively simple and dissolute R&D pipeline, which would help in discovering new things from different perspectives. Big Data has enormous advantages over public health because developing novel strategies for analyzing public health data would require diversified and big data from different sources. Big data analytics enhance disease surveillance by analyzing data from different sources and can enable early detection of disease outbreaks and timely public health interventions. The more the data, the higher the accuracy of the information for targeting the disease, e.g., collecting virulent strains of mycobacterium can help in designing potentially effective drugs or vaccines for the treatment of tuberculosis. Big data analytics has certain applications in public health such as evidence-based medicine, Genome Analytics, Device/Remote monitoring, and patient profile analytics [55]. Establishing a global health data exchange system can facilitate the sharing of data across borders. This collaborative approach can help understand diseases and their determinants.

11.9 Big Data Formats

One major issue is the diversity of biological data. Every new device manufacturer creates its own data format, making data unification an increasingly challenging task. This emphasizes the need for proficient programming abilities in individuals handling a variety of devices so that they can alter current devices or write new scripts to parse data and convert between formats. Traditional standard data storage formats are evolving in the era of big data. Basic data formats (Figure 11.8) have long been developed and regarded as classical for data exchange, such as PDB for protein spatial structures and Fast Alignment (FASTA) for nucleotide and amino acid sequences. New data formats are now available, and the PDB database is one illustration [63, 64, 68].

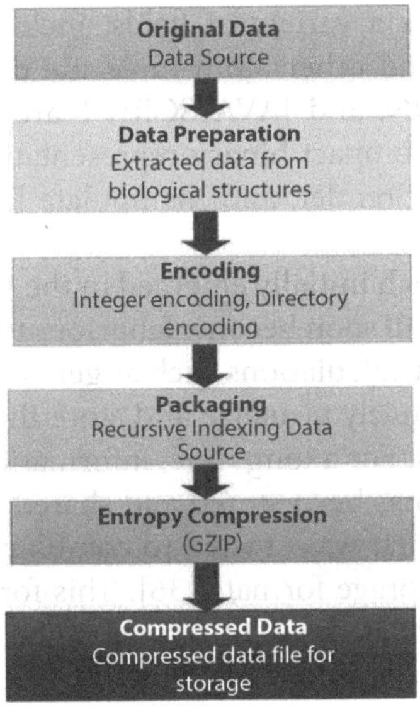

Figure 11.8 Flow chart demonstrating the store, parse normal data file into MMTF data file.

Further developments in structural bioinformatics have resulted in the creation of increasingly complex structures. Thus, it will become tedious to store and parse the data in the databases and perform analysis. The Macromolecular Transmission Format (MMTF), a compact binary format for the storage and transmission of large structural data for quicker visualization and analysis, is another recently proposed binary format for large-scale structures. The remarkable compaction of the data made possible by the binary format allows the entire PDB archive (~29 GB in mmCIF format) to be stored at less than 7 GB. In addition, it requires less time and space and simplifies and eases the analysis. For instance, the HIV viral capsid parsing time (PDB ID: 3J3Q) was calculated to be approximately 400 min using (PDBx/mmCIF (Protein Data Bank Macromolecular Crystallographic Information Framework)) format, which could be performed within the second with MMTF format [68].

Numerous databases containing a wide range of genomic data have been linked to bioinformatics. Currently, the largest available online Molecular Biology Database Collection from Nucleic Acid Research (NAR) comprises approximately 1,900 asset descriptions published in the annual database issue of the journal Nucleic Acids Research (NAR). There were 15 thematic categories and 41 subcategories in the collection [22]. Today's

MMTF format includes a variety of fields, including format, structure, model, chain, group, and other atom-molecule data. To implement this format, JAVA, PYTHON, and JAVA SCRIPT are used as examples (see Figure 11.8). With its compact binary representation, the MMTF format makes it easier to load, render, and manipulate large structural datasets quickly [68].

The PDB format, which initially emerged in the 1970s and gained popularity for data storage, will soon become laborious to store large amounts of 3D structures, carry out calculations such as genomic queries in structural comparisons, and effectively visualize and store the 3D structures of biological macromolecules. For a long time, information regarding the structures of small proteins has been stored and shared using this data format. The PDBx/mmCIF format was created to combine the PDB and mmCIF crystallographic data storage formats [36]. This format officially replaced the PDB format in 2014, as the PDB format is not suitable for large complexes with thousands of amino acids [5].

11.9.1 Quantum Computing

To fully utilize the potential of biological information, new techniques are required in this era of exponential data accumulation. Emerging technology known as quantum computing has the potential to completely change the handling of large amounts of biological data. Quantum computing has the potential to open new vistas in biomedical and genomic research because of its capacity to handle enormous datasets at speeds previously thought to be unachievable. Cutting-edge approaches, big data methods, software, computational tools, and biological databases are being studied to effectively manage the data collected from biological searches. NGS technology has a significant impact on biomedical and genomic research and generates a vast amount of data that can be classified as big data [16].

To fulfil the demands of High-Performance Computing for analysis, NGS experiments must effectively use and create quantum algorithms. The author discussed current methods for managing large datasets in the PDB, NCBI, IEDB, and DDBJ databases by integrating quantum computing technologies with existing ones such as Apache Pig, NoSQL, HBase, Hive using Hadoop, and the MapReduce programming framework. Database management systems with quantum improvements are being developed at unprecedented speeds to store and query massive amounts of data.

Quantum computing is also positioned to play a disruptive role in the healthcare sector, generating an unparalleled amount of data, including clinical operations, patient profiles, care analytics, and medication development. The gathering of enormous amounts of patient profile analytics data has been made possible by rapid improvements in mobile healthcare applications and other monitoring equipment. When it comes to analyzing and drawing conclusions from these data, quantum computing can provide novel solutions that will ultimately drive the development of personalized healthcare and push the limits of medical knowledge [52].

11.10 Conclusion

Biology is one of the main sources that generate a large amount of data in experiments and can be termed big data. Sequencing of the human genome and other genomes also falls under this category. NGS technology has a significant impact on genomic and biomedical research, producing a large amount of anonymous data from various experiments, which can be categorized as big data. The NGS experiment satisfied the HPC requirements by requiring the efficient use and design of a computer algorithm. The use of information technology and the introduction of new DBMS will solve the problem in databases such as PDB, NCBI, IEDB, DDBJ, and IMGT. Databases have petabytes of data, storing, sorting, and managing this huge amount of data is a challenging task and we need to develop algorithms, computational tools, and other data mining techniques with the help of technology such as Apache pig, No-SQL, H-base, Hive using Hadoop and map-reduce programming model frameworks. Technologies, such as XFEL and NMR can producelarge amounts of data from protein crystals. Thousands of structures are deposited every year in the Protein Data Bank (PDB). The advent of technology, such as the development of mobile applications and health monitoring systems or devices, makes it possible to keep the record of patients and help them diagnose in a proper and better way. *In silico* drug synthesis has become viable due to the abundance of molecules in various drug repositories such as drug banks.

Conflict of Interest

The authors declare no conflicts of interest, financial or otherwise.

Acknowledgments

The authors would like to thank the anonymous peer reviewers for their valuable comments and suggestions to further improve the quality of this study. The authors thank Shoolini University. where the idea of writing this manuscript came into mind.

References

1. Abuín, J.M., Pichel, J.C., Pena, T.F., Amigo, J., BigBWA: approaching the Burrows–Wheeler aligner to Big Data technologies. *Bioinformatics*, 31, 24, 4003–4005, 2015.
2. Allam, A., Kalnis, P., Solovyev, V., Karect: accurate correction of substitution, insertion and deletion errors for next-generation sequencing data. *Bioinformatics*, 31, 21, 3421–3428, 2015.
3. Attebury, G., Baranovski, A., Bloom, K., Bockelman, B., Kcira, D., Letts, J., Levshina, T., Lundestedt, C., Martin, T., Maier, W., Hadoop distributed file system for the grid. *2009 IEEE Nuclear Science Symposium Conference Record (NSS/MIC)*, IEEE, 2009.
4. Berlin, K., Koren, S., Chin, C.-S., Drake, J.P., Landolin, J.M., Phillippy, A.M., Assembling large genomes with single-molecule sequencing and locality-sensitive hashing. *Nat. Biotechnol.*, 33, 6, 623–630, 2015.
5. Berman, H., Henrick, K., Nakamura, H., Markley, J.L., The worldwide Protein Data Bank (wwPDB), ensuring a single, uniform archive of PDB data. *Nucleic Acids Res.*, 35, suppl_1, D301–D303, 2007.
6. Bernstein, F.C., Koetzle, T.F., Williams, G.J., Meyer Jr., E.F., Brice, M.D., Rodgers, J.R., Kennard, O., Shimanouchi, T., Tasumi, M., The Protein Data Bank: a computer-based archival file for macromolecular structures. *J. Mol. Biol.*, 112, 3, 535–542, 1977.
7. Bernstein, F.C., Koetzle, T.F., Williams, G.J., Meyer Jr., E.F., Brice, M.D., Rodgers, J.R., Kennard, O., Shimanouchi, T., Tasumi, M., The Protein Data Bank: A computer-based archival file for macromolecular structures. *Eur. J. Biochem.*, 80, 2, 319–324, 1977.
8. Bray, N.L., Pimentel, H., Melsted, P., Pachter, L., Near-optimal probabilistic RNA-seq quantification. *Nat. Biotechnol.*, 34, 5, 525–527, 2016.
9. Buermans, H. and Den Dunnen, J., Next generation sequencing technology: advances and applications. *Biochim. Biophys. Acta (BBA) - Mol. Basis Dis.*, 1842, 10, 1932–1941, 2014.
10. Can, T., Introduction to bioinformatics, in: *miRNomics: MicroRNA biology and computational analysis*, pp. 51–71, 2014.
11. Chang, Y.-J., Chen, C.-C., Chen, C.-L., Ho, J.-M., A de novo next generation genomic sequence assembler based on string graph and MapReduce cloud computing framework. *BMC Genomics*, Springer, 13, 1–7, 2012.
12. Chen, C.-C., Chang, Y.-J., Chung, W.-C., Lee, D.-T., Ho, J.-M., CloudRS: An error correction algorithm of high-throughput sequencing data based on

scalable framework. *2013 IEEE International Conference on Big Data*, IEEE, 2013.
13. Cheng, H., Jiang, H., Yang, J., Xu, Y., Shang, Y., BitMapper: an efficient all-mapper based on bit-vector computing. *BMC Bioinf.*, 16, 1–16, 2015.
14. Chu, J., Sadeghi, S., Raymond, A., Jackman, S.D., Nip, K.M., Mar, R., Mohamadi, H., Butterfield, Y.S., Robertson, A.G., Birol, I., BioBloom tools: fast, accurate and memory-efficient host species sequence screening using bloom filters. *Bioinformatics*, 30, 23, 3402–3404, 2014.
15. Chui, M., Loffler, M., Roberts, R., The internet of things, *McKinsey Quaterly Global Institute*, 2, 1–9, 2010.
16. Dash, S., Shakyawar, S.K., Sharma, M., Kaushik, S., Big data in healthcare: management, analysis and future prospects. *J. Big Data*, 6, 1, 1–25, 2019.
17. Deorowicz, S., Kokot, M., Grabowski, S., Debudaj-Grabysz, A., KMC 2: fast and resource-frugal k-mer counting. *Bioinformatics*, 31, 10, 1569–1576, 2015.
18. El-Metwally, S., Zakaria, M., Hamza, T., LightAssembler: fast and memory-efficient assembly algorithm for high-throughput sequencing reads. *Bioinformatics*, 32, 21, 3215–3223, 2016.
19. Erbert, M., Rechner, S., Müller-Hannemann, M., Gerbil: a fast and memory-efficient k-mer counter with GPU-support. *Algorithms Mol. Biol.*, 12, 1–12, 2017.
20. Fenstermacher, D., Introduction to bioinformatics. *J. Am. Soc. Inf. Sci. Technol.*, 56, 5, 440–446, 2005.
21. Fernandez, E.B., Villarreal, J., Lonardi, S., Najjar, W.A., FHAST: FPGA-based acceleration of Bowtie in hardware. *IEEE/ACM Trans. Comput. Biol. Bioinf.*, 12, 5, 973–981, 2015.
22. Galperin, M.Y., Fernández-Suárez, X.M., Rigden, D.J., The 24th annual Nucleic Acids Research database issue: a look back and upcoming changes. *Nucleic Acids Res.*, 45, D1, D1–D11, 2017.
23. Garapati, S.L. and Garapati, S., Application of big data analytics: an innovation in health care. *Comput. Intell.*, 14, 1, 15–27, 2018.
24. Georganas, E., Buluç, A., Chapman, J., Hofmeyr, S., Aluru, C., Egan, R., Oliker, L., Rokhsar, D., Yelick, K., HipMer: an extreme-scale de novo genome assembler. *Proceedings of the International Conference for High Performance Computing, Networking, Storage and Analysis*, 2015.
25. Ghazi, M.R. and Gangodkar, D., Hadoop, MapReduce and HDFS: a developers perspective. *Proc. Comput. Sci.*, 48, 45–50, 2015.
26. Gonzalez-Dominguez, J., Liu, Y., Schmidt, B., Parallel and scalable short-read alignment on multi-core clusters using UPC++. *PLoS One*, 11, 1, e0145490, 2016.
27. Greene, C.S., Tan, J., Ung, M., Moore, J.H., Cheng, C., Big data bioinformatics. *J. Cell. Physiol.*, 229, 12, 1896–1900, 2014.

28. Heo, Y., Ramachandran, A., Hwu, W.-M., Ma, J., Chen, D., BLESS 2: accurate, memory-efficient and fast error correction method. *Bioinformatics*, 32, 15, 2369–2371, 2016.
29. Jaiswal, V., Chanumolu, S.K., Sharma, P., Chauhan, R.S., Rout, C., EpiCombFlu: exploring known influenza epitopes and their combination to design a universal influenza vaccine. *Bioinformatics*, 29, 15, 1904–1907, 2013.
30. Jones, N.C. and Pevzner, P.A., *An introduction to bioinformatics algorithms*, MIT press, Cambridge, United States, 2004.
31. Kim, D., Langmead, B., Salzberg, S.L., HISAT: a fast spliced aligner with low memory requirements. *Nat. Methods*, 12, 4, 357–360, 2015.
32. Kumar, R. and Sharma, A., Computational strategies and tools for protein tertiary structure prediction, in: *Basic Biotechniques for Bioprocess and Bioentrepreneurship*, pp. 225–242, Elsevier, Cambridge, United States, 2023.
33. Langmead, B., Hansen, K.D., Leek, J.T., Cloud-scale RNA-sequencing differential expression analysis with Myrna. *Genome Biol.*, 11, 1–11, 2010.
34. Langmead, B. and Salzberg, S.L., Fast gapped-read alignment with Bowtie 2. *Nat. Methods*, 9, 4, 357–359, 2012.
35. Lesk, A., *Introduction to bioinformatics*, Oxford University Press, Oxford, England, 2019.
36. Li, D., Liu, C.-M., Luo, R., Sadakane, K., Lam, T.-W., MEGAHIT: an ultra-fast single-node solution for large and complex metagenomics assembly via succinct de Bruijn graph. *Bioinformatics*, 31, 10, 1674–1676, Oxford, England, 2015.
37. Liu, Y., Schmidt, B., Maskell, D.L., DecGPU: distributed error correction on massively parallel graphics processing units using CUDA and MPI. *BMC Bioinf.*, 12, 1–13, 2011.
38. Liu, Y., Schröder, J., Schmidt, B., Musket: a multistage k-mer spectrum-based error corrector for Illumina sequence data. *Bioinformatics*, 29, 3, 308–315, 2013.
39. Maillet, N., Lemaitre, C., Chikhi, R., Lavenier, D., Peterlongo, P., Compareads: comparing huge metagenomic experiments. *BMC Bioinf.*, Springer, 13, 1–10, 2012.
40. Marçais, G. and Kingsford, C., A fast, lock-free approach for efficient parallel counting of occurrences of k-mers. *Bioinformatics*, 27, 6, 764–770, 2011.
41. Martínez, H., Barrachina, S., Castillo, M., Tárraga, J., Medina, I., Dopazo, J., Quintana-Ortí, E.S., Scalable RNA sequencing on clusters of multicore processors. *2015 IEEE Trustcom/BigDataSE/ISPA*, IEEE, 2015.
42. Marx, V., The big challenges of big data. *Nature*, 498, 7453, 255–260, 2013.
43. Medina, I., Tárraga, J., Martínez, H., Barrachina, S., Castillo, M., Paschall, J., Salavert-Torres, J., Blanquer-Espert, I., Hernández-García, V., Quintana-Ortí, E.S., Highly sensitive and ultrafast read mapping for RNA-seq analysis. *DNA Res.*, 23, 2, 93–100, 2016.

44. Melsted, P. and Halldórsson, B.V., KmerStream: streaming algorithms for k-mer abundance estimation. *Bioinformatics*, 30, 24, 3541–3547, 2014.
45. Melsted, P. and Pritchard, J.K., Efficient counting of k-mers in DNA sequences using a bloom filter. *BMC Bioinf.*, 12, 1–7, 2011.
46. Miller, N.A., Farrow, E.G., Gibson, M., Willig, L.K., Twist, G., Yoo, B., Marrs, T., Corder, S., Krivohlavek, L., Walter, A., A 26-hour system of highly sensitive whole genome sequencing for emergency management of genetic diseases. *Genome Med.*, 7, 1, 100, 2015.
47. Morris, G.M., Huey, R., Lindstrom, W., Sanner, M.F., Belew, R.K., Goodsell, D.S., Olson, A.J., AutoDock4 and AutoDockTools4: Automated docking with selective receptor flexibility. *J. Comput. Chem.*, 30, 16, 2785–2791, 2009.
48. Nazipova, N.N., Isaev, E.A.E., Kornilov, V.V., Pervukhin, D.V.E., Morozova, A.A.E., Gorbunov, A.A., Ustinin, M.N., Big Data in bioinformatics. *Математическая биология и биоинформатика*, 13, Suppl, 1–16, 2018.
49. Nordberg, H., Bhatia, K., Wang, K., Wang, Z., BioPig: a Hadoop-based analytic toolkit for large-scale sequence data. *Bioinformatics*, 29, 23, 3014–3019, 2013.
50. Ohashi, H., Hasegawa, M., Wakimoto, K., Miyamoto-Sato, E., Next-generation technologies for multiomics approaches including interactome sequencing. *BioMed. Res. Int.*, 2015, 1–9, 2015.
51. Ondov, B.D., Treangen, T.J., Melsted, P., Mallonee, A.B., Bergman, N.H., Koren, S., Phillippy, A.M., Mash: fast genome and metagenome distance estimation using MinHash. *Genome Biol.*, 17, 1–14, 2016.
52. Outeiral, C., Strahm, M., Shi, J., Morris, G.M., Benjamin, S.C., Deane, C.M., The prospects of quantum computing in computational molecular biology. *Wiley Interdiscip. Rev.: Comput. Mol. Sci.*, 11, 1, e1481, 2021.
53. Pal, T., Padhan, J.K., Kumar, P., Sood, H., Chauhan, R.S., Comparative transcriptomics uncovers differences in photoautotrophic versus photoheterotrophic modes of nutrition in relation to secondary metabolites biosynthesis in Swertia chirayita. *Mol. Biol. Rep.*, 45, 77–98, 2018.
54. Popic, V. and Batzoglou, S., Privacy-preserving read mapping using locality sensitive hashing and secure kmer voting. 046920, 2016, bioRxiv.
55. Raghupathi, W. and Raghupathi, V., Big data analytics in healthcare: promise and potential. *Health Inf. Sci. Syst.*, 2, 1, 3, 2014.
56. Rizk, G., Gouin, A., Chikhi, R., Lemaitre, C., MindTheGap: integrated detection and assembly of short and long insertions. *Bioinformatics*, 30, 24, 3451–3457, 2014.
57. Robinson, J., Soormally, A.R., Hayhurst, J.D., Marsh, S.G., The IPD-IMGT/HLA Database–New developments in reporting HLA variation. *Hum. Immunol.*, 77, 3, 233–237, 2016.
58. Schadt, E.E., Turner, S., Kasarskis, A., A window into third-generation sequencing. *Hum. Mol. Genet.*, 19, R2, R227–R240, 2010.
59. Schmidt, B. and Hildebrandt, A., Next-generation sequencing: big data meets high performance computing. *Drug Discov. Today*, 22, 4, 712–717, 2017.

60. Schneider, D., US supercomputing strikes back. *IEEE Spectr.*, 55, 1, 52–53, 2018.
61. Schultze, J.L., Teaching'big data'analysis to young immunologists. *Nat. Immunol.*, 16, 9, 902–905, 2015.
62. Schulz, M.H., Weese, D., Holtgrewe, M., Dimitrova, V., Niu, S., Reinert, K., Richard, H., Fiona: a parallel and automatic strategy for read error correction. *Bioinformatics*, 30, 17, i356–i363, 2014.
63. Sharma, A., Guleria, V., Jaiswal, V., The Future of Blockchain Technology, Recent Advancement and Challenges, in: *Blockchain and Deep Learning: Future Trends and Enabling Technologies*, pp. 329–349, Springer, Berlin/Heidelberg, Germany, 2022.
64. Sharma, A. and Kumar, R., Recent Advancement and Challenges in Deep Learning, Big Data in Bioinformatics, in: *Blockchain and Deep Learning: Future Trends and Enabling Technologies*, pp. 251–284, Springer, Berlin/Heidelberg, Germany, 2022.
65. Sharma, A., Kumar, R., Jaiswal, V., Classification of heart disease from MRI images using convolutional neural network. *2021 6th international conference on signal processing, computing and control (ISPCC)*, IEEE, 2021.
66. Solomon, B. and Kingsford, C., Fast search of thousands of short-read sequencing experiments. *Nat. Biotechnol.*, 34, 3, 300–302, 2016.
67. Srivastava, A. and Naik, A., Big Data Analysis in Bioinformatics, in: *Advances in Bioinformatics*, pp. 405–429, 2021.
68. Srivastava, P.A., Kalra, S., Yennamalli, R.M., Structural Bioinformatics and Big Data Analytics: A mini-review, *International Journal for Computational Biology*, 6, 1, 25–30, 2017.
69. Tárraga, J., Arnau, V., Martínez, H., Moreno, R., Cazorla, D., Salavert-Torres, J., Blanquer-Espert, I., Dopazo, J., Medina, I., Acceleration of short and long DNA read mapping without loss of accuracy using suffix array. *Bioinformatics*, 30, 23, 3396–3398, 2014.
70. Teng, F., Yu, L., Magoules, F., Simmapreduce: A simulator for modeling mapreduce framework. *2011 Fifth FTRA International Conference on Multimedia and Ubiquitous Engineering*, IEEE, 2011.
71. Vita, R., Overton, J.A., Greenbaum, J.A., Ponomarenko, J., Clark, J.D., Cantrell, J.R., Wheeler, D.K., Gabbard, J.L., Hix, D., Sette, A., The immune epitope database (IEDB) 3.0. *Nucleic Acids Res.*, 43, D1, D405–D412, 2015.
72. Wilton, R., Budavari, T., Langmead, B., Wheelan, S.J., Salzberg, S.L., Szalay, A.S., Arioc: high-throughput read alignment with GPU-accelerated exploration of the seed-and-extend search space. *PeerJ*, 3, e808, 2015.
73. Wood, D.E. and Salzberg, S.L., Kraken: ultrafast metagenomic sequence classification using exact alignments. *Genome Biol.*, 15, 1–12, 2014.
74. Yang, X., Zola, J., Aluru, S., Large-scale metagenomic sequence clustering on map-reduce clusters. *J. Bioinf. Comput. Biol.*, 11, 01, 1340001, 2013.
75. Zhang, Z. and Wang, W., RNA-Skim: a rapid method for RNA-Seq quantification at transcript level. *Bioinformatics*, 30, 12, i283–i292, 2014.

12

Wearable Devices and Health Monitoring: Big Data and AI for Remote Patient Care

S. Kanakaprabha[1]*, G. Ganesh Kumar[2], Bhargavi Peddi Reddy[3], Yallapragada Ravi Raju[4] and P. Chandra Mohan Rai[5]

[1]*Department of Computer Science and Engineering, Rathinam Technical Campus, Anna University, Coimbatore, India*
[2]*Department of Information Technology, Hindusthan Institute of Technology, Coimbatore, India*
[3]*Department of Computer Science and Engineering, Vasavi College of Engineering Ibrahim Bagh, Hyderabad, India*
[4]*Department of Computer Science and Engineering, Madanapalle Institute of Technology and Science, Madanapalle, Andhra Pradesh, India*
[5]*Department of Computer Science and Engineering, Koneru Lakshmaiah Education Foundation, Vaddeswaram, Andhra Pradesh, India*

Abstract
The integration of wearable devices, big data, and artificial intelligence (AI) has revolutionized remote patient care and health monitoring. These technologies enable the continuous and real-time collection of various physiological and behavioral data from individuals, allowing healthcare providers to remotely monitor their health status. Wearable devices such as smartwatches, fitness trackers, and medical sensors offer the ability to track vital signs, physical activity, and sleep patterns. The sheer volume of data generated by these devices, often referred to as big data, presents challenges and opportunities. AI plays a crucial role in deciphering this wealth of information by employing advanced algorithms for data analysis, pattern recognition, and predictive modeling. This synergy between wearable devices, big data, and AI not only empowers patients to actively engage in their own health management, but also enables healthcare professionals to make informed decisions, detect anomalies, and provide timely interventions. This abstract explores the transformative impact of wearable devices and the synergy of big data and AI

**Corresponding author*: skanakaprabha@gmail.com

Neha Sharma, Korhan Cengiz and Prasenjit Chatterjee (eds.) Intelligent Data Analytics for Bioinformatics and Biomedical Systems, (291–312) © 2024 Scrivener Publishing LLC

in enhancing remote patient care, fostering the early detection of health issues, and ultimately improving overall patient outcomes.

***Keywords*:** Artificial intelligence, big data, health monitoring, remote patient, sensors wearable devices

12.1 Introduction

The convergence of wearable devices, big data analytics, and artificial intelligence (AI) has ushered in a new era of healthcare, particularly in the realms of remote patient care and health monitoring. Traditional healthcare models have often been constrained by limited access to real-time patient data and challenges of timely intervention. However, the advent of wearable technologies has broken down these barriers, allowing for the continuous monitoring of patients' physiological and behavioral parameters, irrespective of their geographic location. This transformative shift has been fueled by the proliferation of smartwatches, fitness trackers, biosensors, and other wearable devices equipped with sensors capable of capturing a diverse range of health-related metrics.

Central to this paradigm shift is the concept of big data, the massive volume of information generated by these wearable devices. These data encompass a myriad of variables, including heart rate, blood pressure, temperature, sleep patterns, and physical activity levels. Although the sheer volume of this data can be overwhelming, it holds immense potential for insights that were previously unattainable. This is where the AI steps in as a critical enabler. Advanced machine learning algorithms can sift through data, identify patterns, and extract valuable information, enabling healthcare practitioners to make informed decisions in real time. The integration of AI with big data allows predictive modeling, anomaly detection, and personalized recommendations. For instance, AI algorithms can recognize deviations from a patient's baseline health metrics and issue alerts to both patients and healthcare providers, allowing swift interventions before minor issues escalate into major health concerns. Moreover, continuous monitoring facilitated by wearable devices and AI empowers patients to actively participate in their own healthcare journey, fostering a sense of ownership over their wellbeing.

This chapter delves into the multidimensional impact of wearable devices on remote patient care and highlights the symbiotic relationship between big data and AI. We will explore how wearable technology is reshaping doctor–patient dynamics, enabling proactive healthcare management, enhancing early disease detection, and ultimately revolutionizing the way healthcare is delivered. By analyzing case studies, current trends, and challenges, this study aims to provide a comprehensive understanding of the potential and implications of this transformative synergy. As we navigate this exciting terrain, it becomes clear that wearable devices, big data, and AI are collectively poised to redefine the landscape of remote patient care and herald a new era of patient-centric data-driven healthcare.

Wearable devices have rapidly emerged as pivotal tools in modern healthcare, offering a tangible bridge between medical technology and daily life. These devices, encompassing an array of form factors ranging from smartwatches to adhesive sensors, have redefined how individuals monitor and manage their health. With the increasing focus on preventive and personalized medicine, wearable devices provide a seamless means of continuously gathering and transmitting valuable health data. This information goes beyond traditional sporadic checkups, offering a real-time and comprehensive understanding of an individual's well-being. As we delve into the intricate interplay between these devices and remote patient care, it becomes evident that wearable technology is a cornerstone in the evolution towards more proactive, patient-centric healthcare practices.

12.1.1 Importance of Remote Patient Monitoring

Remote patient monitoring, facilitated by wearable devices, addresses a critical need in modern healthcare by overcoming the limitations of traditional in-person consultations. The ability to gather continuous health data in real time empowers healthcare providers to closely track patients' conditions, detect subtle changes, and intervene promptly. This proactive approach not only enhances patient outcomes, but also minimizes hospital

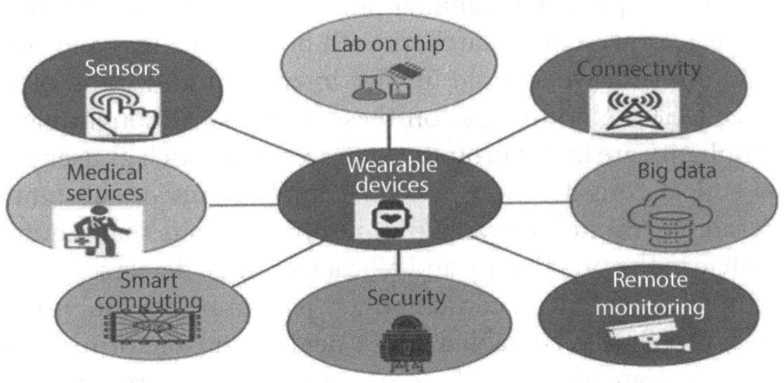

Figure 12.1 An intelligent IoT-based healthcare system.

readmissions and reduces the burden on healthcare systems. By enabling patients to maintain their routines and lifestyles while remaining connected to medical professionals, remote patient monitoring fosters new levels of patient engagement and accountability. Consequently, the integration of wearable devices for remote patient monitoring holds the promise of revolutionizing healthcare delivery, making it more efficient, patient-centered, and responsive to individual needs (see Figure 12.1).

12.1.2 Significance of Big Data and AI in Healthcare

The significance of big data and artificial intelligence (AI) in healthcare cannot be overstated. The vast amount of data generated by wearable devices presents an unprecedented opportunity for deeper insight into patient health patterns and outcomes. AI algorithms excel in processing and interpreting these data, identifying correlations, predicting trends, and even spotting anomalies that might escape human observation. This amalgamation of big data and AI equips healthcare professionals with evidence-based decision-making tools, enabling them to provide more precise diagnoses, personalized treatment plans, and timely interventions. Ultimately, this synergy has the potential to elevate the quality of care, optimize resource allocation, and propel medical research into uncharted territories, transforming the healthcare landscape into a realm of data-driven excellence.

12.2 Related Work

In this study [1], wearable applications have the potential to directly influence clinical choices. It has been argued that wearable technologies could elevate patient care quality while concurrently diminishing care expenses, including off-site patient rehabilitation. The substantial data yielded by wearable devices present researchers with both challenges and prospects, wherein future endeavors could involve intensified utilization of artificial intelligence (AI) methodologies on these datasets. Although many wearable technologies are in the prototype phase, factors such as user adoption, security, ethical considerations, and the implications of substantial data within wearable technology remain unresolved aspects that require attention to enhance the practicality and efficacy of these devices.

This study [2] centers on contemporary patient health monitoring platforms by leveraging IoT-enabled smart devices capable of real-time data collection and transmission. These data are then assessed by healthcare providers, including doctors, hospitals, clinics, and the patients themselves for self-management purposes. The objective was to successfully encapsulate the latest insights concerning approved devices and cutting-edge advancements through a thorough and systematic analysis of the existing literature. In addition, this study explores potential trajectories for the fusion of cloud computing and blockchain, which could potentially herald revolutionary advancements in on-demand medical services. The amalgamation of IoT with real-time remote patient monitoring empowers individuals to take a more proactive role in overseeing their well-being, thereby enabling them to actively track their specific health conditions.

In this study [3], patients can relish tailored medical provisions while the facilitation and dissemination of medical and healthcare services are advanced, propelling the digital transformation of the healthcare sector. This study delves into the utilization and implementation of 5G network technology in the medical realm. It encompasses aspects such as telecare, 5G-enabled remote medical aid, and the deployment of remote robots. Moreover, by amalgamating the attributes of AI applications and the prerequisites of smart healthcare, this study examines the comprehensive strategizing, intelligent adaptation, and customization of 5G network technology in the medical domain. The opportunities and challenges that arise from its application in nursing are also discussed. Ultimately, this study serves as a valuable resource for guiding the evolution and application of 5G network technology in medical services.

In this study [4], the article underscores the pivotal role of big data and AI-ML in the formulation of digital twins (DTs) or DT-based systems across diverse industrial sectors is examined. This is done by shedding light on current cutting-edge implementations. Through a comprehensive approach, we conducted a systematic review that encompassed various interdisciplinary electronic bibliographic databases as well as existing patents within the domain. Additionally, we pinpointed development tools that can streamline the creation of digital twins at various levels. Furthermore, we devised a reference architecture fueled by big data and enriched by AI that guides developers toward the realization of a comprehensive DT-enabled system. In conclusion, we brought to the fore the research potential of AI-ML in the realm of digital twinning, shedding light on challenges and current prospects.

In this study [5], Cognitive Computing (CC), a subset of AI, emerged as a potent remedy for addressing these challenges, offering a pivotal role in facilitating knowledge-rich automation endeavors. Acquiring an understanding of the latest advancements and contemporary landscape of CC is an initial step necessary for researchers to advance in this field. In this light, this study delivers an all-encompassing overview of preceding research within the domain of CC, encompassing not only the challenges and solutions, but also outlining future research trajectories. More specifically, this study delves into CC-driven techniques that tackle practical issues across four extensively explored application domains: healthcare, cybersecurity, big data, and IoT. These applications have been meticulously examined while elucidating unresolved research quandaries.

In this study [6], the procedure for selecting articles encompassed five sequential phases: initial planning and study identification, evaluation of articles, extraction of outcomes, summarization, and distribution of audit findings. A total of 93 documents were included in this study. Our findings underscore that the attainment of efficient patient-centric healthcare depends on the handling, analysis, and integration of an extensive array of health data. Such an approach holds the potential for expedited and more accurate diagnoses while optimizing the allocation of healthcare resources. However, fully harnessing the advantages of digitization and technological advancement necessitates the reconfiguration of conventional operational and strategic methodologies, in tandem with the acquisition of novel proficiencies.

The literature reflects [7] the boundless possibilities facilitated by AI-based telemedicine in promoting healthcare development through its inherent flexibility and adaptability. The progression of telerobotic surgery and the significance of the Internet of Robotic Things (IoRT) have been briefly examined. Additionally, this study delves into the specifics of available wearable devices designed for biomedical and healthcare applications. These devices are adept at gathering data, which are then analyzed using established protocols by machine intelligence to forecast health-related concerns. In conclusion, this narrative explores the eventual proliferation and transformation of these technologies within the modern healthcare system and biomedical research landscape. This trajectory encompasses a spectrum ranging from personalized drug design to precise drug administration and extends beyond.

In this study [8], the escalating global population has amplified the demand for technologies, computerized algorithms, and intelligent devices capable of monitoring and aiding patients at any time and place, thereby empowering them to maintain autonomous lifestyles. Real-time remote patient monitoring is as a crucial aspect of the telemedicine landscape. Within the realm of healthcare provision, patient prioritization poses a formidable hurdle due to the intricate decision-making entailed when patients are regarded as "big data." To the best of our knowledge, no study has illuminated the correlation between the attributes of "big data" and the process of real-time remote healthcare monitoring in the context of patient prioritization, along with the inherent challenges this process entails.

In this study [9], in an era of contemporary technological advancements, industries across the spectrum are undergoing transformations to enhance the quality of their offerings, with the goal of satisfying clients. Healthcare leverages modern technology to revolutionize the approach to patient care and treatment. Within this technological epoch, the healthcare ecosystem's objective surpasses that of disease management, encompassing the comprehensive well-being of patients. By integrating sensor-equipped IoT-based smart healthcare systems with artificial intelligence, the harmonious orchestration of healthcare services has emerged. This empowers healthcare professionals to oversee patients' daily routines in real-time, thus facilitating timely responses to healthcare requirements.

This achievement is due to the utilization of AI [10], which efficiently handles vast volumes of data to forecast forthcoming occurrences. Currently, deep learning-based AI has garnered substantial global attention and has significantly influenced the healthcare sector. Deep learning has found extensive application in image recognition, speech recognition, and natural language processing. It has the potential to be a conduit for transforming extensive biomedical data into enhancements in human well-being. This study undertakes a literature review aimed at identifying the pivotal technologies, methodologies, algorithms, and models that underpin smart health systems. Furthermore, it explores the primary application domains and challenges associated with the smart health realm.

12.3 Wearable Technologies in Healthcare

Wearable technologies have become integral to healthcare, bridging the gap between medical science and daily life. Ranging from smartwatches and fitness trackers to advanced biosensors, these devices offer continuous monitoring of vital signs, physical activity, etc. This real-time data collection not only empowers individuals to actively manage their health but also enables healthcare providers to offer more personalized and proactive care. Wearable technologies are shaping a new era of preventive medicine, transforming the way we perceive and engage with well-being.

12.3.1 Types of Wearable Devices (Smartwatches, Fitness Trackers, Medical-Grade Wearables, etc.)

Wearable devices encompass a diverse range of technologies tailored to monitor various aspects of health and well-being. Smartwatches, with their multifunctional capabilities, offer features such as heart rate tracking, activity monitoring, and electrocardiograms (ECGs). Fitness trackers focus predominantly on physical activity metrics such as steps taken, distance traveled, and calories burned. Medical-grade wearables, designed with precision and accuracy in mind, can measure vital signs, such as blood pressure, blood glucose levels, and oxygen saturation. These devices often adhere to stringent regulatory standards to ensure their reliability in clinical settings. Moreover, specialized wearables cater to niche applications such as continuous glucose monitoring for diabetes management or wearable patches for medication delivery. The diversity within wearable devices underscores their adaptability to a spectrum of health-monitoring needs, making them pivotal tools in modern healthcare.

12.3.2 Applications in Monitoring Vital Signs (Heart Rate, Blood Pressure, Temperature, etc.)

Wearable devices have revolutionized the monitoring of vital signs, offering a convenient and continuous method to track key health indicators. Heart rate monitoring, a common feature of most wearables, provides insights into cardiovascular health and helps users gauge their fitness

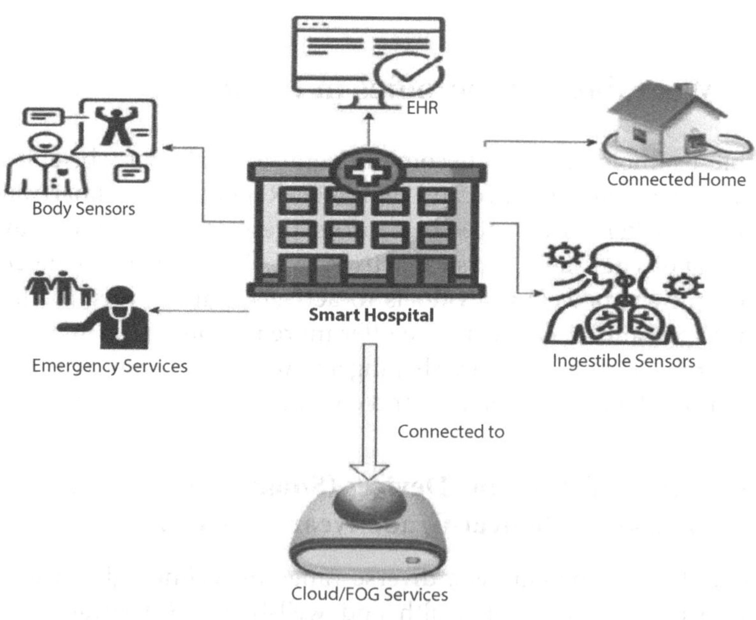

Figure 12.2 Assisted wearable sensor systems for healthcare monitoring.

levels. Blood pressure tracking, once limited to medical facilities, is now possible through wearables, enabling hypertension management and the early detection of anomalies. Temperature monitoring aids in identifying fevers or fluctuations that could signify the underlying health issues. These devices also contribute to sleep analysis by recording the sleep patterns and cycles. With wearables, individuals can proactively manage their well-being, and healthcare providers can gain access to a more comprehensive picture of their patients' health, enabling timely interventions and personalized treatment plans (see Figure 12.2).

12.3.3 Wearables for Tracking Physical Activity and Sleep Patterns

Wearables play a pivotal role in promoting active lifestyles and improving sleep quality by allowing precise tracking of physical activity and sleep patterns. Fitness trackers, equipped with accelerometers and gyroscopes, monitor steps taken, distance traveled, and calories burned, providing users with insight into their daily activity levels. These devices also offer goal-setting features and real-time feedback, which motivates individuals to maintain healthier routines. Additionally, wearables can analyze sleep duration, sleep cycles, and even the quality of sleep through movement and heart rate data. By tracking these parameters, users can identify sleep trends and make informed adjustments to enhance sleep hygiene. This integration of activity and sleep monitoring not only promotes holistic well-being but also aids in the early detection of potential health issues stemming from sedentary behavior or sleep disturbances.

12.4 Remote Patient Monitoring

Remote patient monitoring enabled by wearable devices presents a transformative approach to healthcare delivery. It allows healthcare providers to continuously gather real-time health data from patients outside traditional clinical settings. This capability is particularly advantageous for individuals with chronic conditions, postoperative recovery, and those who require consistent monitoring. By receiving accurate and up-to-date information about vital signs, physical activity, and other health metrics, healthcare professionals can promptly identify any deviations from the baseline and intervene proactively. This not only enhances patient outcomes but also reduces hospital readmissions and healthcare costs. Remote patient monitoring empowers patients to actively engage in health management, thereby promoting a sense of ownership and accountability. As wearable technology advances and integrates with sophisticated data analytics, remote patient monitoring is poised to revolutionize healthcare by fostering patient-centered care, early intervention, and improved overall wellness.

12.4.1 Definition and Benefits of Remote Patient Monitoring

Remote patient monitoring (RPM) refers to the use of wearable devices and other technologies to collect and transmit patients' health data from a distance, thereby allowing healthcare providers to monitor their conditions remotely. This approach offers numerous benefits to both patients and healthcare systems. RPM enables timely tracking of vital signs, symptoms, and treatment adherence, facilitating the early detection of potential health issues and reducing the need for frequent in-person visits. Patients experience greater convenience as they can continue their daily activities while remaining under medical surveillance. This proactive monitoring enhances chronic disease management, reduces hospitalization, and improves overall patient outcomes. Additionally, RPM optimizes resource allocation by focusing on patients who truly need immediate attention, thereby reducing the strain on healthcare facilities. In essence, remote patient monitoring is a pivotal shift towards personalized, efficient, and patient-centric healthcare delivery (see Figure 12.3).

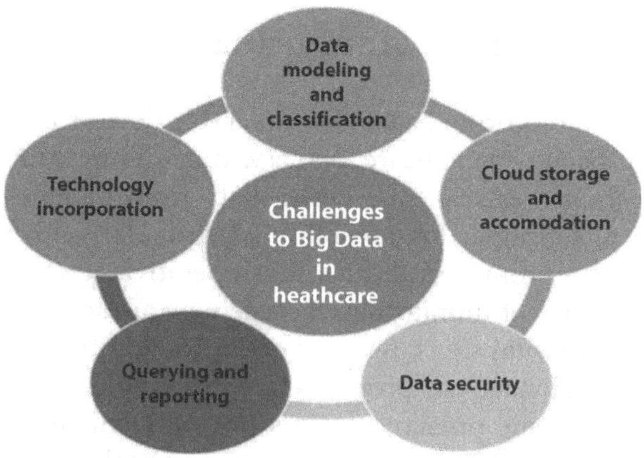

Figure 12.3 Big data analytics for healthcare.

12.5 Use Cases: Chronic Disease Management, Post-Operative Care, Elderly Care, Etc.

Remote patient monitoring (RPM) encompasses a range of applications across various healthcare scenarios and offers tailored solutions for improved patient care and outcomes.

1. **Chronic Disease Management:** RPM is particularly valuable for managing chronic conditions, such as diabetes, hypertension, and heart disease. Patients can track their vital signs, blood sugar levels, and medication adherence, whereas healthcare providers receive real-time data to make informed treatment adjustments and provide timely interventions.
2. **Postoperative Care:** After surgical procedures, RPM allows healthcare professionals to closely monitor patients' recovery progress, detect any complications early, and guide them through the healing process. This reduces the risk of postoperative complications and readmissions.
3. **Elderly Care:** RPM plays a vital role in elderly care by monitoring seniors' health parameters, activity levels, and medication schedules. This enables caregivers and family members to ensure their well-being and promptly address concerns.
4. **Maternal Health:** Pregnant women can benefit from RPM by tracking their maternal health indicators and fetal well-being. Healthcare providers can identify potential risks and provide personalized care plans throughout pregnancy.
5. **Respiratory Conditions:** Patients with respiratory disorders, such as asthma or chronic obstructive pulmonary disease (COPD), can use RPM to monitor lung function and receive guidance on managing their condition effectively.
6. **Cardiac Monitoring:** RPM aids in continuous monitoring of cardiac patients' heart rhythms, detecting irregularities or abnormalities that might require medical attention.
7. **Remote Rehabilitation:** Patients undergoing physical therapy or rehabilitation can be monitored remotely, ensuring that they follow prescribed exercises and routines for optimal recovery.

8. **Weight Management:** RPM helps individuals manage their weight and lifestyle by tracking their physical activity, nutrition, and overall progress.
9. **Wellness and Prevention:** Even individuals without chronic conditions can benefit from RPM by staying proactive about their health. Regular monitoring of vital signs and health metrics can help detect the early signs of potential issues.

In each of these cases, RPM offers personalized care, reduces healthcare costs, minimizes the need for in-person visits, and empowers patients to take an active role in managing their health. Data-driven insights provided by wearable devices contribute to better-informed medical decisions and ultimately lead to improved patient outcomes.

12.6 Challenges of Traditional In-Person Care vs. Remote Monitoring

Traditional in-person healthcare encounters have long been the cornerstone of medical practice, offering direct interaction between patients and healthcare providers. However, this model has several challenges. Patients often experience inconveniences and time constraints associated with traveling to clinics or hospitals. Moreover, in-person visits are sporadic, making it challenging to accurately monitor health trends. Diagnosis and intervention may be delayed due to limited access to real-time data, potentially affecting patient outcomes. Additionally, healthcare systems can be strained by a high volume of patients seeking in-person care, leading to longer waiting times and a reduced quality of care.

On the other hand, while remote patient monitoring (RPM) overcomes many of these challenges, it also introduces its own set of complexities. Ensuring patient compliance and adherence to regular use of wearable devices can be a hurdle. Technical issues, data security concerns, and the digital divide among older populations can pose obstacles to the implementation of RPM. Healthcare providers must adapt to interpret remote data and effectively identify meaningful trends. Striking a balance between automated data analysis and personalized human oversight is essential. Furthermore, RPM might not be suitable for all medical conditions or patient preferences, requiring a nuanced approach that integrates both remote monitoring and in-person care, where necessary. Addressing these challenges is pivotal to realizing the full potential of RPM while ensuring

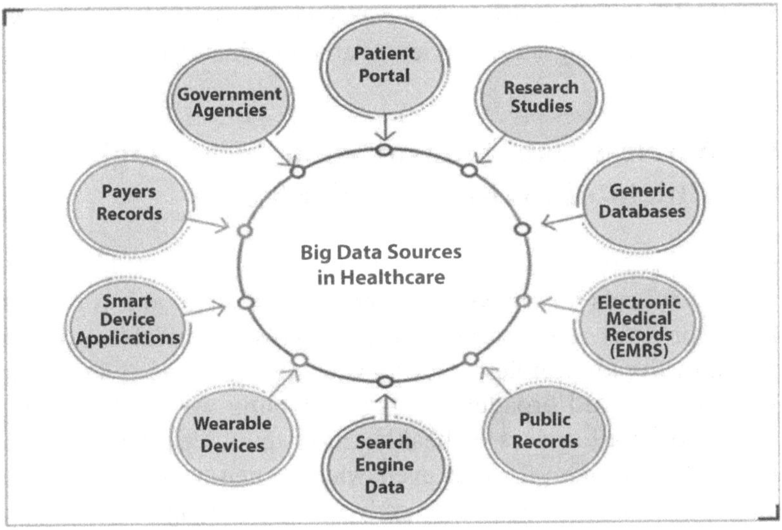

Figure 12.4 Big data and predictive analytics in healthcare.

that patients receive the best possible care. Figure 12.4 illustrates the diversity of big data sources in healthcare [11].

12.7 Data Collection and Transmission

Wearable devices gather diverse health data through sensors, including heart rate, temperature, and activity levels. These data are transmitted wirelessly to cloud-based platforms, where they are processed and analyzed. Real-time data transmission enables healthcare providers to monitor patients' health remotely, facilitating prompt intervention and informed medical decisions.

12.7.1 Sensors and Data Collection Methods in Wearables

Wearable devices leverage various sensors to collect comprehensive health data. Accelerometers and gyroscopes track movement and orientation, offering insight into physical activity and posture. Optical sensors measure the heart rate, blood oxygen levels, and even blood pressure. Temperature sensors provide information about body temperature fluctuations. Electrodes facilitate electrocardiogram (ECG) measurements, whereas galvanic skin response sensors monitor stress levels. Some wearable devices incorporate a GPS for location tracking. These sensors collectively enable continuous collection of health metrics, ensuring a holistic view of an individual's well-being.

12.8 Wireless Data Transmission Technologies (Bluetooth, Wi-Fi, Cellular, Etc.)

Wearable devices use various wireless technologies to transmit health data to remote platforms for analysis and monitoring. Bluetooth is commonly employed for short-range communication between wearables and smartphones, allowing for seamless data transfer. Wi-Fi connectivity facilitates higher data rates and broader coverage, enabling wearables to transmit data to cloud-based servers or healthcare systems. Cellular connectivity, including 4G and 5G, offers an even wider range of data transmission, enabling wearables to send data directly without relying on other devices. Additionally, technologies such as near-field communication (NFC) enable quick and secure data exchange, particularly for tasks such as sharing medical records. The choice of wireless technology depends on factors such as data volume, distance, and power consumption, ensuring the effective and efficient transmission of health data.

12.8.1 Ensuring Data Security and Privacy

Maintaining robust data security and privacy is paramount in the realm of wearable devices and health data. As wearables gather sensitive health information, stringent encryption protocols are essential to safeguard the data during transmission and storage. Adherence to regulatory standards such as HIPAA and GDPR is vital to protect patient privacy and control data access. Multifactor authentication, secure data servers, and regular security audits bolster the protection of collected data from unauthorized access. Transparent communication with users regarding data usage and sharing practices fosters trust and informed consent. Ultimately, a comprehensive approach encompassing technology safeguards, legal compliance, and ethical considerations is vital to uphold data security and preserve patient privacy in the wearable healthcare landscape.

12.8.2 Big-Data Analytics in Healthcare

Big-data analytics has emerged as a transformative tool in healthcare, leveraging large and complex datasets, including those generated by wearable devices, to extract valuable insights. This approach involves advanced algorithms and machine learning techniques to uncover patterns, trends, and correlations within the data. In healthcare, big data analytics can aid early disease detection, predictive modeling, personalized treatment recommendations, and resource optimization. Healthcare professionals can make informed decisions, tailor interventions, and improve patient outcomes by analyzing vast amounts of health information, including vital signs, genetics, and lifestyle factors. The integration of big data analytics with wearable-generated data enhances the precision and efficiency of healthcare delivery, fostering a data-driven approach that enhances medical research and ultimately transforms the way we understand and manage health.

12.8.3 Role of Big Data in Healthcare Decision-Making

Big data empower healthcare decision-making by providing comprehensive and real-time insights into patient health, treatment effectiveness, and population health trends. Analyzing vast datasets from wearable devices and other sources enables evidence-based decisions, personalized treatment plans, and the early identification of health risks, ultimately improving patient care and shaping more efficient healthcare strategies.

12.8.4 Handling and Processing Large Volumes of Wearable-Generated Data

Managing the substantial influx of data from wearable devices requires robust infrastructure and data-processing techniques. Cloud computing offers scalable storage and computational resources to efficiently handle these large volumes. Data preprocessing involves cleaning, filtering, and normalizing the raw data for analysis. Advanced data analytics tools and machine learning algorithms were then employed to extract meaningful insights, identify patterns, and predict health outcomes. Additionally, techniques such as data aggregation and compression optimize storage and transmission while ensuring real-time data analysis for timely healthcare interventions.

12.8.5 Data Storage, Integration, and Interoperability

Data storage, integration, and interoperability play pivotal roles in wearable-generated data management. Robust storage systems, which are often cloud-based, accommodate vast volumes of data. The effective integration of diverse data sources, including wearables, electronic health records, and clinical data, enhances comprehensive patient profiles. Ensuring interoperability through standardized formats and APIs facilitates seamless data exchange between systems, enabling holistic healthcare insights.

12.8.6 AI and Machine Learning in Health Monitoring

AI and machine learning have revolutionized health monitoring by analyzing wearable-generated data. These technologies can identify subtle patterns, detect anomalies, and predict health trends. By continuously learning from the data, AI assists in early disease detection, personalized treatment recommendations, and real-time interventions, ultimately enhancing the accuracy and effectiveness of remote patient care (see Figure 12.5). Figure 12.5 demonstrates remote patient monitoring using artificial intelligence.

12.9 Introduction to AI and ML Applications in Healthcare

The application of Artificial Intelligence (AI) and Machine Learning (ML) in healthcare resulted in transformative advancements. AI algorithms process vast datasets from wearables, electronic health records, and medical

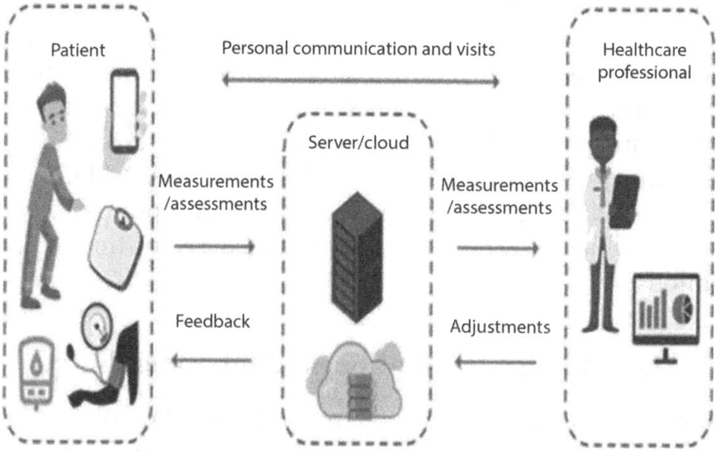

Figure 12.5 Remote patient monitoring using artificial intelligence.

imaging, thereby enabling accurate diagnosis, risk prediction, and treatment optimization. ML models learn from these data to identify nuanced patterns, aiding early disease detection and personalized medicine. These technologies empower healthcare professionals with data-driven insights, improve patient outcomes and transform healthcare into a proactive, precise, and patient-centric paradigm.

12.9.1 Predictive Analytics for Early Disease Detection

Predictive analytics powered by AI and ML have revolutionized early disease detection. By analyzing historical patient data from wearable devices and other sources, these models can identify subtle changes that precede overt symptoms. Through pattern recognition and correlation analysis, predictive algorithms can flag deviations from individual health baselines, thereby enabling timely intervention. Such technology is particularly impactful in chronic conditions such as diabetes, where predictive models can forecast blood sugar fluctuations. This approach shifts healthcare from reactive to proactive, enabling healthcare providers to initiate preventive measures, personalize treatment plans, and significantly improve patient outcomes by catching diseases at their earliest stages.

12.9.2 Real-Time Anomaly Detection and Alerts

Real-time anomaly detection and alerts in wearable health monitoring involve leveraging AI and ML to continuously analyze incoming data for deviations from the expected patterns. When unusual or potentially concerning changes are detected, such as sudden spikes in the heart rate or abnormal sleep patterns, immediate alerts are generated. These alerts can be transmitted to healthcare professionals and patients, enabling timely intervention and proactive management of health conditions. This dynamic approach enhances patient safety, improves early detection of health issues, and empowers individuals to take prompt action in response to critical changes in their well-being.

12.9.3 Clinical Decision Support Systems

Clinical Decision Support Systems (CDSS) powered by AI and data analytics provide healthcare professionals with evidence-based insights to aid in diagnosis, treatment planning, and patient care. By integrating wearable-generated data and electronic health records, the CDSS offers personalized recommendations, drug interaction alerts, and risk assessments. By processing vast amounts of patient information, these systems enhance medical decision making, reduce errors, and ensure adherence to best practices, ultimately improving the quality and safety of healthcare delivery.

12.9.4 Integration of AI Insights into Clinical Workflows

The integration of AI insights into clinical workflows has transformed healthcare practices. AI-driven analytics, fueled by wearable-generated data, offers valuable information to healthcare providers within their existing processes. For instance, AI algorithms can assist in diagnosing conditions based on wearables' real-time data, aiding clinicians in making more accurate and timely decisions. By seamlessly incorporating AI-generated insights into electronic health records and treatment plans, clinical workflows become more efficient and patient-centered, enhancing the quality of care and enabling healthcare professionals to harness the power of data-driven medicine.

12.9.5 Enabling Personalized Treatment Plans Based on Wearable Data

Utilization of wearable data enables the creation of personalized treatment plans through AI-driven insights. AI algorithms can identify individual health trends, triggers, and responses by analyzing comprehensive health data collected from wearables. This information empowers healthcare providers to tailor treatment regimens according to patients' unique needs and responses. Whether by adjusting medication dosages, recommending lifestyle modifications, or suggesting specific interventions, these personalized treatment plans optimize outcomes by aligning medical decisions with the patient's real-time health status and evolving health patterns.

12.9.6 Enhancing Healthcare Professional Decision-Making

AI-powered insights derived from wearable data significantly enhance professional healthcare decision-making. AI algorithms provide comprehensive insights into patient health trends, risk factors, and potential complications by analyzing diverse health metrics over time. This will empower clinicians to provide evidence-based recommendations for diagnosis, treatment, and patient management. Real-time alerts and predictive analytics enable proactive interventions, reduce errors, and streamline clinical decisions. This amalgamation of AI-generated insights with clinical expertise optimizes patient care, fostering more informed, timely, and effective decision making across the healthcare continuum.

12.9.7 Challenges and Ethical Considerations in Using Patient-Generated Data

Utilization of patient-generated data from wearables presents a range of challenges and ethical considerations. Ensuring data privacy and security is paramount because sensitive health information is involved. Data accuracy and reliability must also be addressed as wearables can produce errors or inconsistencies. The potential for data overload requires effective strategies to filter and prioritize relevant information for healthcare professionals. In addition, issues surrounding consent, ownership, and data sharing must be navigated transparently to uphold patient autonomy. Balancing the benefits of wearables with these challenges requires a framework that upholds patient rights, establishes data governance, and maintains the highest ethical standards for the collection, use, and protection of patient-generated data.

12.10 Future Directions and Trends

The trajectory of wearable devices, big data, and AI in remote patient care holds immense promise for transformative advancement. Wearables are expected to become more seamlessly integrated into everyday life, with increased focus on comfort, aesthetics, and long-term wearability. Big-data analytics will evolve to handle even larger and more diverse datasets, enabling more accurate predictive models and refined insights. AI algorithms will become more sophisticated and capable of deciphering intricate health patterns and offering real-time context-aware recommendations.

In the future, wearable devices could extend beyond monitoring physiological parameters to encompass mental health, cognitive function, and early signs of neurodegenerative disorders. The integration of wearables with telemedicine and virtual reality could enable immersive remote consultation and personalized rehabilitation programs. Ethical considerations and regulatory frameworks will continue to evolve, to ensure patient privacy and data protection.

Furthermore, advancements in wearables, big data, and AI will drive collaboration among healthcare professionals, data scientists, engineers, and designers, thereby fostering interdisciplinary innovations. The synergy of these technologies will redefine the boundaries of remote patient care, enabling proactive interventions, preventing diseases before symptoms manifest, and ultimately creating a more patient-centered and data-driven healthcare landscape. As these advancements unfold, the future of wearable devices and health monitoring promises to reshape the way we perceive and manage health, transcending the boundaries of traditional healthcare paradigms.

12.11 Conclusion

The convergence of wearable devices, big data, and artificial intelligence has ushered in a new era of remote patient care, thereby revolutionizing the healthcare landscape. The ability to continuously monitor health metrics through wearables and harness the power of big data analytics and AI has transformed how patients engage with their health and healthcare professionals deliver care. Wearable devices have evolved from mere accessories to integral tools for real-time health monitoring, thereby enabling proactive interventions and early disease detection. The synergy between big data and AI provides insights that are previously unattainable, thereby enhancing clinical decision-making and personalizing treatment plans. This data-driven approach not only empowers patients to take charge of their well-being, but also enables healthcare providers to deliver more precise and personalized care. The future holds the promise of wearables becoming more sophisticated and seamlessly integrated into our lives. Big data analytics and AI will continue to evolve, enabling healthcare to move beyond reactive responses to more proactive, predictive, and preventive approaches. However, this transformation is not without challenges, including data privacy, ethical considerations, and technical hurdles, which must be carefully navigated.

For wearable devices, big data and AI have united to reshape the future of remote patient care. This fusion of technology has the potential to enhance patient outcomes, improve healthcare efficiency, and empower individuals to prioritize and actively manage their health. With continued innovation and collaboration, the vision of data-driven, patient-centric healthcare systems powered by wearable technology is steadily becoming a reality.

References

1. Tuegel, E.J., Ingraffea, A.R., Eason, T.G., Spottswood, S.M., Reengineering aircraft structural life prediction using a digital twin. *Int. J. Aerosp. Eng.*, 2011, 1–14, Aug. 2021.
2. Lu, Y., Liu, C., Wang, K., II, Huang, H., Xu, X., Digital twin-driven smart manufacturing: Connotation reference model applications and research issues. *Robot. Comput.-Integr. Manuf.*, 61, Feb. 2020.
3. Qi, Q. and Tao, F., Digital twin and big data towards smart manufacturing and industry 4.0: 360 degree comparison. *IEEE Access*, 6, 3585–3593, 2018.
4. Rasheed, A., San, O., Kvamsdal, T., Digital twin: Values challenges and enablers from a modeling perspective. *IEEE Access*, 8, 21980–22012, 2020.
5. Okoli, C. and Schabram, K., A guide to conducting a systematic literature review of information systems research. *Communications of the Association for Information Systems*, 37, 879–910, 2015, [online] Available: http://dx.doi.org/10.2139/ssrn.1954824.
6. Grieves, M. and Vickers, J., Digital twin: Mitigating unpredictable undesirable emergent behavior in complex systems, in: *Transdisciplinary Perspectives on Complex Systems*, pp. 85–113, Springer, Cham, Switzerland, 2017.
7. Glaessgen, E. and Stargel, D., The digital twin paradigm for future NASA and US air force vehicles. *Proc. 53rd AIAA/ASME/ASCE/AHS/ASC Struct. Struct. Dyn. Mater. Conf. 20th AIAA/ASME/AHS Adapt. Struct. Conf. 14th AIAA*, p. 1818, 2022.
8. Söderberg, R., Wärmefjord, K., Carlson, J.S., Lindkvist, L., Toward a digital twin for real-time geometry assurance in individualized production. *CIRP Ann.*, 66, 1, 137–140, 2017.
9. Dong, R., She, C., Hardjawana, W., Li, Y., Vucetic, B., Deep learning for hybrid 5G services in mobile edge computing systems: Learn from a digital twin. *IEEE Trans. Wirel. Commun.*, 18, 10, 4692–4707, Oct. 2019.
10. Björnsson, B., Borrebaeck, C., Elander, N., Gasslander, T., Gawel, D.R., Gustafsson, M. *et al.*, Digital twins to personalize medicine. *Genome Med.*, 12, 1, 1–4, Dec. 2020.

13

Disease Biomarker Discovery with Big Data Analysis

G. Venu Gopal[1], Kanakaprabha S.[2*], Gangavarapu Moahana Rao[3], Yallapragada Ravi Raju[4] and G. Ganesh Kumar[5]

[1]*Department of Computer Science and Engineering, KL education Foundation, Guntur, India*
[2]*Department of Computer Science and Engineering, Rathinam Technical Campus, Anna University, Coimbatore, India*
[3]*Department of Computer Science and Engineering, Rajiv Gandhi University of Knowledge Technology, Nuzividu, Andhra Pradesh, India*
[4]*Department of Computer Science and Engineering, Madanapalle Institute of Technology and Science, Madanapalle, Andhra Pradesh, India*
[5]*Department of Information Technology, Hindusthan Institute of Technology, Coimbatore, India*

Abstract

In the pursuit of enhancing disease diagnosis, prognosis, and treatment, the integration of big data analytics and biomarker discovery has emerged as a pivotal approach. This abstract provides a concise overview of the intricate interplay between disease biomarker identification and the utilization of large-scale data analysis techniques. The chapter emphasizes the imperative role of machine learning in deciphering multi-omics data, illuminating challenges, methodologies, and case studies, while also addressing ethical considerations. By delving into the amalgamation of diverse omics data, this chapter underscores the potential to unveil novel insights, transforming healthcare through personalized medicine paradigms.

***Keywords*:** Approach, disease, diagnosis, healthcare, medicine, personalized

**Corresponding author*: skanakaprabha.@gmail.com

Neha Sharma, Korhan Cengiz and Prasenjit Chatterjee (eds.) Intelligent Data Analytics for Bioinformatics and Biomedical Systems, (313–330) © 2024 Scrivener Publishing LLC

13.1 Introduction

In the period of care drug, the identification of reliable disease biomarkers holds immense potential for revolutionizing healthcare practices. The convergence of big data analysis and biomarker discovery has emerged as a formidable approach to unearth hidden patterns and unveil molecular signatures indicative of various diseases. This chapter delves into the synergistic relationship between disease biomarker identification and the control of big data analytics. By harnessing the wealth of information generated by high-throughput technologies across multiple omics domains, including genomics, proteomics, metabolomics, and transcriptomics, researchers can gain deeper insights into the underlying molecular mechanisms of diseases [1]. This introduction sets the stage for an exploration of advanced machine learning techniques that enable the extraction of expressive data from multi-omics data, ultimately leading to the discovery of robust and clinically relevant biomarkers.

13.1.1 The Need for Multi-Omics Data Integration in Biomarker Discovery

Traditional biomarker discovery often relied on single-dimensional data, limiting the comprehensive understanding of disease complexities. With the advent of multi-omics technologies, researchers are now equipped to capture a holistic view of biological systems. However, this integration presents challenges arising from data heterogeneity, dimensionality, and noise. Overcoming these hurdles is imperative to harness the full potential of multi-omics data for accurate biomarker identification (refer to Figure 13.1).

13.1.2 Role of Machine Learning in Multi-Omics Data Analysis

Machine learning algorithms have demonstrated their prowess in handling complex and high-dimensional facts. In the framework of multi-omics data, machine learning offers the means to uncover intricate relationships, classify disease states, and predict treatment outcomes [2]. This chapter will delve into various machine learning approaches, including traditional methods, deep learning architectures, and network-based models, which collectively provide the toolkit for integrating, analyzing, and interpreting multi-omics data (refer to Figure 13.2).

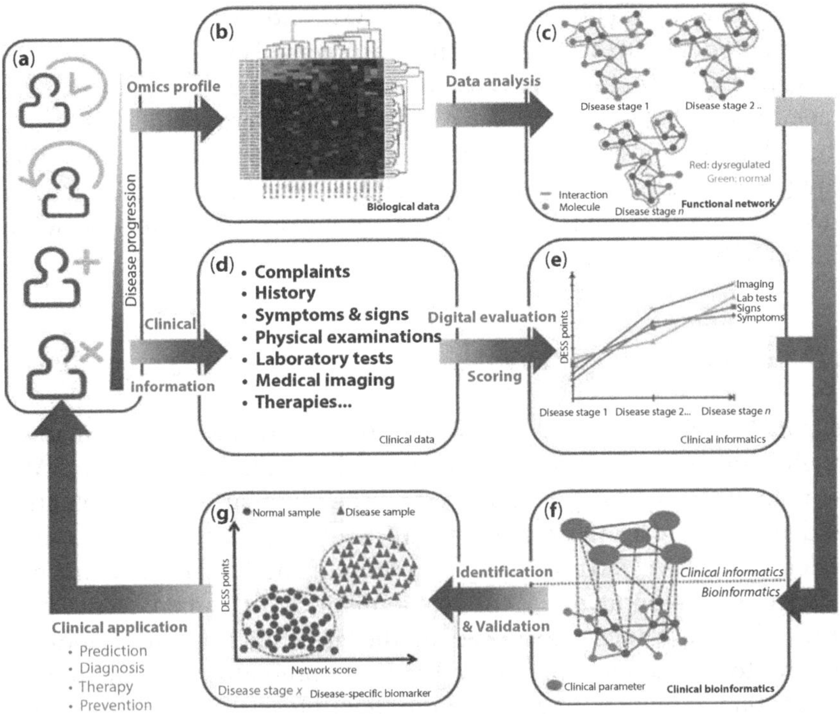

Figure 13.1 Bioinformatics clinical informatics.

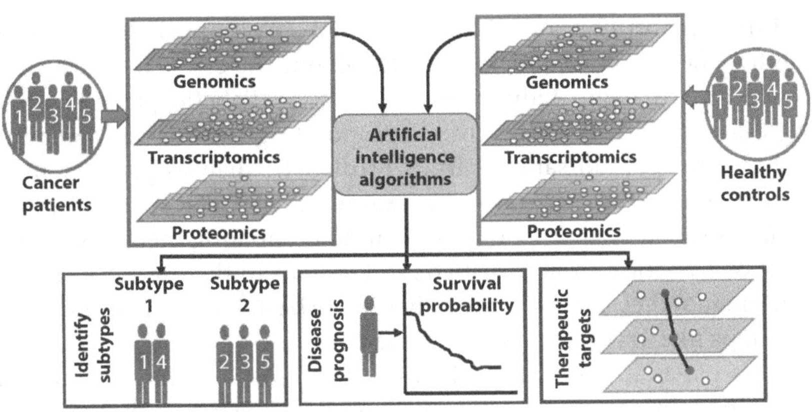

Figure 13.2 Multi-omics data analysis.

By marrying the fields of big data analysis and biomarker discovery, this chapter underscores the transformative potential of unraveling disease heterogeneity, advancing diagnostic accuracy, and guiding personalized therapeutic interventions. Through a systematic exploration of challenges, methodologies, case studies, and ethical considerations, this chapter aims to equip researchers, clinicians, and bioinformaticians with the insights needed to navigate the intricate landscape of disease biomarker discovery in the era of big data analytics [3].

13.2 Literature Survey

This paper showcases the efficacy of utilizing structured information through a practical illustration involving a biomarker use case. [1] We present an extensive compilation of established biomarkers and potential candidates sourced from existing literature. Our approach employs four prevalent neuropsychiatric disorders to exemplify both shared and distinctive biomarker components. We illustrate distinct enrichment trends and offer insights into tactics for uncovering the latest and innovative findings conducive to biomarker exploration. Lastly, we present a novel and inventive taxonomy grounded in brain region identifiers, significantly enhancing the capacity for comprehensive and intricate information retrieval in the domain of neuroscience research.

The study comprises two main aspects: firstly, it involves a thorough analysis aimed at identifying metabolite profiles that differentiate between individuals with diabetes in the Emirates and their healthy counterparts. [2] This analysis entails the examination of blood samples from 50 diabetic Emiratis and 42 healthy individuals to uncover metabolite variations. Secondly, the study conducts a metabolomic investigation comparing patients with diabetic kidney disease to non-diabetic patients undergoing dialysis, with the objective of pinpointing distinctive biomarkers. To achieve this, blood samples from 11 diabetic dialysis patients and 25 non-diabetic dialysis patients were examined. The research successfully identifies a substantial array of potential differentiating metabolites in the context of diabetic and non-diabetic individuals in the Emirates. The discerned metabolites are systematically categorized, including classification into groups like Tryptophan and Purines.

In this paper [3] Biomarker investigation holds promising prospects within the realms of atopic dermatitis and psoriasis research. Despite the existence of various efficacious treatments, substantial challenges persist pertaining to diagnosis precision, targeted therapeutic development, as well as ethical and societal considerations [4]. This paper leverages a comprehensive evaluation of existing literature and rational analysis to delve into the ethical and societal discourse surrounding biomarker exploration in the context of atopic dermatitis and psoriasis. The examination encompasses subjects including the advantages and drawbacks of segmenting patient cohorts, ethical implications linked to extensive data and advanced analytics for biomarker integration in atopic dermatitis and psoriasis.

The rise of genomic sketching skills and focused molecular embattled remedies has amplified the significance of biomarkers in the clinical care of individuals with cancer. Single gene/protein assessments as well as multigene "signature" analyses have been introduced to gauge specific disruptions in molecular pathways, [4] offering guidance for therapeutic choices as predictive biomarkers. Moreover, genome-based predictive biomarkers are accessible for numerous cancer types, with the possible to be integrated into clinical extrapolative staging schemes or practice strategies. However, a substantial disparity persists between the original unearthing of biomarkers and their actual clinical implementation, owing to the contests inherent in the journey of cancer biomarker advancement.

In this paper we present an overview of the latest progress in utilizing big data analyses within the realms of precision medicine and health informatics. As technological strides enable the collection of molecular and medical information, we have entered the realm of "Big Data" within the fields of biology and medicine. These expansive datasets hold immense potential for advancing precision medicine. [5] We delineate primary challenges encountered in precision medicine and detail recent breakthroughs in methods that integrate data to extract personalized insights from the extensive datasets generated by diverse omics studies. We review current integrative techniques for disease classification, biomarker identification, and drug repurposing, while also enumerating the available tools for experts in the field. Given the incessant growth of these vast datasets, we underscore the critical challenges that big data integration methods are poised to confront.

In this paper [6] Earlier approaches utilized "triangular strategies" that focused on identifying individual biomarker candidates within limited cohorts, succeeded by traditional immunoassays conducted on significantly larger validation cohorts. In contrast, we introduce a "rectangular" approach to plasma proteome profiling. Here, the proteomic profiles of extensive cohorts are linked with their health and disease phenotypes. Implementing such concepts in clinical settings entails restructuring various aspects of diagnostic decision-making. We explore initial strides taken in this direction.

In this paper it was ongoing discovery of novel proteins and metabolites with potential as biomarkers, alongside patient genetic, [7] clinical, and environmental data, including microbiota information, is paving the way for cutting-edge clinical decision support systems (CDSSs) driven by machine learning models, tailored for personalized ASD-focused medication. In this context, we delve into innovative computational solutions aimed at evaluating the viability of new ASD biomarker candidates within the proteome and metabolome domains. This assessment takes into account their frequency of occurrence in existing literature and feasibility in laboratory medicine. Furthermore, we explore the utilization of CDSS empowered by artificial intelligence as a potent avenue to seamlessly participate omics data into electronic health/medical records (EHR/EMR), potentially adding substantial value in the foreseeable coming to the experimental management of ASD.

In this paper Comprehensive integration was achieved by amalgamating well-linked details encompassing molecular attributes, experimental biology, gene expression patterns, overall survival data, functional substantiation, [8] tumor staging, and clinical applicability. This research, operating under a data-driven and literature-informed paradigm for biomarker exploration, not only presented corroborative analyses but also identified 36 promising molecules, with IGF1R and FRS2 emerging as the most potent prognostic biomarkers. Consequently, ExoBCD stands as the inaugural extensively validated knowledge repository for exosomal investigations in breast cancer. Beyond laying the groundwork for subsequent inquiries, it bolsters endeavors aimed at unraveling molecular mechanisms, pinpointing biomarkers, and advancing meaningful clinical utility.

In this paper [9] the emergence of artificial intelligence, notably machine learning, alongside systems biology, has provided a pathway for the streamlined amalgamation and elucidation of vast datasets, facilitating the discovery of clinically relevant insights. Within this narrative review, we explore the utilization of big data integration and machine learning within the context of translational research focused on IBD. Methods like machine learning offer the potential to refine patient classification, predict disease evolution, and anticipate therapy responses, thereby optimizing treatment choices and positively affecting cost, well-being, and safety. Additionally, we delineate the challenges and prospects presented by machine learning and big data in the realm of clinical IBD research.

In this study paper [10] facilitated the identification of key attributes within medical big data, their utilization within the domain of cardiology, and the analytical approaches applied to this extensive data. The outcomes of this investigation reveal a significant body of research dedicated to therapeutic big data in the context of cardiology. This research serves to consolidate and structure the prevailing literature based on predefined keywords and explore inquiries. The findings of this investigation stand to enhance clinical decision-making, providing a basis for more reliable choices that can be leveraged as substantial evidence in the treatment of individuals afflicted with cardiovascular conditions.

13.3 Challenges in Multi-Omics Data Integration

The combination of multi-omics data for disease biomarker discovery is a promising avenue but is accompanied by a range of challenges that necessitate careful consideration and innovative solutions [11].

13.3.1 Data Heterogeneity and Integration Challenges

Multi-omics datasets encompass diverse molecular layers, such as genomics, transcriptomics, proteomics, and metabolomics. Each layer exhibits distinct characteristics, including different data types, scales, and sources. Integrating these heterogeneous datasets requires addressing issues of data alignment, normalization, and integration. Mismatched resolutions and missing values across omics layers can introduce biases that hinder the accurate extraction of meaningful information.

13.3.2 Dimensionality Reduction and Feature Selection

Multi-omics datasets are often high-dimensional, leading to the "curse of dimensionality. "High-dimensional data exacerbates computational complexity, increases noise, and may lead to overfitting. Dimensionality lessening techniques, such as principal component analysis (PCA) and t-distributed stochastic neighbor embedding (t-SNE), are working to transform the data into lower-dimensional spaces. Additionally, selecting relevant features across omics layers is critical for reducing noise and extracting essential information, necessitating robust feature selection strategies [12].

13.3.3 Feature Representation and Integration Techniques

The integration of multi-omics data is navigated through a spectrum of techniques. Early fusion merges disparate omics data at the outset, aiming to capture collective information, while late fusion maintains data separation until later stages, harmonizing results at the integration point. Network-based methods exploit biological interactions to prioritize features, revealing dysregulated modules. Deep learning architectures leverage neural networks to unveil intricate patterns in raw data, accommodating hierarchical relationships. These approaches collectively empower researchers to transcend data heterogeneity, unearth biologically meaningful biomarkers, and enhance disease understanding with unprecedented depth and accuracy.

13.3.4 Early Fusion vs. Late Fusion Approaches

In the pursuit of effectively integrating multi-omics data, researchers employ either initial fusion or late fusion strategies. Primary fusion involves combining raw or preprocessed data from different omics layers at the outset, creating a unified representation. This approach seeks to capture shared information across omics types but can be challenged by differences in data scales and distributions. In contrast, late fusion maintains separate processing of each omics layer until a later stage, where integrated features are combined for analysis. While potentially mitigating heterogeneity challenges, late fusion requires additional steps to synthesize information. Selecting the optimal fusion strategy depends on the specific research objectives and the extent to which cross-omics relationships need to be captured [13].

13.3.5 Network-Based Integration Methods

Network-based integration leverages biological knowledge to facilitate the integration of multi-omics data. By constructing molecular interaction networks that represent relationships between genes, proteins, and other molecules, these methods provide a framework to prioritize biologically relevant features and identify key regulatory elements. Nodes and edges in the network correspond to molecular entities and their interactions, enabling the identification of modules or clusters that are dysregulated in diseases. Network-based integration empowers the discovery of biomarkers within a context of biological pathways and interactions, enhancing the interpretability of the results [14].

13.4 Deep Learning Architectures for Multi-Omics Data

Deep learning has emerged as a formidable tool for multi-omics data analysis due to its aptitude to mechanically learn complex representations from

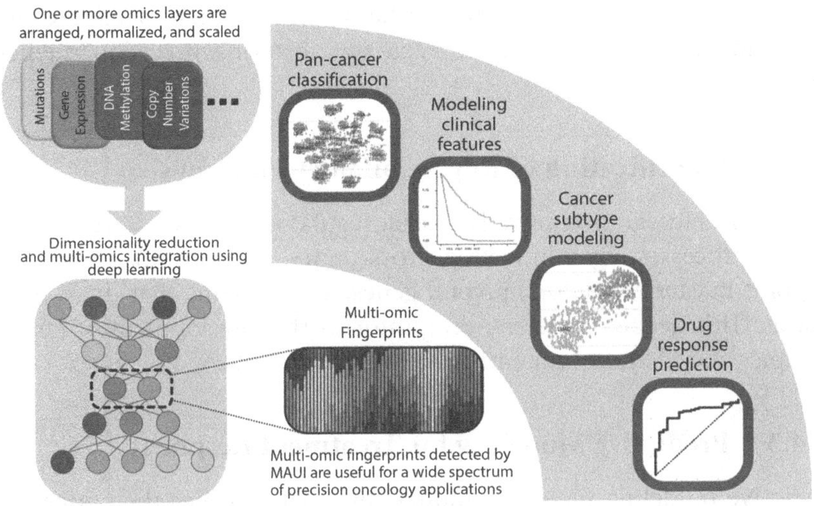

Figure 13.3 Deep learning architectures for multi-omics data.

raw data. Deep neural networks, including autoencoders, convolutional neural networks (CNNs), and recurrent neural networks (RNNs), enable the extraction of hierarchical and abstract features from multi-omics data. These architectures capture intricate patterns and relationships, enabling the discovery of hidden biomarkers. Transfer learning and generative adversarial networks (GANs) further extend the utility of deep learning by transferring knowledge from one omics domain to another and generating synthetic data samples, respectively (refer to Figure 13.3).

While powerful, the application of deep learning methods necessitates substantial data and computational resources and demands careful regularization to avoid overfitting. Collectively, these feature representation and integration techniques offer a range of strategies to harmonize diverse omics data sources and extract meaningful insights. The high-quality of approach be contingent on the nature of the data, the explore areas, and the computational resources available, ultimately contributing to the discovery of robust disease biomarkers with enhanced accuracy and clinical relevance.

13.4.1 Disease Subtyping and Stratification

Integrative analysis of multi-omics data offers a transformative perspective on disease subtyping and stratification. By capturing intricate molecular signatures across omics layers, researchers can delineate distinct disease subtypes with unique underlying mechanisms. This enables tailored treatments and enhances prognostic accuracy, fostering precision medicine paradigms.

13.4.2 Identification of Key Regulatory Pathways

Multi-omics integration unveils crucial regulatory pathways orchestrating disease processes. By unraveling cross-omics relationships, researchers pinpoint master regulators, pivotal genes, and proteins that drive pathogenesis. This deeper understanding informs the development of targeted therapies and identifies potential intervention points.

13.4.3 Predictive Modeling for Treatment Response

Predictive modeling fueled by multi-omics data enables the anticipation of patient response to treatments. By discerning predictive biomarkers, researchers can optimize therapeutic strategies, minimize adverse effects, and elevate patient outcomes. This empowers clinicians to make informed decisions based on molecular insights.

The integrative analysis of multi-omics data empowers researchers to transcend conventional boundaries, catalyzing disease understanding, treatment personalization, and biomarker-driven healthcare advancements.

13.4.4 Cancer Biomarker Discovery Using Multi-Omics Data

The application of multi-omics data integration in cancer biomarker discovery has revolutionized our understanding of this complex disease. By combining genomics, transcriptomics, proteomics, and metabolomics data, researchers can decipher the intricate landscape of molecular alterations driving tumorigenesis (refer to Figure 13.4).

Through integrative analyses, distinctive molecular subtypes within cancers can be unveiled, aiding in prognosis and treatment decisions. Case studies demonstrate how cross-omics interactions expose novel biomarkers, shedding light on early detection, personalized therapy, and improved patient outcomes.

13.4.5 Neurological Disorder Classification through Integration

Neurological disorders present intricate challenges due to their multifaceted etiologies. Integrative analysis of multi-omics data offers a hopeful avenue to dissect these complexities. By amalgamating genomics,

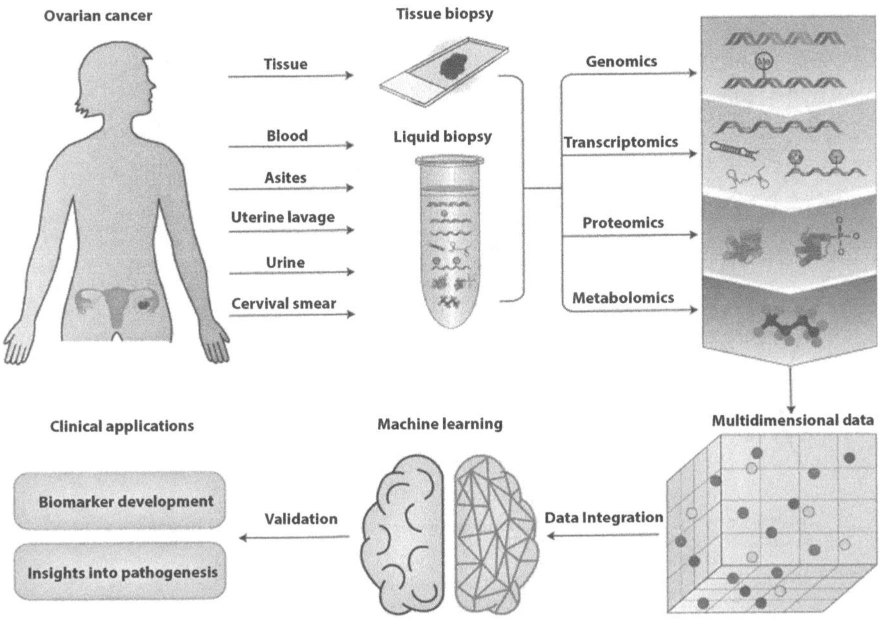

Figure 13.4 Cancer biomarker discovery using multi-omics data.

transcriptomics, and other omics layers, researchers can identify shared molecular pathways across disorders, paving the way for accurate classification and differential diagnosis.

Case studies showcase how machine learning algorithms leverage integrated data to distinguish subtypes within neurological disorders, unraveling crucial insights for tailored interventions and advancements in neurological healthcare. These case studies exemplify the transformative potential of multi-omics data integration, showcasing how it not only enhances disease understanding but also shapes clinical practices and therapeutic strategies across diverse medical domains [15].

13.5 Evaluation Metrics and Validation Strategies

In the realm of multi-omics data analysis, meticulous evaluation and validation are paramount. Cross-validation techniques, like k-fold and stratified cross-validation, tailor the assessment of predictive models to the complexities of multi-omics data, ensuring robustness and mitigating overfitting. Complementary to this, assessing the robustness and generalizability of biomarker models through methods such as bootstrapping and

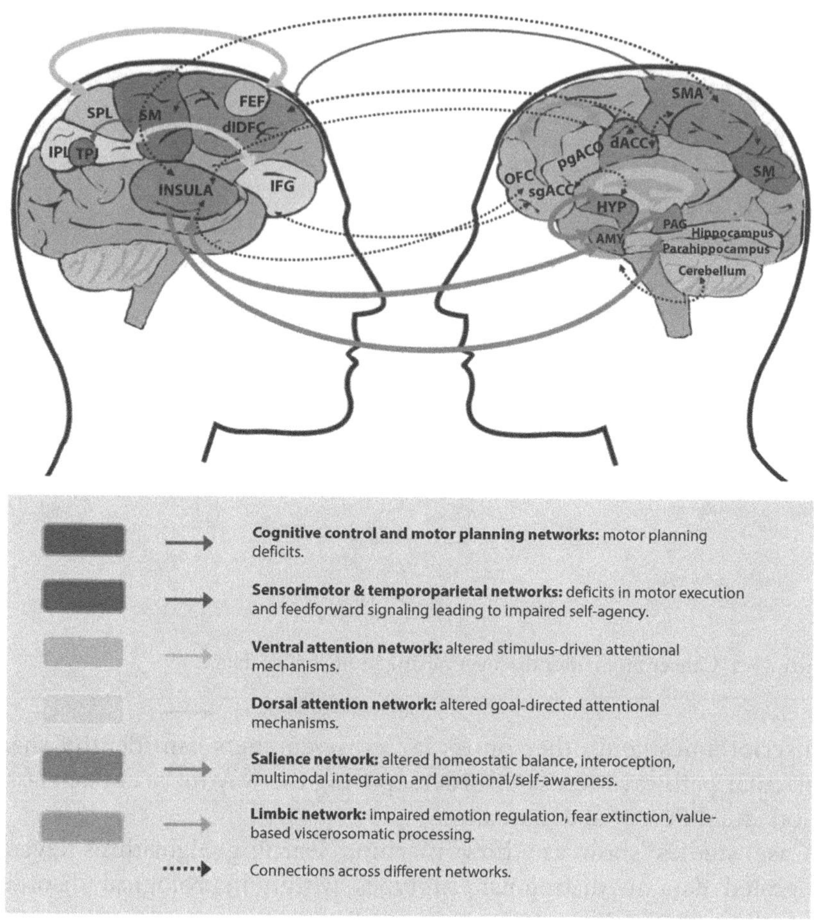

Figure 13.5 Neurological disorder classification.

external validation validates their reliability and applicability in diverse contexts [16]. Together, these strategies provide a solid foundation for confident biomarker discovery, offering insights that transcend the intricacies of multi-omics datasets and guiding their potential translation into clinical practice. Figure 13.5 shows the evidence of the improved performance of the algorithm when applied to the dataset, demonstrating a significant reduction in error rates compared to previous models.

13.5.1 Cross-Validation Techniques for Multi-Omics Data

The evaluation of predictive models derived from multi-omics data necessitates specialized validation techniques. Cross-validation, such as k-fold and stratified cross-validation, divides the dataset into subsets, allowing each subset to serve as both training and validation data [17]. This mitigates the risk of overfitting and provides a more accurate estimation of model performance across different omics layers. Cross-validation ensures that the model's predictive capacity is robust and capable of handling the inherent complexities of multi-omics data.

13.5.2 Assessing Robustness and Generalizability of Biomarker Models

Ensuring the reliability and applicability of biomarker models demands rigorous assessment. Bootstrapping and permutation tests gauge the stability of selected biomarkers by repeatedly resampling the dataset and observing the consistency of identified features. Additionally, external validation using independent datasets or data from different cohorts validates the model's ability to generalize beyond the training data. This evaluation safeguards against overfitting and validates the clinical utility of biomarkers in diverse contexts. By employing cross-validation and robustness assessment techniques, researchers can confidently ascertain the performance, reliability, and generalizability of biomarker models derived from multi-omics data. These strategies bolster the credibility of biomarker discoveries and pave the way for their integration into clinical practice, thereby enhancing disease management and patient care [18].

13.6 Ethical Considerations in Biomarker Discovery

Ethical considerations are integral to the advancement of biomarker discovery in the context of multi-omics data analysis. As researchers harness vast amounts of personal and health-related information, critical ethical dimensions come into play.

13.6.1 Privacy and Security of Patient Data

Preserving the privacy and security of patient data constitutes a cornerstone of ethical multi-omics biomarker discovery. As multi-omics data contains intimate health-related information, safeguarding patient identities and sensitive details is paramount. Employing robust anonymization techniques and encryption safeguards data against unauthorized access. Adherence to stringent data protection regulations, such as HIPAA and

GDPR, establishes a strong framework to ensure that patient trust remains uncompromised and the potential benefits of biomarker discoveries are achieved while respecting individual privacy.

13.6.2 Bias and Fairness in Machine Learning Models

The integration of machine learning in biomarker discovery necessitates vigilant attention to potential biases within multi-omics data. These biases can perpetuate discriminatory outcomes, reinforcing inequalities across different population groups. Ensuring fairness requires rigorous assessment and mitigation of biases in data collection, preprocessing, and algorithm design. Transparent reporting of bias-mitigation efforts and continuous monitoring during model deployment fosters equitable biomarker discoveries that can be applied across diverse populations, contributing to the advancement of inclusive healthcare practices.

13.6.3 Integration of Single-Cell Omics Data

The addition of single-cell omics statistics holds immense promise for advancing biomarker discovery. Single-cell technologies provide unprecedented resolution, enabling the characterization of cellular heterogeneity within tissues. Integrating single-cell genomics, transcriptomics, and proteomics data can unravel intricate disease mechanisms at a cellular level,

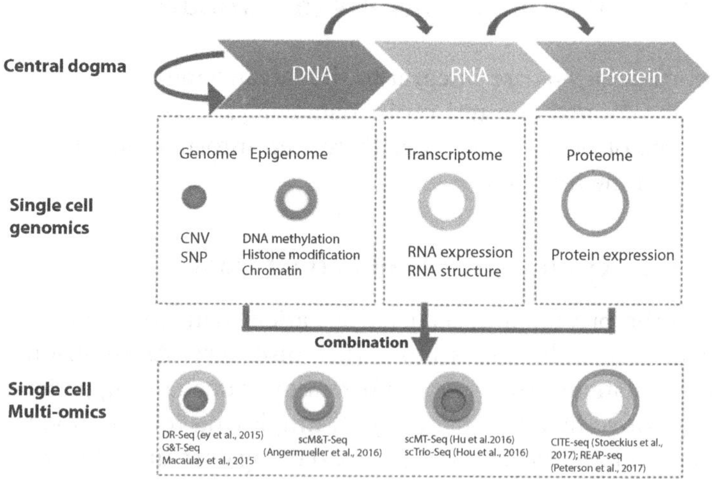

Figure 13.6 Single-cell omics data.

facilitating the identification of rare cell populations, cell states, and their contributions to disease progression (refer to Figure 13.6).

However, this integration presents novel challenges, including data sparseness and noise inherent to single-cell measurements. Innovative methodologies that account for these challenges will be essential to attach the full potential of single-cell omics data and ambition biomarker discovery toward a deeper understanding of disease biology.

13.6.4 Explainable AI for Biomarker Discovery

As AI methods become integral to biomarker discovery, ensuring transparency and interpretability of these models gains significance. Explainable AI (XAI) techniques aim to demystify the decision-making process of complex machine learning models. In biomarker discovery, XAI can elucidate how specific omics features are contributing to predictions, enabling researchers and clinicians to understand the biological context and rationale behind identified biomarkers. By providing insights into the relationships between input features and model outputs, XAI enhances trust, facilitates model validation, and fosters the integration of AI-driven biomarkers into clinical practice. As biomarker discovery transitions from data-driven insights to actionable knowledge, the adoption of XAI will play a pivotal role in bridging the gap between computational predictions and biological interpretation.

13.6.5 Personalized Medicine and Biomarker-Based Therapies

The mixing of multi-omics data holds the key to unlocking the potential of personalized medicine and biomarker-driven therapies. By comprehensively characterizing individual patients' molecular profiles, multi-omics data enable the identification of unique biomarker signatures that guide tailored treatment strategies. These signatures can inform decisions about drug selection, dosages, and treatment regimens, optimizing therapeutic outcomes while minimizing adverse effects (refer to Figure 13.7).

Furthermore, the integration of real-time patient data allows for dynamic treatment adjustments, ensuring interventions remain aligned with patients' evolving molecular landscapes. As technology advances and our understanding of disease complexity deepens, multi-omics-driven personalized medicine stands poised to reshape healthcare by offering precise, effective, and patient-centered therapeutic interventions.

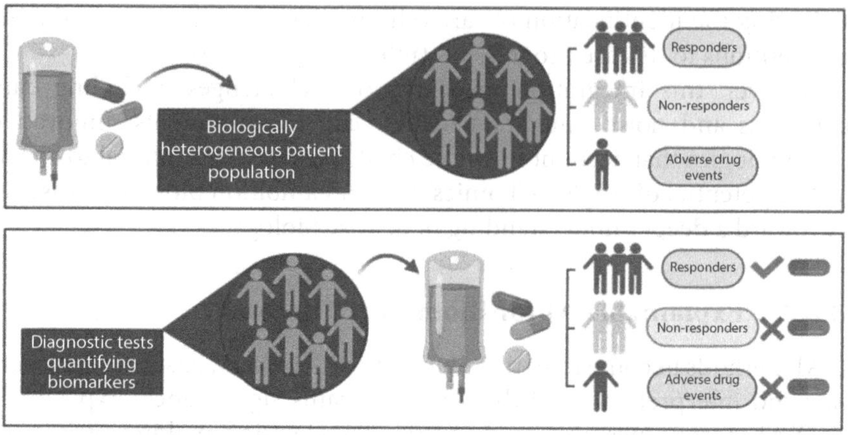

Figure 13.7 Personalized medicine and biomarker therapies.

13.7 Conclusion

The journey of disease biomarker discovery with big data analysis has illuminated new avenues for unraveling the complexities of diseases and transforming healthcare paradigms. This exploration has underscored the remarkable synergy between cutting-edge technologies and innovative methodologies, showcasing how multi-omics data integration, machine learning, and ethical considerations collectively reshape the landscape of biomarker identification. By addressing challenges in data integration, feature representation, and validation strategies, researchers have unlocked the potential to decode intricate molecular signatures underlying diseases. The presented case studies have highlighted the tangible impact of these approaches in enhancing diagnostics, prognosis, and treatment strategies across diverse medical domains.

Ethical considerations, such as privacy preservation and fairness in AI, have been emphasized as integral facets of responsible biomarker discovery. As advancements continue, the integration of single-cell omics data promises to add granularity to our understanding of diseases, while explainable AI ensures that the knowledge gained remains transparent and interpretable. The future, illuminated by the prospect of personalized medicine and biomarker-based therapies, holds the promise of revolutionizing patient care. The alignment of individual molecular profiles with tailored treatment strategies offers the potential to maximize therapeutic efficacy, minimize adverse effects, and ultimately redefine the standard of healthcare distribution. As we stand at the junction of data-driven discovery and health care alteration, the synergy of big data analysis and biomarker exploration offers a roadmap to a future where diseases are detected earlier, treated more effectively, and personalized medicine becomes a reality. This journey, while challenging, underscores the indomitable spirit of scientific inquiry and the potential of human ingenuity to reshape the medical landscape for the better.

References

1. Unkovic, P. and Basuray, A., Heart failure with recovered EF and heart failure with mid-range EF: Current recommendations and controversies. *Curr. Treat. Options Cardiovasc. Med.*, 20, 35, Apr. 2021.
2. Kitchenham, B., Brereton, O.P., Budgen, D., Turner, M., Bailey, J., Linkman, S., Systematic literature reviews in software engineering—A systematic literature review. *Inf. Software Technol.*, 51, 7–15, Jan. 2019.
3. Goyal, J., Sharma, N., Kumar, A., Anand, A., Prabha, C., Classifying Diabetes Using Artificially Intelligent Techniques: A Comparative Analysis. *2023 IEEE 2nd International Conference on Industrial Electronics: Developments & Applications (ICIDeA)*, IEEE, pp. 353–358, 2023, September.
4. Rumsfeld, J.S., Joynt, K.E., Maddox, T.M., Big data analytics to improve cardiovascular care: Promise and challenges. *Nat. Rev. Cardiol.*, 13, 6, 350–359, Mar. 2020.
5. Davarzani, N., Wijk, S.S.-V., Maeder, M.T., Rickenbacher, P., Smirnov, E., Karel, J. *et al.*, Novel concept to guide systolic heart failure medication by repeated biomarker testing—Results from TIME-CHF in context of predictive preventive and personalized medicine. *EPMA J.*, 9, 2, 161–173, 2020.
6. Srivastav, G., Rashid, M., Singh, R., Gehlot, A., Sharma, N., Breast Cancer Detection in Mammogram Images using Machine Learning Methods and CLAHE Algorithm, in: *2022 5th International Conference on Contemporary Computing and Informatics (IC3I)*, IEEE, pp. 1187–1192, 2022, December.
7. Kinkorová, J. and Topolčan, O., Biobanks in Horizon 2020: Sustainability and attractive perspectives. *EPMA J.*, 9, 345–353, Dec. 2018.
8. Golubnitschaja, O., Kinkorova, J., Costigliola, V., Predictive Preventive and Personalised Medicine as the hardcore of 'Horizon 2020': EPMA position paper. *EPMA J.*, 5, 1, 1–29, 2021.
9. Kumar, A., Sharma, N., Chauhan, R., Khare, A., Anand, A., Sharma, M., A Stack Ensemble Approach for Early Alzheimer Classification Using Machine Learning Algorithms, in: *International Conference on Recent Trends in Image Processing and Pattern Recognition*, pp. 82–96, Springer Nature Switzerland, Cham, 2023, December.
10. Golubnitschaja, O., Watson, I.D., Sandberg, S., Ferrari, M., Costigliola, V., Position paper of the EPMA and EFLM: A global vision of the consolidated

promotion of an integrative medical approach to advance health care. *EPMA J.*, 4, 1, 12, 2019.

11. Mitra, D., Sharma, N., Rashid, M., Singh, R., Classification Rules based Breast Cancer Detection using Machine Learning Approach, in: *2022 5th International Conference on Contemporary Computing and Informatics (IC3I)*, IEEE, pp. 1274–1278, 2022, December.
12. Scruggs, S.B., Watson, K., Su, A., II, Hermjakob, H., Yates, J.R., Lindsey, M.L. *et al.*, Harnessing the heart of big data. *Circulat. Res.*, 116, 7, 1115–1119, 2019.
13. Sharma, N., Chakraborty, C., Kumar, R., Optimized multimedia data through computationally intelligent algorithms. *Multimed. Syst.*, 29, 5, 2961–2977, 2023.
14. Vaishali, G. and Kalaivani, V., Big data analysis for heart disease detection system using map reduce technique. *Int. Conf. Comput. Technol. Intell. Data Eng. (ICCTIDE)*, 2020.
15. Sharma, N. and Batra, U., An enhanced Huffman-PSO based image optimization algorithm for image steganography. *Genet. Program. Evolvable Mach.*, 22, 189–205, 2021.
16. Seth, D., Biswas, N., Ghosh, D., Big health data: Cardiac remodelling and functional interactions of big brain based implications in body sensor networks. *7th Int. Conf. Commun. Syst. Netw. Technol.*, 2021.
17. Lutimath, N.M., Sharma, N., Byregowda, B.K., Prediction of heart disease using random forest, in: *2021 Emerging Trends in Industry 4.0 (ETI 4.0)*, IEEE, pp. 1–4, 2021, May.
18. Lutimath, N.M., Ramachandra, H.V., Raghav, S., Sharma, N., Prediction of heart disease using genetic algorithm, in: *Proceedings of Second Doctoral Symposium on Computational Intelligence: DoSCI 2021*, pp. 49–58, Springer, Singapore, 2022.

14

Real-Time Epilepsy Monitoring and Alerting System Using IoT Devices and Machine Learning Techniques in Blockchain-Based Environment

Mohsen Ghorbian[1] and Saeid Ghorbian[2]*

[1]*Department of Computer Engineering, Qom Branch, Islamic Azad University, Qom, Iran*

[2]*Department of Molecular Genetics, Ahar Branch, Islamic Azad University, Ahar, Iran*

Abstract

Epilepsy patients are constantly at risk of an attack. Epileptic attacks are unpredictable and can result in irreparable damage; when they happen in high-risk environments, patients can be caused die. It is crucial to anticipate epileptic attacks before they occur to reduce patients' risks. The use of new technologies can predict the occurrence of epileptic attacks to a great extent. This chapter proposes an intelligent alert mechanism using new technologies such as Internet of Things (IoT), Machine Learning (ML), and blockchain. The proposed mechanism includes three phases. The first phase of the proposed mechanism involves continuously gathering brainwave data through sensors embedded in IoT devices and storing it in the Hyperledger Fabric (HLF) blockchain using the Accessibility mechanism. In the second phase, which includes the analysis of the gathered data, the intelligent analysis mechanism, using powerful ML algorithms, attempts to analyze and predict epilepsy attacks. In the third phase, the Alert mechanism attempts to notify the patient's relatives and predetermined medical centers in case of the prediction of possible epileptic attacks by sending an alerting message. With the proposed mechanism, epileptic attacks can be predicted to a great extent, reducing both the physical damage and psychological impact of such attacks. The proposed mechanism allows all communication processes to be secured using the HLF blockchain,

**Corresponding author*: ghorbian20@gmail.com

Neha Sharma, Korhan Cengiz and Prasenjit Chatterjee (eds.) Intelligent Data Analytics for Bioinformatics and Biomedical Systems, (331–356) © 2024 Scrivener Publishing LLC

which is expected to reduce concerns associated with the security of communication processes significantly.

Keywords: Hyperledger fabric blockchain, machine learning, Internet of Things, epilepsy attacks, intelligent alert mechanism

14.1 Introduction

Epilepsy attack is a neurological condition with many causes. Epilepsy attacks can be triggered by brain damage. In other words, damage to the brain has been identified as one of the causes of epilepsy attacks. The electrical activity of the patient's brain changes abnormally with the onset of epileptic attacks, as reflected in the brain waves. Hence, the brain wave pattern varies and is heterogeneous during epileptic attacks. Epilepsy is characterized by two types of brain waves: ictal waves, which occur during the active phase of the seizures. These patterns are usually powerful and irregular due to abnormal nerve cell activity. EEG electrodes record these brain waves to diagnose and characterize epileptic attacks. Interictal waves are observed during the relaxation phase between epileptic attacks. They also indicate abnormal nerve cell activity but are weaker and more regular than excitatory waves. EEG analysis of brain waves is an important method for diagnosing and treating epilepsy [1]. IoT is a technological phenomenon involving the communication and interaction between various physical objects. Sensors, electronic devices, and Internet-connected devices are examples of these objects. As a result of the ability of these objects to collect and transmit data and information to central systems, the IoT allows organizations and users to remotely control objects, analyze data, and make data-driven decisions. There are many types of IoT, such as smart home automation, smart cities, Industry 4.0, and e-health. IoT plays an important role in improving efficiency, enhancing resource management, and providing innovative services in each of these areas. It is possible to use the IoT to diagnose epileptic attacks by continuously monitoring brain activity and recording brain waves using sensors and related devices. Therefore, IoT devices can transmit gathering data to central systems [2]. ML is an artificial intelligence (AI) area that allows algorithms to learn connections and relationships between inputs and outputs using training data from observations, experiences, measurements, environmental interactions, and other sources. Hence, using this data, algorithms can be trained to predict, make decisions, and perform specific tasks with new data without requiring detailed planning. This technology is widely used in various fields and applications due to its powerful ability to analyze large and complex data, identify patterns and hidden relationships in data, predict and make accurate decisions, adapt to changes, and be continuously improved. ML technology can complement the data-gathering process by IoT by processing them as part of the process. By analyzing the data gathered by IoT devices, patterns, trends, and behaviors associated with epileptic attacks can be identified, allowing predictions of future attacks to be made [3]. Blockchain is a distributed technology that stores and manages information through interconnected blocks. Each block contains a set of transactions linked to the previous block. All transactions carried out in the blockchain are accessible to all participants and are visible to them. Blockchain technology can contribute significantly to the security of the IoT. In the IoT, different devices are contributed and share sensitive information, and this subject makes data security extremely important. Hence, blockchain technology makes it possible to ensure that information sent between devices does not change and that all data in the form of transactions can be traced. Additionally, blockchain can efficiently and effectively authenticate devices and secure access [4]. This chapter uses the unique capabilities and features of new technologies such as IoT, ML, and blockchain to predict epilepsy attacks. Thus, an intelligent alert mechanism for epileptic attacks has been proposed using these technologies. In the proposed mechanism, three phases are defined, and each of these technologies will play an essential role in each phase. Hence, the proposed mechanism relies on IoT technology for monitoring, gathering, and transmitting data. ML technology attempts to analyze the collected data and predict potential attacks. The communication process between IoT and ML is carried out through blockchain technology, which ensures the security of the proposal mechanism, communication, and data exchange.

The structure of this chapter is as follows: As a starting point, the first part describes the necessary prerequisites, such as an Overview of IoT technology, Blockchain technology, ML technology, and epilepsy disease. The second part of IoT and ML in healthcare examines the HLF architectural framework as a permission-based blockchain, epilepsy detection procedures, and various approaches to ML. The third part comprehensively examines Incorporating ML whit IoT in the blockchain. In the fourth part of this chapter, an intelligent alert mechanism in IoT healthcare is proposed in three phases: Data gathering, transmission, and storage, Analyzing stored data, and Sending an alert message. Finally, the fifth section concludes this discussion.

14.2 Preliminaries

This section provides information on ML, epilepsy disease, the IoT, and blockchain technology. Using IoT technology, abnormal electrical activity in the brain can be controlled and monitored. Abnormal electrical activity in the brain can be considered one of the possible symptoms of epilepsy. The data collected by IoT technology can be analyzed using mechanisms based on AI technologies. ML is a subset of AI that can obtain the pattern of normal electrical activity in the brain and investigate and compare abnormal electrical activity with normal electrical activity. Moreover, AI-based mechanisms can predict the likelihood of epilepsy and notify the sick individual, their relatives, or nearby medical centers by sending a message through an intelligent alert mechanism (IAM). Since the people who use these technologies communicate with each other via the internet, all communication between them is secured using blockchain technology.

14.2.1 Overview of IoT Technology

IoT is an ecosystem of electronic devices and physical objects communicating with one another and the Internet network. There are many types of these devices, including sensors, medical devices, smart cars, home and industrial devices, and electronic devices related to smart cities. In this ecosystem, devices collect data with sensors and send it to cloud servers or central devices using programmed instructions. Thus, this data is transformed and analyzed using AI mechanisms that are considered for data analysis and can be analyzed and used to make optimal decisions and improve processes. The IoT is currently utilized in many fields, including smart cities, industries, agriculture, transportation, and the environment. These are some of the applications and features of the IoT in these fields:

- **Smart City:** In a smart city, the IoT collects and analyzes various data about the city's state with various sensors and devices, such as CCTV cameras, meteorological sensors, etc. It includes traffic conditions, air pollution levels, parking conditions, etc.
- **Smart Industry:** The IoT is used to monitor and control production processes, reduce production costs, increase productivity, and improve product quality. Sensors and smart devices collect detailed data regarding the status of production devices and production lines.

- **Smart Agriculture:** The IoT in agriculture collects data using various sensors and devices, including weather and soil sensors, and is used to improve the quality of products, reduce production costs, and optimize natural resource management. Hence, it is possible to optimize the management of water, soil, and fertilizer using the IoT [5].

The IoT has been employed in healthcare to collect various data regarding people's physical condition and health with the help of sensors, wearable devices, and medical devices. The data collected includes heart rate, blood pressure, blood sugar, and body temperature. The collected data is then analyzed and checked using AI-based mechanisms, and when any disease or health problem is detected, doctors and medical centers are notified. Using the IoT to examine brain waves is one of the exciting applications of the IoT in healthcare. Using electroencephalography (EEG) technology, doctors can record a person's brain waves and then analyze them using mechanisms based on AI-based. Using this application, mental disorders, such as depression, anxiety, insomnia, and others, can be evaluated and treated more effectively. Therefore, diagnosing and treating these disorders more effectively is possible by examining how a person's brain functions [6].

14.2.2 Blockchain Technology

Blockchain technology rapidly evolves with applications in various fields, including data security, finance, transportation, and health. Blockchain is based on distributed networks, in which each node (computer) contains the information it requires to verify transactions and records. Each block contains information about the transactions and other information, such as the time and date of the block creation, the hash of the previous block, etc. One of the most important characteristics of blockchain technology is its high degree of security. In blockchain, transactions are verified by a network of nodes without an intermediary or center. The network nodes take part in this process and, by combining their processing powers with those of other nodes, verify and verify transactions that are to be added to the chain. Hence, this prevents people and abusers from accessing and modifying the blockchain in any way. In blockchain, each block contains a hash used as a token or proof that the information in the block has not been changed. As a result, any attempt to change a block causes changes in subsequent blocks that automatically identify the attempt to change the block because the previous block data is encrypted in the new hash of the new block [7]. For this reason, blockchains are a safe and transparent means of storing and combining information used in various fields, including finance, transportation, and even voting. In the blockchain, each block contains a new transaction added to the previous block. These blocks are continuously added to the network, hence the name blockchain. To add a new transaction to the chain, it is necessary for the network nodes to first verify the transaction and then add the transaction as a new block to the chain. Hence, to achieve this goal based on the type of blockchain, network nodes compete against one another. For instance, in permissionless blockchains such as Bitcoin, The process is known as block mining. Those nodes that confirm transactions quicker can mine the new block and receive bitcoins as a reward. Meanwhile, to create a new block in permission-based blockchains such as HLF, no fees are paid for creating blocks. Therefore, blockchain is an innovative and advanced technology that provides high levels of security and transparency and is widely used in various industries, including finance, transportation, and even elections. In addition to the private sector, the public sector can review and enhance trust between individuals and organizations [8].

14.2.3 Overview of ML Technology

ML is one of the branches of AI that allows computer systems to automatically extract patterns and rules using input data, analyze the data, and provide more accurate and better answers. This method allows computers to analyze large and complex data to provide the best answer to issues with sufficient and accurate information.ML also enables computers to automatically extract patterns and rules based on input data from existing sensors on IoT devices and use them to reach improved decisions. ML constantly evolves and improves due to its wide range of applications [9]. With the advancement of technology and the growth of smart devices, the world produces enormous amounts of data, requiring more advanced methods to analyze and utilize that data. This technology is used in various fields. The following are some of the applications of this technology:

- **Imaging:** ML is one of the most important applications in the imaging field. The technology is used to recognize faces, patterns, objects, etc. For instance, ML models recognize faces from video images in facial recognition applications.
- **Natural language processing (NLP):** ML is used in NLP to process and extract information from texts and web content.

This technology is used in machine translation, sentiment analysis, automatic question-and-answer systems, etc.

- **Intrusion detection:** ML approaches can be utilized in cyber security as a practical technology. ML models are used in intrusion detection to detect unauthorized patterns in user behavior in computer networks and websites [10].

ML in healthcare is one of the most critical and practical technologies, as it improves performance and accuracy in diagnosing and treating diseases and improving patients' health. Hence, using ML algorithms can identify and diagnose diseases, including cancer, heart disease, diabetes, infectious diseases, etc. Moreover, by utilizing this technology, it is possible to enhance the accuracy of diagnostics, determine the appropriate treatment, and determine a patient's recovery method. Health systems management and disease prevention are other applications of ML By analyzing health data, it is possible to diagnose diseases early, prevent the spread of diseases, and develop new treatment and prevention methods. Therefore, ML in the health field is one of the most widely used and effective methods for improving the quality of health care and people's general health [11].

14.2.4 Epilepsy Disease

Epilepsy is a chronic neurological disorder characterized by seizures, changes in consciousness and behavior, and irregular movements. In addition to genetic factors, epilepsy can also be caused by various other factors, including head trauma, brain infection, medications, environmental factors, etc. Epilepsy can affect anyone at any age and can last a lifetime. A seizure is the primary symptom of epilepsy, a sudden reaction in the nervous system that occurs during a seizure. Images obtained from Magnetic Resonance Imaging (MRI) and EEG methods can be useful in the diagnosis of epilepsy as well as in assisting doctors in the diagnosis and treatment of epilepsy patients. During seizures, the intensity and duration of body movements, behavior, and states of consciousness can change. Epilepsy treatment methods include anticonvulsant drugs, surgical procedures, psychological treatments, and supplements [12]. Doctors will determine the appropriate treatment method based on the type and severity of the patient's condition. However, some factors can make seizures in epileptic patients more severe. For instance, stress, fatigue, increased alcohol consumption, certain medications, etc., can increase seizures. Epileptic patients should therefore avoid these agents and adhere to the anticonvulsant drugs prescribed by their physician to reduce the severity of attacks.

Epilepsy can psychologically and socially impact a patient and his family. Therefore, psychological and social support is crucial for the patient and his family. Additionally, epilepsy can negatively affect a patient's daily life, so education and counseling are important to support the patient [13].

14.3 IoT and ML in Healthcare

Healthcare is one of the fields in which, due to the growth of the population and the increase in life expectancy, more requirements are placed for monitoring, caring for, preventing, and predicting factors affecting human health. In this field, ML and the IoT can have an important impact on the well-being and health of people. ML technology can be used to analyze data and predict and treat diseases. Hence, using ML approaches by analyzing the data relating to various diseases, predicting the diseases' behavior and the appropriate treatment options is possible. In the field of IoT, various objects such as sensors, medical devices, and wearable devices are connected to Internet networks. These devices collect data about an individual's health throughout the day, and in the next step, these data are transmitted to healthcare data systems. Hence, doctors and other health professionals can use this data to design effective treatment and prevention programs for each individual [14]. Combining ML and IoT technologies can be highly effective in diagnosing and treating diseases. ML approaches can analyze medical records and X-ray images to identify patterns and likely diagnoses based on big data. The ability to use this capability can help physicians diagnose patients more accurately and develop a personalized treatment plan. Therefore, ML approaches can be used to analyze X-ray and MRI images to detect cancer and other diseases in their early stages. In addition, ML and IoT technologies can contribute to improved patient outcomes and reduced healthcare costs. Automating routine tasks and improving administrative processes reduces the misuse of time and resources to provide health services. Overall, integrating ML and IoT technologies in healthcare has great transformational potential in delivering healthcare and can help improve patient outcomes. However, it is important to note that these technologies are also associated with risks and challenges, including data privacy concerns [15].

14.3.1 HLF Architectural Framework

HLF is an open-source, cryptocurrency-independent blockchain framework used collaboratively to solve problems and provide solutions in various industries. This blockchain facilitates user access to blockchain data and the development of blockchain applications using technologies such as smart contract architecture. Using methods such as multiple signatures and authentication networks, HLF solves problems such as security, privacy, reliability, and performance, and its high flexibility makes it appropriate for a wide range of applications. One of the critical characteristics of the HLF blockchain is its internal structure. In typical blockchains, such as public blockchains, transaction processing is slow, and block distribution is heterogeneous. By using an appropriate and optimized internal structure, the HLF minimizes these problems. The HLF blockchain is structured to process transactions simultaneously and in parallel, increasing transaction processing speed and reducing transaction costs [16]. Also, to increase the security of the HLF blockchain, a hybrid system of public and private cryptography is employed. Transactions sent privately using this system are inaccessible to others using public encryption algorithms and can only be viewed by those with a private key. The HLF blockchain is structured as a network where each block has a unique identifier. These identifiers allow for the tracking of transactions and the verification of their authenticity. The HLF blockchain is structured as a network where to create each block in this network must make a unique identifier. These identifiers allow for the tracking of transactions and the verification of their authenticity. This blockchain uses a distributed system to generate blocks. In this system, groups work together to produce blocks and confirm transactions. The HLF blockchain uses a Byzantine Fault Tolerance (BFT) protocol to increase efficiency. This protocol minimizes network attacks and transaction inconsistencies, and the blockchain network is stable and secure. Additionally, HLF uses an intensive processing system to reduce processing costs and increase efficiency [17]. This system compresses transactions into blocks and requires less network space. HLF is an independent blockchain that can connect with other blockchains. The interledger protocol and other mechanisms, such as Atomic Swaps, provide this capability. Interledger Protocol is a network protocol for sending and receiving transactions between blockchains. In other words, the protocol allows different blockchains to communicate with one another and send and receive transactions. Also, HLF blockchains utilize powerful encryption algorithms to protect transaction privacy. Using this mechanism, all related transactions and information are coded using strong cryptographic algorithms, and only authorized people with the right to access the information can use them. Hence, all persons and organizations participating in HLF blockchain activities are authenticated to prevent unauthorized or fraudulent activities [18]. The HLF is structured in a modular manner. The structure of HLF is illustrated in Figure 14.1. There are several important components of the HLF structure, including:

- **Ledger:** A ledger is a system for recording transactions and events occurring in the HLF network. In other words, it records all transactions and logs within the HLF network in a secure, integrated, and specific manner [19].
- **Endorsement:** An endorsement in HLF means approval or approval of transactions by network members who are authorized and capable of approving and executing transactions. Endorsement is one of the key mechanisms used in HLF to ensure transaction integrity and health and improve the network's efficiency and speed.
- **Chaincode:** A chaincode is a type of smart contract that can run programming codes in the network. Chaincode is a primary component of HLF and is used to perform many network operations [20].

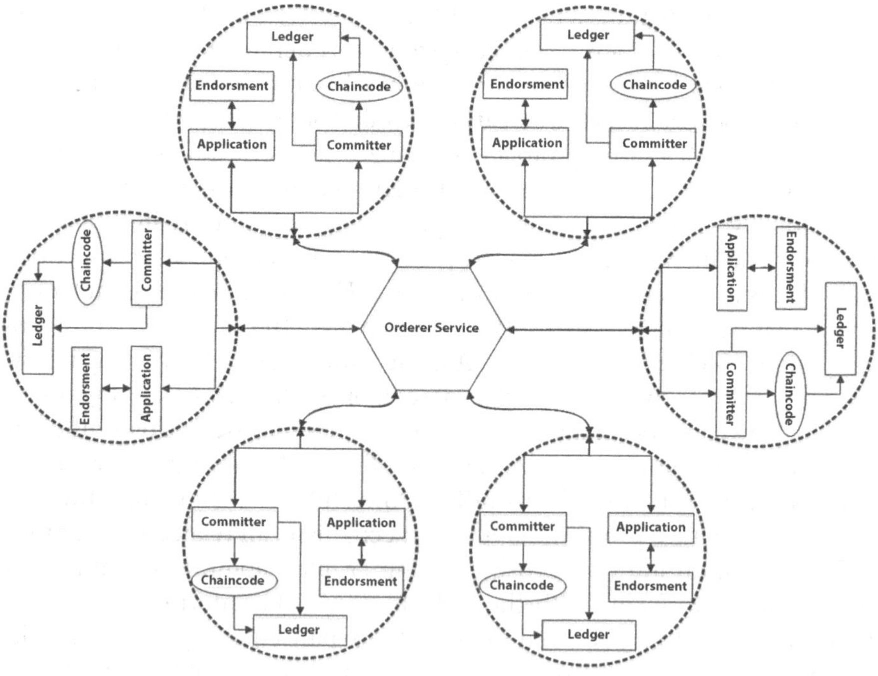

Figure 14.1 The HLF structure framework.

- **Committer:** A committer in HLF refers to a network member responsible for confirming and recording transactions that endorsers have approved. In other words, the HLF committers are responsible for executing and recording approved transactions [21].
- **Application:** An application in HLF is software that can communicate with the HLF network and perform operations such as sending and receiving transactions, managing user identities, and executing smart contracts. Applications in HLF provide communication between the network and users in general.
- **Orderer Service:** An Orderer service in HLF means the service of sorting and arranging transactions that are performed in the HLF network (refer Figure 14.1). In other words, the Orderer service is responsible for managing and setting the order and priority of transactions within the HLF network [22].

14.3.2 Epilepsy Detection Procedures

Epilepsy is a neurological condition characterized by sudden and involuntary seizures. Several types of seizures may occur, including clonic (muscle movement disorder), tonic (muscle contraction), myoclonic (muscle twitching), and absence (sudden disappearance through inactivity). As a result of seizures, some individuals may also experience symptoms such as blurred vision, confusion, headaches, and irritability. In most cases, epilepsy occurs in children and adolescents but can occur at any age. Epilepsy is often treated with anticonvulsant medications, dietary changes, and stress management. As medical methods and technology have developed, new methods of diagnosis and treatment for epilepsy have become available [23]. The following are a few of these methods.

- **EEG:** An EEG is one of the most important diagnostic methods in epilepsy. Hence, electrodes placed on the head record the brain's electrical activity in this method. An individual with epilepsy will exhibit a very different pattern of electrical activity in their brain than an individual with a healthy brain.
- **MRI:** An MRI is one of the most effective methods for diagnosing epilepsy. Doctors with an MRI can obtain an image

of the brain structure and detect any changes occurring therein [24].

- **Positron Emission Tomography (PET):** A PET involves injecting a radioactive substance into the active cells of the brain. Doctors use this method to identify the brain's most active parts during seizures.
- **AI methods:** In this method, by using AI and ML methods, a model is created to diagnose epilepsy and predict seizures. With the help of these methods, doctors can diagnose and predict epilepsy based on imaging and clinical data [25].

Generally, the diagnosis of epilepsy involves clinical imaging, AI methods, etc., and depending on the severity and type of the disease, it may be necessary to use more than one of these techniques.

14.3.3 Various Approaches to ML

ML is one of AI's main concepts, allowing machines to learn from their experiences and use specially designed algorithms to recognize patterns and predict outcomes more accurately. In addition to disease diagnosis, data analysis, and even the creation of music and images, this technology has a wide variety of applications. Hence, training data is supplied to the machine to implement ML technology, and then the machine is trained using specific algorithms, such as neural networks, using training data. The machine analyzes training data and identifies patterns related to a specific situation. After training, the machine displays its readiness to recognize patterns when entering new data. ML technology can detect complex patterns and predict results more accurately than traditional methods. Due to its practicality in many fields of application, this technology is considered one of the most crucial AI tools [26]. With further research in this area, it can be used to solve complex problems and improve the efficiency of various systems, particularly in the healthcare field. ML includes several different approaches and methods. Some of these significant approaches include:

- **Supervised Learning:** In this approach, input data is classified into two categories (for instance, positive and negative). All training data is labeled, and the algorithms use the labeled training data to predict new input data [27].
- **Unsupervised Learning:** In this approach, the algorithms must identify patterns in the training data without knowing

the labels. An instance of this approach includes a clustering mechanism [28].

- **Reinforcement Learning:** In this approach, the algorithm is trained by interacting with the environment and receiving rewards or punishments. In this approach, the algorithm can utilize its past experiences to make the correct decision regarding handling and interacting with the environment [29].
- **Semi-Supervised Learning:** In this approach, some data is labeled, while others are unlabeled. The machine is trained using labeled and unlabeled data [30].
- **Semi-Unsupervised Learning:** In this approach, some training data is labeled while the remaining data is unlabeled. Therefore, the algorithm is trained with labeled data while exploiting unlabeled data [31].
- **Neural Networks:** In this approach, inputs are connected to the output layer via hidden layers, and several neurons are used to connect the inputs to the output layer. It is the function of each neuron to convert the input into output by using a weight and activation function [32].

Using ML in the healthcare field provides many opportunities to improve the health of individuals and society. As a result of using this technology, more accurate diagnosis and prediction of diseases, design of medicine, recovery plans, and disease prevention will be possible. Additionally, by analyzing large and important amounts of data, it is possible to understand disease causes and treatment results better and make more accurate decisions accordingly.

14.4 Incorporating ML with IoT in the Blockchain

With the advancement of technology and the development of the IoT, particularly in the healthcare sector, it is possible to incorporate ML with the IoT in the blockchain process. Incorporating ML technology and the IoT in permission-based blockchains such as HLF is used in healthcare can be used to improve healthcare services' quality, reduce healthcare costs, enhance patient management, and improve disease diagnosis. As a result of this integration, a massive amount of data will be gathered and stored in a distributed communication network. The data collected by medical sensors and other devices include temperature, heart rate, blood pressure, blood sugar level, and other medical information. These data are then added to chain blocks and analyzed and interpreted using ML to improve healthcare services [33]. In this mechanism, blockchains act as a distributed database, and the information is encoded in blocks using cryptographic algorithms to protect data and privacy. Several advantages of this structure include its speed, security, accuracy in diagnosing diseases, improved patient management, and cost-effectiveness. However, to implement this mechanism, medical and technical experts must cooperate, hardware and software costs will be high, and some legal and privacy issues will be problematic in some countries [34]. The following are some of the advantages and disadvantages of this merger. The advantages of incorporating ML, IoT, and blockchain technology in healthcare are as follows:

- **Easier access to medical data:** Using the IoT, medical data can be collected from various devices, including sensors, applications, and medical devices. Blockchain technology enables this data to be encrypted and stored securely.
- **Medical data analysis:** Medical data collected by the IoT and stored in the blockchain can be processed by ML algorithms, improving disease diagnosis and treatment [35].
- **Medical data sharing:** With the help of blockchain technology, medical data can be shared safely, with the permission of their owners, and feasible to provide a safe connection between patients and doctors.
- **Improving medical data security:** Using blockchain technology for storing and accessing medical data can help improve data security and protect patients' privacy [36].

The disadvantages of incorporating ML, IoT, and blockchain technology in healthcare are as follows:

- **Complex implementation:** Implementing and incorporating ML, IoT, and blockchain technologies can be complex.
- **Need for advanced knowledge:** Incorporating ML, IoT, and blockchain in healthcare requires advanced technology and know-how, which may not be available to all organizations.
- **Scope of data analysis:** Incorporating ML and the IoT presents challenges for analyzing and understanding complex medical data, and the results obtained from the analysis could be affected. Additionally, storing large quantities and

dimensions of data in blockchains can slow down access to data [37].

Incorporating ML, IoT, and blockchain technology in healthcare can significantly improve health and treatment services. It is important, however, for these technologies to be utilized optimally that health organizations, doctors, and technologists cooperate and ensure that patient privacy and medical information are protected.

14.5 Intelligent Alert Mechanism in IoT Healthcare

EEG is the primary method of diagnosing cerebral epilepsy. This method involves using electrodes placed on the person's head to record their brain's electrical activity over time. EEG is a non-invasive method of recording electrical activity in the brain. Brain waves refer to the brain's electrical activity, which occurs at different frequencies and patterns. These brain waves can be categorized into four types that include:

- **Beta waves:** The beta waves are associated with awake and focused mental activity (for example, between 12 and 30 Hz). They are usually amplified when the brain solves problems, focuses on cognitive tasks, or performs mental functions.
- **Alpha waves:** This wave usually occurs in a calm and thoughtless state with a medium frequency (for example, 8-12 Hz). Alpha waves are amplified during relaxation, meditation, or rest.
- **Theta waves:** The theta waves have a low frequency (for example, between 4 and 8 Hz) and are associated with sleep activity and integrated mental states. A person's theta wave activity is predominant during deep sleep, as is the case during rapid eye movement sleep.
- **Delta waves:** The delta wave has a shallow frequency (less than 4 Hz) associated with deep sleep and significant brain diseases. Delta waves can also be observed in certain disease states, such as epilepsy [38].

During epilepsy attacks, the brain's normal patterns of electrical activity are altered abnormally. These changes may include:

- **Increasing or decreasing the frequency of brain waves:** There are some diseases in which brain wave frequency may be increased or decreased. For example, in some epilepsy disorders, beta and alpha waves may increase, or delta and theta waves may decrease [39].
- **Abnormal brain wave production:** Epilepsy attacks may produce abnormal brain wave patterns, including sharp and spike waves. These are some of the unusual patterns seen in some forms of epilepsy attacks [40].
- **Increased undesirable or irregular activity:** During some epilepsy attacks, the brain's electrical activity may become irregular or undesirable. Hence, this may include irregular patterns of brain waves with different frequencies and a pattern that cannot be adjusted [41].

EEG analysis of epilepsy attacks requires the expertise and experience of doctors specializing in neurophysiology or neurology. EEG analysis is a non-invasive diagnostic method. As a result of epilepsy attacks, created patterns include different waves which change over time. A doctor specializing in neurophysiology or neurology may be able to obtain valuable information by analyzing EEG patterns to determine the electrical activity in the brain. These professionals examine brain patterns to identify abnormal changes that may indicate epileptic attacks. Furthermore, Epileptic attacks are unpredictable, so doctors cannot predict them [42].

This chapter attempts to propose an early detection mechanism for epileptic attacks by using IoT, ML, and blockchain technologies. In this proposed mechanism, brain waves are received through sensors. Hence, due to the capacity and capabilities of IoT technology, the process of gathering, receiving, and sending brain waves can be accomplished. The waves gathering whit embedded sensors on the IoT Devices are transmitted to an intelligent mechanism responsible for processing and analyzing brain waves using ML technology. Hence, this intelligent mechanism uses powerful ML algorithms to investigate, analyze, and predict any changes or potential changes. In this case, the intelligent mechanism can interpret the changes in frequency as an indication that an epileptic attack is imminent. Therefore, the proposed mechanism warns those near the patient, the patient, and even medical centers before the onset of an epileptic attack. It is important to note that epileptic attacks can bring irreparable complications due to the incapacity of the sufferer to control his activities when they occur, which makes any alerting before their occurrence a major advantage. The use of the IoT has brought concerns about the security of the data transfer process and misuse of the transferred data. It has therefore been attempted to secure all information exchange processes through permission-based blockchains such as HLF in the proposed mechanism. Applying this technology to sensitive fields, such as healthcare, can provide the foundation for the safest application of IoT technology while alleviating existing concerns. Following is a describing of the steps of the proposed mechanism, as illustrated in Figure 14.2, accompanied by details. The proposed mechanism architecture is presented in Figure 14.3. There are three main phases to the intelligent early alerting system of an epileptic attack, which include:

- Data gathering, transmission, and storage
- Analyzing stored data
- Sending an alert message

14.5.1 Data Gathering, Transmission, and Storage

During the first phase of the proposed mechanism, sensors will be embedded in IoT devices to receive brain signals continuously. After receiving these waves, these sensors transmit them to devices associated with the IoT (step 1). The proposed mechanism incorporates a component known as the Accessibility mechanism to facilitate safe communication and prevent data misuse. This mechanism is a gateway between IoT devices and blockchain networks, providing an early warning system for epileptic attacks. In this manner, only authenticated IoT devices can be granted access to the system under this mechanism. The IoT devices must store the sensors' data; in other words, they must send gathering data to the mechanism and store them. It is, therefore, necessary for them to verify their authenticity before sending data. The IoT devices request the Accessibility mechanism to confirm their identity (step 2). Upon receiving the request from the IoT devices, the accessibility mechanism attempts to authenticate the requesting device (step 3). When the IoT devices are authenticated, the accessibility mechanism generates a response and sends it to the IoT devices (step 4). After confirming their authenticity, IoT devices try to store the data they receive from the sensors through a transaction or transactions through the accessibility mechanism. Hence, they present a request to register their desired transactions through the Accessibility mechanism (step 5). As soon as the accessibility mechanism receives the transaction-based requests, it sends them to the Endorser component (step 6). During this step, the Endorser evaluates the sent transactions for approval (step 7). After the Endorser has approved and validated the transactions sent, a response is sent from the

Endorser to the Accessibility mechanism (step 8). The Accessibility mechanism, which serves as an application in the Hyperledger Fabric blockchain, sends the request to register the transactions approved by the Endorser to the Orderer Service section (step 9). Next, the Orderer service creates a queue to queue up the received transactions for registration in the blockchain and send them in order. The Orderer service requests Chaincode to record the transactions (step 10). As soon as Chaincode receives the Orderer service request, it attempts to create a Query to request the insertion of transactions and sends it to the Ledger (step 11). Upon receiving a request from Chaincode, Ledger attempts to store the requested transaction; in other words, Ledger attempts to store the requested data (step 12). As soon as the ledger has stored the transactions or the data, it creates a response and sends it to Chaincode to notify it of successful data storage (step 13). After receiving a successful response for data storage, Chaincode generates a response for the Accessibility mechanism (step 14). Next, the Accessibility mechanism attempts to notify IoT devices of successful data storage by creating a response (step 15).

14.5.2 Analyzing Stored Data

With the completion of stage 15, the first phase of the intelligent early warning mechanism for epileptic attacks, which includes gathering, sending, and storing data, is complete. In the continuation of the implementation of other steps and the beginning of the second phase of the intelligent early warning mechanism of epileptic attacks, which involves the analysis of the stored data, the intelligent analysis component will be responsible for analyzing the data gathered. Data is analyzed by the intelligent analysis component using ML techniques and algorithms, and the results are compared with previous patterns stored in a database. The Intelligent Analysis section, therefore, requests access to the stored data from the Orderer. It should be noted that sending requests to the Endorser is also implemented in the same manner as phase one, so to minimize complications in the proposed mechanism, it has been eliminated (step 16). When the Orderer service receives the request to read the data, it places the request in the execution queue. Orderer then sends the queued requests to Chaincode for execution (step 17). When Chaincode receives a request, it creates a Query and sends it to the Ledger (step 18). Ledger attempts to prepare the requested data after receiving the request from Chaincode (step 19). When the data is prepared, Ledger generates a response and sends it to Chaincode (step 20). After receiving a response from the ledger regarding preparing the requested data, Chaincode created a response and sent it to the intelligent analysis component (step 21). As soon as the Intelligent Analysis component receives the requested information, it attempts to implement ML techniques and algorithms on the information. After reviewing and analyzing the data, the patterns obtained are compared with those of existing patterns in the data bank (step 22).

14.5.3 Sending an Alert Message

After the completion of stage 22, the second phase of the intelligent early alert mechanism for epileptic attacks ends. In the third phase of this proposed mechanism, if epileptic attacks are predicted in the previous phase, Alerting messages will be sent to the people and centers identified in advance. Hence, the third phase of the proposed mechanism is developed based on the results and predictions made in the second phase to provide people with the necessary alerting. Upon completion of the second phase, the results are sent to the Alert Mechanism section (step 23). Upon receiving the results of the intelligent analysis, the alert mechanism attempts to notify predetermined individuals of an epileptic attack as soon as possible. The system sends an alert message to the medical centers and individuals

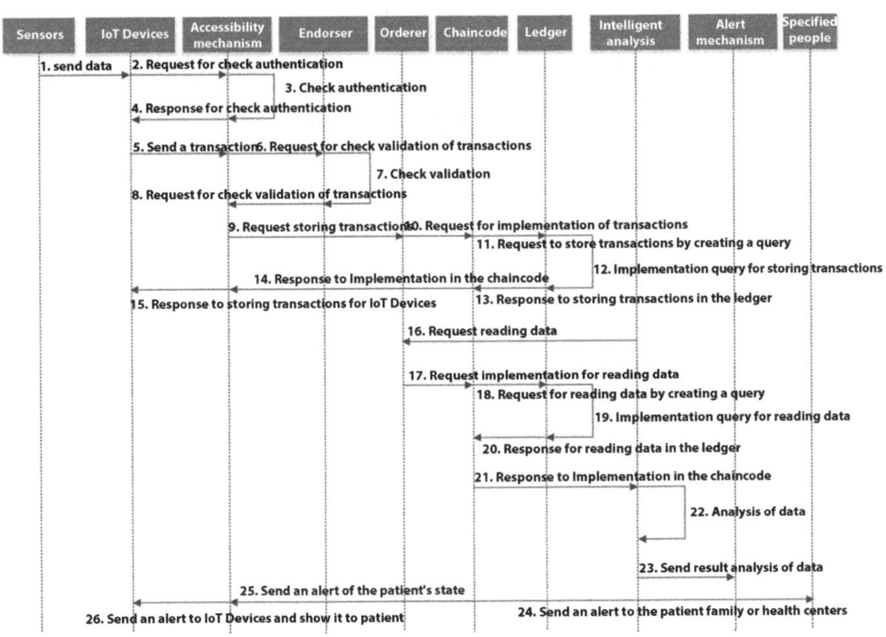

Figure 14.2 An intelligent early warning system for epilepsy attacks based on IoT, ML, and blockchain technology.

near the patient determined in advance (step 24). Additionally, the Alert mechanism generates a message simultaneously with the execution of step 24 and sends it to the Accessibility mechanism (step 25). As soon as the accessibility mechanism receives the alerting message, it attempts to notify the patient of the possibility of epileptic attacks by generating a warning message through the IoT (step 26) (refer to Figure 14.2).

Consequently, people with epilepsy cannot maintain their control of body parts, and it is possible that if they are in inappropriate places during these attacks, they may suffer irreparable injuries or even die. As a result, the intelligent early alerting mechanism for epilepsy attacks can significantly reduce the complications caused by epilepsy attacks to a great extent by analyzing brain waves and predicting the likelihood of epileptic attacks by providing timely and early alerts. Hence, the patients, or those close to them, can prepare for an epileptic attack, thereby saving their life (refer to Figure 14.3).

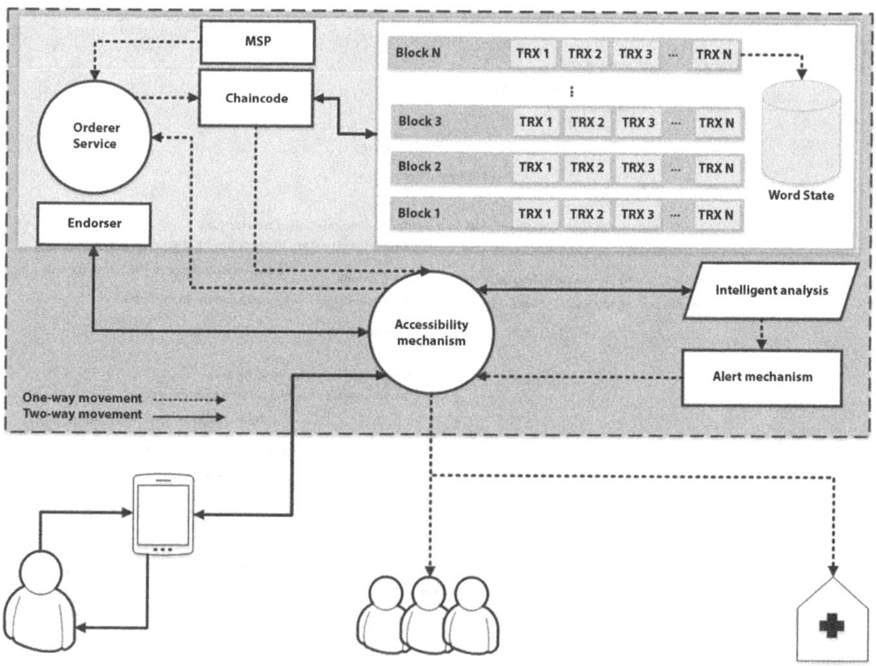

Figure 14.3 An intelligent alert mechanism in IoT healthcare.

14.6 Conclusion

People with epilepsy suffer from unpredictable attacks that can have various side effects. The patient's during epileptic attacks result in almost no control over their body activities, making it impossible to maintain their balance. Hence, when they are in a dangerous environment, these attacks can result in death. In recent years, the use of new technologies to solve challenges and problems has increased in various fields, particularly healthcare. Therefore, by incorporating new technology into the field of predicting epileptic attacks, doctors can be able to reduce the risks associated with this uncontrollable disease. This chapter proposed an intelligent, alert mechanism for solving this problem. A proposed mechanism uses several different technologies, such as IoT, ML, and blockchain, in three different phases. The proposed mechanism utilizes IoT technology in its first phase to gather brain wave data from epileptic patients and will store the gathered data by employing different components embedded within the blockchain system. During the second phase of the proposed mechanism, it has been attempted to analyze the collected data using ML techniques. In the second phase, the intelligent analysis component implements ML techniques on the collected data. This section analyzes the results and attempts to find patterns in the patient's brain waves. The pattern obtained is then compared with other patterns in the data bank available in intelligent analysis. In the third phase, the Alert mechanism attempts to notify the patient, their family members and medical centers identified in advance when an epileptic attack is predicted in the second phase of the proposed mechanism. As the proposed mechanism is based on permissioned blockchain HLF, by embedding an accessibility mechanism, it has been attempted to base all communication processes between IoT devices on authentication. A vital component of the proposed mechanism is the accessibility mechanism, which serves as a gateway for data exchange between the system and the patients. The purpose of this component is to prevent the misuse of the patient's information and unauthorized access to it. Therefore, using this intelligent alert mechanism can help reduce the side effects of these attacks by predicting the possibility of attacks and informing the patient in advance, and even in the case of challenging environments can save the patient's life.

In the future, the possibility of using other new technologies, such as serverless computing, will allow for resource consumption in IoT devices to be managed efficiently and to maximize the efficiency of the resources available. On the other hand, reducing the complexity caused by this mechanism's implementation process will also be considered since combining several technologies into one mechanism is always a challenge, and creating coordination between them is very difficult.

References

1. Amin, U. and Benbadis, S.R., The role of EEG in the erroneous diagnosis of epilepsy. *J. Clin. Neurophysiol.*, 36, 4, 294–297, 2019.
2. Jagtap, P.T. and Bhosale, N.P., IOT based epilepsy monitoring using accelerometer sensor, in: *2018 International Conference on Information, Communication, Engineering and Technology (ICICET)*, IEEE, pp. 1–3, 2018, August.
3. Al-Hajjar, A.L.N. and Al-Qurabat, A.K.M., An overview of machine learning methods in enabling IoMT-based epileptic seizure detection. *J. Supercomput.* 79, 16017–16064, 2023.
4. Reyna, A., Martín, C., Chen, J., Soler, E., Díaz, M., On blockchain and its integration with IoT. Challenges and opportunities. *Future Gener. Comput. Syst.*, 88, 173–190, 2018.
5. Haras, M. and Skotnicki, T., Thermoelectricity for IoT–A review. *Nano Energy*, 54, 461–476, 2018.
6. Laport, F., Dapena, A., Castro, P.M., Vazquez-Araujo, F.J., Iglesia, D., A prototype of EEG system for IoT. *Int. J. Neural Syst.*, 30, 07, 2050018, 2020.
7. Mingxiao, D., Xiaofeng, M., Zhe, Z., Xiangwei, W., Qijun, C., A review on consensus algorithm of blockchain, in: *2017 IEEE international conference on systems, man, and cybernetics (SMC)*, IEEE, pp. 2567–2572, 2017, October.
8. Helliar, C.V., Crawford, L., Rocca, L., Teodori, C., Veneziani, M., Permissionless and permissioned blockchain diffusion. *Int. J. Inf. Manage.*, 54, 102136, 2020.
9. Merenda, M., Porcaro, C., Iero, D., Edge machine learning for ai-enabled iot devices: A review. *Sensors*, 20, 9, 2533, 2020.
10. Khan, M.A., HCRNNIDS: Hybrid convolutional recurrent neural network-based network intrusion detection system. *Processes*, 9, 5, 834, 2021.
11. Qayyum, A., Qadir, J., Bilal, M., Al-Fuqaha, A., Secure and robust machine learning for healthcare: A survey. *IEEE Rev. Biomed. Eng.*, 14, 156–180, 2020.
12. Elwan, S., Alexopoulos, A., Silveira, D.C., Kotagal, P., Lateralizing and localizing value of seizure semiology: Comparison with scalp EEG, MRI and PET in patients successfully treated with resective epilepsy surgery. *Seizure*, 61, 203–208, 2018.
13. Aydin, Ü., Rampp, S., Wollbrink, A., Kugel, H., Cho, J.H., Knösche, T.R., Grova, C., Wellmer, J., Wolters, C.H., Zoomed MRI guided by combined EEG/MEG source analysis: a multimodal approach for optimizing presurgical

epilepsy work-up and its application in a multi-focal epilepsy patient case study. *Brain Topogr.*, 30, 417–433, 2017.
14. Sworna, N.S., Islam, A.M., Shatabda, S., Islam, S., Towards development of IoT-ML driven healthcare systems: A survey. *J. Netw. Comput. Appl.*, 196, 103244, 2021.
15. Khalid, H., Hussain, M., Al Ghamdi, M.A., Khalid, T., Khalid, K., Khan, M.A., Fatima, K., Masood, K., Almotiri, S.H., Farooq, M.S., Ahmed, A., A comparative systematic literature review on knee bone reports from mri, x-rays and ct scans using deep learning and machine learning methodologies. *Diagnostics*, 10, 8, 518, 2020.
16. Antwi, M., Adnane, A., Ahmad, F., Hussain, R., ur Rehman, M.H., Kerrache, C.A., The case of HyperLedger Fabric as a blockchain solution for healthcare applications. *Blockchain: Res. Appl.*, 2, 1, 100012, 2021.
17. Sousa, J., Bessani, A., Vukolic, M., A byzantine fault-tolerant ordering service for the hyperledger fabric blockchain platform, in: *2018 48th annual IEEE/IFIP international conference on dependable systems and networks (DSN)*, IEEE, pp. 51–58, 2018, June.
18. Barger, A., Gorgadze, V., Belenov, A., Frolovicheva, E., Atomyze-The Scalable Hyperledger Fabric-Powered Blockchain Platform Revolutionizing Asset-Backed Tokenization, in: *2023 IEEE International Conference on Omni-layer Intelligent Systems (COINS)*, IEEE, pp. 1–8, 2023, July.
19. Sukhwani, H., Wang, N., Trivedi, K.S., Rindos, A., Performance modeling of hyperledger fabric (permissioned blockchain network), in: *2018 IEEE 17th international symposium on network computing and applications (NCA)*, IEEE, pp. 1–8, 2018, November.
20. Baliga, A., Solanki, N., Verekar, S., Pednekar, A., Kamat, P., Chatterjee, S., Performance characterization of hyperledger fabric, in: *2018 Crypto Valley conference on blockchain technology (CVCBT)*, IEEE, pp. 65–74, 2018, June.
21. Kim, Y., Kim, K.H., Kim, J.H., Power trading blockchain using hyperledger fabric, in: *2020 International Conference on Information Networking (ICOIN)*, IEEE, pp. 821–824, 2020, January.
22. Honar Pajooh, H., Rashid, M., Alam, F., Demidenko, S., Hyperledger fabric blockchain for securing the edge internet of things. *Sensors*, 21, 2, 359, 2021.
23. Lowrie, M. and Garosi, L., Classification of involuntary movements in dogs: myoclonus and myotonia. *J. Vet. Intern. Med.*, 31, 4, 979–987, 2017.
24. Sebastiano, D.R., Tassi, L., Duran, D., Visani, E., Gozzo, F., Cardinale, F., Nobili, L., Del Sole, A., Rubino, A., Dotta, S., Schiaffi, E., Identifying the epileptogenic zone by four non-invasive imaging techniques versus stereo-EEG in MRI-negative pre-surgery epilepsy patients. *Clin. Neurophysiol.*, 131, 8, 1815–1823, 2020.
25. Borbély, K., Emri, M., Kenessey, I., Tóth, M., Singer, J., Barsi, P., Vajda, Z., Pál, E., Tóth, Z., Beyer, T., Dóczi, T., Pet/Mri in the presurgical evaluation of patients with epilepsy: a concordance analysis. *Biomedicines*, 10, 5, 949, 2022.

26. Wang, C., Tan, X.P., Tor, S.B., Lim, C.S., Machine learning in additive manufacturing: State-of-the-art and perspectives. *Addit. Manuf.*, 36, 101538, 2020.
27. Alexopoulos, K., Nikolakis, N., Chryssolouris, G., Digital twin-driven supervised machine learning for the development of artificial intelligence applications in manufacturing. *Int. J. Comput. Integr. Manuf.*, 33, 5, 429–439, 2020.
28. Usama, M., Qadir, J., Raza, A., Arif, H., Yau, K.L.A., Elkhatib, Y., Hussain, A., Al-Fuqaha, A., Unsupervised machine learning for networking: Techniques, applications and research challenges. *IEEE Access*, 7, 65579–65615, 2019.
29. Arulkumaran, K., Deisenroth, M.P., Brundage, M., Bharath, A.A., Deep reinforcement learning: A brief survey. *IEEE Signal Process. Mag.*, 34, 6, 26–38, 2017.
30. Van Engelen, J.E. and Hoos, H.H., A survey on semi-supervised learning. *Mach. Learn.*, 109, 2, 373–440, 2020.
31. Zhang, Z., Zhang, P., Wang, P., Sheriff, J., Bluestein, D., Deng, Y., Rapid analysis of streaming platelet images by semi-unsupervised learning. *Comput. Med. Imaging Graphics*, 89, 101895, 2021.
32. Chen, M., Challita, U., Saad, W., Yin, C., Debbah, M., Artificial neural networks-based machine learning for wireless networks: A tutorial. *IEEE Commun. Surv. Tutorials*, 21, 4, 3039–3071, 2019.
33. Kundu, N., Rani, G., Dhaka, V.S., Machine learning and iot based disease predictor and alert generator system, in: *2020 Fourth International Conference on Computing Methodologies and Communication (ICCMC)*, IEEE, pp. 764–769, 2020, March.
34. Ghorbian, M. and Ghobaei-Arani, M., A Blockchain-Enabled Serverless Approach for IoT Healthcare Applications, in: *Serverless Computing: Principles and Paradigms*, pp. 193–218, Springer International Publishing, Cham, 2023.
35. Neelakandan, S., Beulah, J.R., Prathiba, L., Murthy, G.L.N., Irudaya Raj, E.F., Arulkumar, N., Blockchain with deep learning-enabled secure healthcare data transmission and diagnostic model. *Int. J. Model. Simul. Sci. Comput.*, 13, 04, 2241006, 2022.
36. Kumar, R., Kumar, P., Tripathi, R., Gupta, G.P., Islam, A.N., Shorfuzzaman, M., Permissioned blockchain and deep learning for secure and efficient data sharing in industrial healthcare systems. *IEEE Trans. Ind. Inf.*, 18, 11, 8065–8073, 2022.
37. Ghazal, T.M., Hasan, M.K., Alshurideh, M.T., Alzoubi, H.M., Ahmad, M., Akbar, S.S., Al Kurdi, B., Akour, I.A., IoT for smart cities: Machine learning approaches in smart healthcare—A review. *Future Internet*, 13, 8, 218, 2021.
38. Wen, T.Y. and Aris, S.M., Electroencephalogram (EEG) stress analysis on alpha/beta ratio and theta/beta ratio. *Indones. J. Electr. Eng. Comput. Sci.*, 17, 1, 175–182, 2020.
39. Wolinski, N., Cooper, N.R., Sauseng, P., Romei, V., The speed of parietal theta frequency drives visuospatial working memory capacity. *PloS Biol.*, 16, 3, e2005348, 2018.

40. Vaca, G.F.B. and Park, J.T., Focal EEG abnormalities and focal ictal semiology in generalized epilepsy. *Seizure*, 77, 7–14, 2020.
41. Kanner, A.M. and Bicchi, M.M., Antiseizure medications for adults with epilepsy: a review. *JAMA*, 327, 13, 1269–1281, 2022.
42. Juárez-Martinez, E.L., Nissen, I.A., Idema, S., Velis, D.N., Hillebrand, A., Stam, C.J., van Straaten, E.C., Virtual localization of the seizure onset zone: Using non-invasive MEG virtual electrodes at stereo-EEG electrode locations in refractory epilepsy patients. *NeuroImage: Clin.*, 19, 758–766, 2018.

15

Integrating Quantum Computing in Bioinformatics and Biomedical Research

Prasad Selladurai[1], Ruby Dahiya[2], Baskar Kandasamy[3]* and Venkateswaran Radhakrishnan[4]

[1]*Department of Chemistry, Pachaiyappa's, College for Men, Kanchipuram, Tamil Nadu, India*
[2]*Department of Computer Science and Engineering, School of Computing Science and Engineering, Galgotias University, Greater Noida, India*
[3]*Department of AI&DS, Kongunadu College of Engineering and Technology, Trichy, Tamil Nadu, India*
[4]*Cyber and Information Security, College of Computing and Information Sciences, University of Technology and Applied Sciences, Salalah, Oman*

Abstract

The integrated application of quantum computing into bioinformatics and biomedical research marks a paradigm change in our approach to complicated biological and medical challenges. This confluence has the ability to unleash tremendous computational power and revolutionary algorithms, revolutionizing the analysis and interpretation of biological data and speeding up the pace of discovery in the life sciences. This chapter presents a brief description of the current quantum computing environment in bioinformatics and biomedical research, outlining the fundamental concepts of quantum computing and its unique potential. We look at the important uses of quantum computing in various fields, such as modeling complex biological systems and drug development, as well as improving large-scale genomic data processing and protein folding predictions. We also examine the difficulties and limits of quantum computing, such as hardware constraints and the necessity for quantum software development adapted to specific biological applications. In addition, we discuss ongoing research efforts and potential advancements in the field, such as quantum-inspired machine learning models

**Corresponding author*: drkbaskarphd@gmail.com; ORCID: 0000-0003-4294-8206
Ruby Dahiya: ORCID: 0000-0001-9492-2054
Venkateswaran Radhakrishnan: ORCID: 0000-0003-1096-0278

Neha Sharma, Korhan Cengiz and Prasenjit Chatterjee (eds.) Intelligent Data Analytics for Bioinformatics and Biomedical Systems, (357–380) © 2024 Scrivener Publishing LLC

and hybrid quantum-classical techniques. These developments have the ability to bridge the gap between present classical computing approaches and quantum computing transformational potential in bioinformatics and medicinal research. Finally, combining quantum computing into bioinformatics and biomedical research provides an enticing way for solving complicated issues in genomes, proteomics, and drug discovery. While this integration is still in its early stages, the synergy between quantum computing and life sciences holds enormous potential for speeding up scientific discovery and propelling improvements in illness detection and treatment. This chapter builds the foundation for grasping the current state and future possibilities of quantum computing in bioinformatics and medicinal research.

***Keywords*:** Quantum computing, bioinformatics, biomedical, biological systems, qubits

15.1 Introduction

Bioinformatics and biomedical research have long been at the forefront of scientific investigation, as they attempt to uncover the complexity of life, sequence the human genome, and develop innovative illness therapies. Over the last few decades, the increase in computer capacity has been critical in driving the advancement of these fields. However, as biological and medical databases grow in size and complexity, there is an increasing demand for more powerful computer resources and novel algorithms to analyze, interpret, and model this wealth of data. In this environment, quantum computing is emerging as a disruptive technology with the ability to redefine the limits of computational capability in the biological sciences [9]. Quantum computing utilizes quantum physics concepts to do tasks that were previously considered to be beyond the capabilities of traditional computers.

It has the ability to solve issues considerably quicker than their traditional equivalents, which is very useful when dealing with complex biological and medical data. Quantum computing ushers in a paradigm change that has the potential to alter the way we approach fundamental biological problems, investigate the complexities of genetics, and accelerate pharmaceutical development. This study investigates the incorporation of quantum computing into bioinformatics and biomedical research, focusing on the enormous influence that this fledgling technology threatens to have on the life sciences as shown in Figure 15.1. We will start by explaining the underlying concepts of quantum computing and why it is useful in biological and medical realms. Following that, we will examine the several applications and use cases where quantum computing has the potential to make a difference, ranging from modeling biological systems at new levels

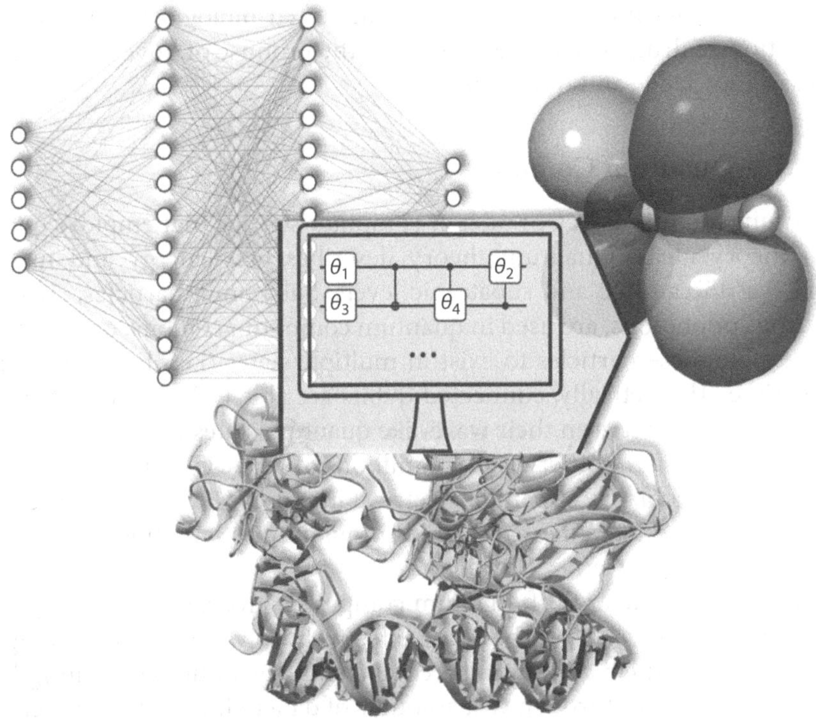

Figure 15.1 Quantum computing in bioinformatics.

of precision to revolutionizing drug development procedures and optimizing genetic data processing.

Furthermore, we will discuss the existing hurdles and limits of quantum computing while acknowledging ongoing efforts in hardware development and quantum software creation. Quantum computing in bioinformatics and biomedical research is not without challenges, but the potential rewards are enormous, spanning from drug discovery acceleration to medical treatment personalization This study explores the synergies between quantum computing and the life sciences, as well as providing a pathway for understanding the present status and future possibilities of using quantum computing in bioinformatics and medicinal research [5]. The possibilities are tremendous as quantum technologies grow, and the merging of quantum computing with these domains promises to open up new horizons in our knowledge of biology and the creation of medical treatments.

The integration of quantum computing into bioinformatics and biomedical research marks an important turning point in computational life sciences. The unique capabilities of quantum computing have the ability to expedite data processing, model complicated biological systems, and revolutionize drug development, offering the promise of huge advances in disease knowledge and treatment.

15.1.1 Quantum Computing

Quantum computing is a branch of computer science that employs quantum theory ideas. Quantum theory describes how energy and matter behave at the atomic and subatomic levels. Subatomic particles, such as electrons or photons, are used in quantum computing. Qubits, or quantum bits, enable these particles to exist in multiple states (i.e., 1 and 0) at the same time. Theoretically, connected qubits are able to "take advantage of the interference between their wave-like quantum states to carry out computations that might otherwise take millions of years. Classical computers nowadays use a binary stream of electrical impulses (1 and 0) to represent information in bits. When compared to quantum computing, this limits their processing power.

In the 1980s, the area of quantum computing arose. Certain computer problems were revealed to be more effectively solved by quantum algorithms than by their conventional equivalents. Quantum computing has the capacity to filter through vast amounts of data to find viable answers to complicated issues and challenges. Whereas traditional computers utilize bits with either 0s or 1s to store information, quantum computers employ qubits. Qubits contain information in a quantum state that interacts with 0 and 1 in several dimensions [6]. The Wall Street Journal is an American newspaper. "Google Aims for Commercial-Grade Quantum Computer by 2029." Many of the world's most renowned corporations have expressed interest in the huge computing capacity and predicted market size for its utilization. IBM, Microsoft, Google, D-Waves Systems, Alibaba, Nokia, Intel, Airbus, HP, Toshiba, Mitsubishi, SK Telecom, NEC, Raytheon, Lockheed Martin, Rigetti, Biogen, Volkswagen, and Amgen are among the companies involved.

Supporting in Quantum Computing Research

Since quantum computing technology remains in its early stages, it is fast advancing, and many intriguing applications are on the horizon. Simulating complicated molecules, for example, is incredibly difficult with today's computers, taking over a century of processing time. In contrast, a quantum computer might theoretically complete such a task in a few of hours. Climate analysis, transit planning, biology, financial services, encryption, and code breaking are all predicted to gain from quantum computing.

Everyone delighted to be a valued partner to numerous quantum research initiatives and organizations, including OpenSuperQPlus, MUNIQC-SC, IQM, Q-NEXT, Chicago Quantum Exchange (CQE), and ETH Zurich. We continue to push advances in quantum computing research and play an important role in influencing the development of this transformational technology through these collaborations.

Supporting Quantum Computer in Bioinformatics Research
Much has been said about quantum computing promise for a wide range of applications, yet there have been few examples of a quantum advantage for real-world issues of practical significance. Quantitative methods to biological problem solving have grown increasingly important. Two types of computational approaches, in particular, are at the heart of biological research:

- Techniques based on the physicochemical features of molecules, organisms, and systems, as well as Computer science approaches for navigating massive data that characterize genomics, proteomics, interactomics, and so on.

Both IBM and Microsoft refer to chemistry as the initial application for quantum computing, a fundamentally new type of computer that currently being developed. Chemistry, without a doubt, has several bioinformatics application opportunities. Quantum chemistry has applications in agriculture, epigenetics, and a variety of other fields [13]. Quantum computers may be utilized to create novel pharmaceuticals, novel materials, and to investigate catalytic and molecular interactions. Among the initial interesting challenges that quantum computers are likely to handle are simulations of tiny molecules or chemical processes. The computers may then be used to hasten the hunt for novel medications or to kickstart the creation of energy-saving catalysts that accelerate chemical processes.

15.1.2 The Role of Quantum Computing in Bioinformatics

Quantum computing has the potential to alter bioinformatics by providing novel answers to challenging computational issues in genomics, proteomics, and other fields of life sciences. Here are some of the main functions that quantum computing can play in bioinformatics:

- **Accelerated Sequence Alignment and Searching:** Quantum methods like Grover's algorithm may dramatically speed up database searching and sequence alignment activities. This is especially useful for exploring big genetic datasets quickly, detecting sequence similarities, and extracting significant genetic information.

- **Analysis of Genomic Data:** Quantum computing can efficiently process and analyze large genomic datasets. Quantum algorithms for activities such as genome assembly, variant calling, and phylogenetic analysis have the ability to accelerate genomics research and pave the way for personalized treatment.
- **Molecular Modeling and Drug Discovery:** Quantum computing allows for very precise simulations of molecular interactions and quantum chemistry. This is useful in drug development because it allows researchers to model and analyze molecular behavior, create novel medications, and anticipate how diverse compounds interact with biological targets.
- **Protein Folding and Structural Predictions:** In bioinformatics, understanding protein folding is critical. By mimicking the quantum nature of molecular interactions, quantum computing can give more exact protein folding predictions, which classical computers frequently struggle to represent effectively.
- **Biomarker Recognition:** Quantum algorithms can help in biomarker identification and categorization. Quantum computing can help detect possible illness indicators and forecast disease outcomes more effectively by processing and analyzing large-scale biological data at a faster rate.
- **Network Analysis and Systems Biology:** Complex biological networks and systems may be analyzed using quantum techniques. They can aid in the identification of critical regulatory nodes in gene networks, the mapping of complex biological pathways, and the prediction of how perturbations in these networks impact overall system behavior.
- **Personalized Medicine:** By swiftly processing and analyzing patient-specific genetic and medical data, quantum computing might pave the path for personalized medicine. This allows for personalized treatment plans, medication regimens, and diagnostics based on a person's unique genetic composition.

- **Optimization in Bioinformatics:** Many bioinformatics activities include optimization, such as determining which method is most effective to align sequences or selecting the optimum combination of parameters in a biological model. The optimization capabilities of quantum computing can assist bioinformaticians in finding optimum solutions more quickly and correctly.
- **Hybrid Quantum-Classical techniques:** Hybrid quantum-classical techniques can handle difficult bioinformatics challenges by combining the strengths of classical and quantum computers. This synergy takes use of the speed of quantum computing in specialized tasks while depending on classical computing for more general processes, providing a balanced solution.
- **Quantum Machine Learning:** Quantum machine learning models can improve bioinformatics applications such as protein-protein interaction prediction, drug design optimization, and high-dimensional biological data analysis.

In quantum computing has the potential to transform bioinformatics by speeding up data processing, simulation, and optimization processes. Its distinct characteristics, such as quantum parallelism and interference, offer the possibility of solving some of the most difficult computer problems in the biological sciences. The relevance of quantum computing in bioinformatics is projected to grow as quantum technologies progress.

15.1.3 Application of Quantum Technologies

Quantum impacts are already present in our daily lives. Modern Smartphone's, for example, have billions of transistors that regulate currents and voltages using the quantum mechanical features of semiconductors. This is the initial generation of quantum technology, which uses natural quantum phenomena. The second phase, on the other hand, is concerned with the creation and control of individual quantum states. Our considerable knowledge in RF technology, as well as the outstanding efficiency of our devices, contributes to the progress of quantum research [12]. Zurich Instruments will join the Rohde & Schwarz family in July 2021. Zurich Instruments offers a diverse variety of quantum technology products that complement the Rohde & Schwarz T&M portfolio.

The three main domains of quantum technology are:

- Quantum computing - Quantum computing is a critical field of quantum technology. Unlike traditional systems that handle data sequentially using binary code, quantum computers (QC) save time by processing data in parallel. This enables them to handle complicated issues that traditional computers find difficult to solve. QCs might render public key encryption systems outdated, forcing investigation into potential future attack scenarios.
- Quantum communication - This is where quantum communications enter the picture. QKD is a cryptographic method that allows two parties to safely exchange a secret encryption key over a public channel. Any eavesdropping effort disrupts the quantum state and warns the communication parties. Unlike quantum computing, QKD is nearing completion. Rohde & Schwarz and Zurich Instruments are active participants in this process, working on projects like OpenQKD to incorporate quantum-safe technologies into current systems.
- Quantum sensor technology - Another key use of quantum technology is sensing. Quantum sensing offers enormous possibilities for high-precision radar systems, which can identify small, slow-moving objects like drones, something traditional radar technology fails to do. Rohde & Schwarz has helped the UK Quantum Technology Hub Sensors and Timing project evaluate quantum clocks for this purpose. We are additionally a part of the Quarate (Quantum Radar Team) project, which is investigating quantum radar at microwave frequencies.

15.1.4 Characteristics of Quantum Computing in Bioinformatics

Quantum computing has numerous distinguishing features that make it highly appealing for bioinformatics, especially for solving difficult computational issues in genomics, proteomics, and other life science areas [14]. Here are some of the important features of quantum computing in bioinformatics:

- Quantum Parallelism: Because quantum bits, or qubits, may exist in superpositions, quantum computers can process numerous possibilities at the same time. This intrinsic parallelism is useful in activities such as scanning vast databases or optimizing complicated biological systems, where many viable solutions must be investigated.
- Exponential Speedup: For some situations, quantum algorithms can yield an exponential speedup over their conventional equivalents. This can significantly reduce the time necessary for sophisticated data analysis, modeling, and optimization, allowing bioinformaticians to get insights faster.
- Machine Learning Advancements: Quantum machine learning models leverage quantum principles to enhance bioinformatics tasks, such as predicting protein-protein interactions, optimizing drug discovery, and making sense of high-dimensional biological data more effectively.
- High-Dimensional Data Processing: Quantum computing can efficiently process high-dimensional biological data, which is often encountered in gene expression analysis, omics data, and network modeling. This capability enables more comprehensive and accurate data analysis.
- Personalized Medicine: Quantum computing can process patient-specific genetic and medical data rapidly, paving the way for personalized medicine. This enables healthcare professionals to develop tailored treatment plans and diagnostics based on individual genetic profiles.
- Hybrid Quantum-Classical techniques: Using hybrid techniques that combine the benefits of classical and quantum computing, bioinformaticians may use quantum computing's speed for specialized tasks while depending on classical computing for more general operations.
- Quantum Security: Quantum cryptography and quantum-resistant algorithms provide increased data security, which is crucial in bioinformatics for securing sensitive medical and genetic information.
- Biomarker Identification: Quantum computing can help researchers find possible illness indicators and predict disease outcomes more efficiently, allowing for earlier diagnosis and treatment.

- Complicated Network Analysis: Quantum algorithms can handle complicated biological networks including gene regulatory networks and protein-protein interaction networks, which are important in systems biology and network analysis.

Finally, the unique properties of quantum computing, such as quantum parallelism, exponential speedup, and the capacity to mimic quantum systems, make it a great tool for solving the computational issues inherent in bioinformatics [1]. The application of quantum computing in bioinformatics is predicted to lead to substantial discoveries in genomics, drug discovery, and personalized medicine as quantum technologies improve.

15.1.5 What are the Tools Used in Quantum Computing in Bioinformatics?

As of my last knowledge update in September 2021, quantum computing was still in its early stages of development and not widely integrated into bioinformatics tools. However, there has been growing interest in exploring the potential of quantum computing in bioinformatics [8]. Some of the tools and platforms used for quantum computing in bioinformatics at that time included:

- Qiskit: Qiskit is an open-source quantum computing platform developed by IBM. It offers a quantum development environment for researchers to experiment with quantum algorithms and build applications, which might include bioinformatics activities.
- Cirq: Cirq is a quantum computing framework that was created by Google's Quantum AI team. It is intended for the development of quantum algorithms pertinent to bioinformatics, as well as the creation and optimization of quantum circuits.
- Microsoft Quantum Development Kit: The Quantum Development Kit from Microsoft is a collection of tools for writing quantum algorithms. Q# (Q-sharp), a quantum programming language, may be used by researchers to investigate quantum computer applications, including those in biology.

- Amazon Braket is a quantum computing service that gives users access to quantum hardware and simulators. It may be used by researchers to conduct research with quantum algorithms and investigate possible applications in a variety of fields, notably bioinformatics.
- Rigetti Forest: Rigetti is well-known for giving people access to quantum computers and quantum simulators. The Rigetti Forest platform provides quantum software development tools and libraries for bioinformatics issues.
- Xanadu PennyLane: PennyLane by Xanadu is a quantum machine learning library that integrates quantum computing with machine learning frameworks such as TensorFlow and PyTorch. PennyLane can be used by researchers to do quantum-enhanced machine learning in bioinformatics.
- IBM Quantum Experience: The IBM Quantum Experience platform provides access to cloud-based quantum computing resources. Researchers can test quantum circuits, create quantum algorithms, and investigate possible biology applications.

It's worth noting that the subject of quantum computing is fast expanding, and new tools and platforms may have developed since my previous update. Researchers interested in bringing quantum computing to bioinformatics should remain up to date on the latest discoveries and investigate the available tools and platforms. Collaboration between quantum physicists, computer scientists, and bioinformaticians is also essential for driving the development of tools and solutions adapted to the special problems of bioinformatics [17].

15.2 Novel Approaches of Quantum Computing in Bioinformatics

15.2.1 Quantum Chemistry for Drug Discovery

Because quantum computing allows for precise simulations of molecular interactions and chemical processes, drug discovery time and resources are substantially reduced. Quantum chemistry techniques have the potential to change the face of pharmaceutical research.

The IBM Quantum Experience platform gives users access to cloud-based quantum computing capabilities. Researchers may put quantum circuits to the test, develop quantum algorithms, and look at potential biological applications. It's noteworthy that the field of quantum computing is rapidly evolving, and novel platforms and tools may have emerged since my last update [18]. Researchers interested in using quantum computing to bioinformatics should stay current on new discoveries and study existing tools and platforms. Collaboration between quantum physicists, computer scientists, and bioinformaticians is also critical for pushing the creation of tools and solutions tailored to bioinformatics' unique difficulties.

According to specialists in drug research, quantum computing methods may bring value to antibody research and development by generating a unique antibody structure. Integrating quantum algorithms with today's conventional tools may occur organically when developing knowledge and planning to tackle the challenge. Using various algorithms, hybrid algorithms, and techniques, the optimum quantum instrument to meet the objective may be determined. On the future are countless possible quantum applications. It is predicted to play an important role in drug development, as well as in the testing and synthesis of compounds for use in medicine, among other uses. The bio-medical imaging revolution has the potential to change detection and diagnostics in the direction of novel medication development using Figure 15.2 drug discovery.

Biogen, an American biotechnology company, is experimenting with quantum to aid in the treatment of neurological illnesses. According to The Quantum Insider, quantum-enabled optimization, sampling, and machine learning algorithms can be utilized to speed drug development.

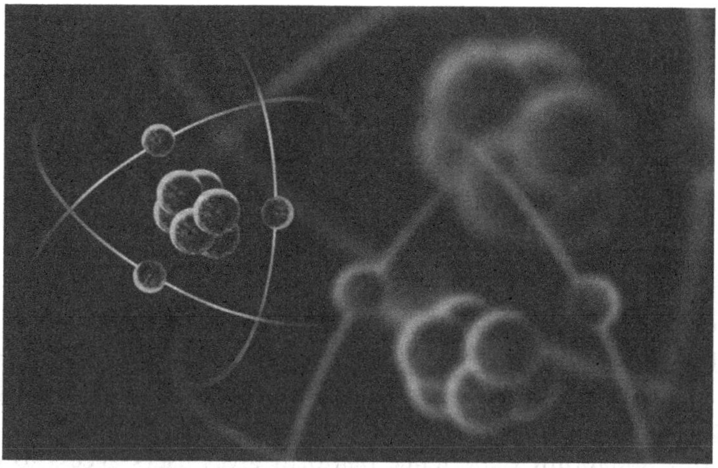

Figure 15.2 Drug discovery.

Another pharmaceutical business pioneering quantum computing to expedite and optimize healthcare services and solutions is Boehringer Ingelheim, a Google Quantum AI partner for the past three years. Their long-term objective is to create unique and cutting-edge new medications. Harnessing the potential of quantum physics is a complex and sensitive process, with many challenges still ahead. Qubits are sensitive, and a secure environment is necessary to keep them in superposition and entanglement. If the qubits are not kept in severe conditions, the entire system will fail.

15.2.2 A Quantum Advance in Genetics

The exponential development of genomic data necessitates improved computer capabilities. Quantum algorithms for genetic data analysis offer quicker and more efficient processing, resulting in greater understanding of genomics and personalized treatment [15]. In the future, the discipline of genetics, which studies genes, heredity, and genetic diversity, may be inextricably linked to quantum computing. Among the most exciting uses is DNA sequence analysis. Traditional genetic data analysis approaches are computationally demanding and sometimes limited in scope. Quantum computers have the potential to speed up DNA sequence alignment, the development of phylogenetic trees, and the discovery of genetic markers linked with illnesses.

These computational developments have the potential to have a huge impact on health, such as speedier illness screening, more personalized medication, and perhaps the elimination of some hereditary disorders. In addition, quantum computers' capacity to model interactions between molecules and assembling at the quantum level should lead to a better understanding of protein structures and medication interactions. This has the potential to revolutionize drug discovery and development, resulting in more accurate and effective therapies. Companies such as Polarisqb, ODE L3C, and Quantinuum are already striving to use quantum computing methods to model and evaluate specific chemical compounds. Their study might have an impact on the future of medication development.

Genetics: A Quantum Future?

Interactions between quantum computers and genomics might usher in a new era of scientific discovery. The collaboration of two seemingly unrelated domains has the potential to transform our understanding of genetics and bioinformatics. As quantum computing evolves and its capabilities expand, we may expect dramatic advances that will revolutionize medical research, medication development, and our understanding of life's complexities [10, 16]. While hurdles exist, the idea of gaining previously unachievable insights and capabilities through the combination of quantum computing and biology remains enticing. The world awaits the next chapter in the tale of science's grand confluence as researchers continue to study this juncture.

15.2.3 Hybrid Quantum-Classical Approaches

Researchers are investigating hybrid quantum-classical techniques to handle complex biological issues by combining the characteristics of conventional and quantum computers, perhaps giving more efficient solutions. Drug discovery applications benefit greatly from hybrid quantum-classical machine learning. The researchers proved that hybrid architectures that integrate quantum computers with deep conventional networks may be used for drug discovery applications [3]. They created a tiny but powerful model, small enough to fit on a cutting-edge D-Wave quantum annealer, and trained it using a subset of the ChEMBL dataset of physiologically active chemicals.

To handle complicated issues in bioinformatics, hybrid quantum-classical techniques use the strengths of both quantum and traditional computers. Quantum computers use quantum bits, or qubits, which may exist in several states at the same time, allowing them to do certain operations far quicker than traditional computers. Quantum computers, on the other hand, are still in their infancy and confront technological limits. Hybrid techniques combine quantum processors with conventional computers, resulting in a synergy that overcomes both systems' limits.

Applications in Bioinformatics:

- Molecular Simulations: Quantum computers are ideal for modeling the quantum behavior of molecules. They can, for example, precisely anticipate molecular interactions and optimize drug candidates in drug development. To represent complicated biomolecular systems more effectively, hybrid techniques integrate quantum simulations with conventional methods.
- Protein Structure Prediction: Protein structure prediction is a key challenge in bioinformatics [11]. Quantum computers can effectively search for a protein's lowest energy conformation, which is an important step in structure prediction. These quantum optimization techniques are used in hybrid

approaches to improve accuracy and minimize processing time.

- Genomics: Analyzing huge genomic datasets, such as DNA sequencing data, requires a significant amount of time and effort. By outsourcing computationally costly components to quantum computers, hybrid techniques can speed up activities like sequence alignment, variant calling, and metagenomics analysis.
- Quantum machine learning techniques: provide the benefits in feature selection and optimization. In bioinformatics, hybrid techniques can be utilized for tasks such as illness categorization, biomarker development, and treatment response prediction.

Challenges and Considerations

While hybrid quantum-classical techniques have enormous potential, they also pose difficulties:

- Limitations of Quantum Hardware: Quantum computers are currently constrained by means of qubit count and error rates. The integration of these technologies with traditional systems needs careful resource management.
- Algorithm Development: The creation of quantum algorithms and their integration into current bioinformatics pipelines necessitates multidisciplinary collaboration among quantum physicists, computer scientists, and biologists.
- Data Handling: Because quantum computing requires accurate data encoding and decoding, large-scale data handling can be difficult.

Quantum computers are not yet publicly available, and most research in this field is done in specialized quantum labs or through cloud-based quantum computing services [4]. Despite these obstacles, hybrid quantum-classical techniques have significant potential in bioinformatics. We should expect revolutionary contributions to the sector as quantum technology evolves and algorithmic improvements continue, leading to speedier drug development, more precise protein structure predictions, and enhanced genomics analysis. The exciting frontier of hybrid quantum-classical bioinformatics promises to change our understanding of biology and speed up the creation of life-changing solutions in healthcare and industry.

15.2.4 Quantum-Inspired Machine Learning

These models incorporate quantum concepts into conventional machine learning, providing better capabilities for analyzing biological and medical data. Quantum Machine Learning in Bioinformatics: Transforming Data Analysis in Life Sciences [7]. Bioinformatics, or the analysis of biological data using computer and statistical methods, is critical in modern life sciences. It has a wide range of applications, ranging from genomics and proteomics to drug development and clinical diagnostics. With the proliferation of biological data, there is a growing demand for novel computational tools to analyze and extract relevant insights. Quantum-inspired machine learning is developing as a paradigm shift in bioinformatics, having the ability to greatly improve data processing and speed biological discoveries.

What Is Quantum-Inspired Machine Learning in Bioinformatics?
Quantum-inspired machine learning is a synthesis of quantum computing with classical machine learning techniques. While it does not use actual quantum computers, it uses quantum physics to construct algorithms that are capable of handling complicated biological data more effectively than traditional machine learning approaches [7, 18]. To address bioinformatics issues, this technique employs principles like as superposition, entanglement, and quantum annealing.

Applications in Bioinformatics:

- Sequence Analysis: In genomics, quantum-inspired machine learning may be utilized to speed up sequence alignment, pattern identification, and variant calling. These methods aid in the discovery of genetic mutations, structural changes, and regulatory regions in DNA and RNA sequences.
- Determining the three-dimensional structures: Proteins is a difficult issue with important consequences for drug development. Quantum-inspired machine learning can optimize energy landscapes and investigate various protein conformations, which can help in structure prediction and medication formulation.
- Drug Discovery: Quantum-inspired approaches can speed up virtual screening of chemical compounds towards target proteins, allowing researchers to uncover possible drug

candidates more quickly and affordably. This speeds up the drug-development process.

- Biological Network Analysis: Quantum-inspired algorithms that improve data clustering, community identification and network modeling may be used to analyze biological networks such as protein-protein interaction networks or metabolic pathways.
- Illness Prediction: By processing high-dimensional data and capturing intricate correlations in patient records, quantum-inspired machine learning can enhance illness prediction models.

Challenges and Considerations:

- Algorithm Development: Developing quantum-inspired machine learning algorithms necessitates multidisciplinary collaboration among quantum physicists, computer scientists, and bioinformaticians. These methods must be customized for certain bioinformatics applications.
- Data Integration: It is critical to integrate with current bioinformatics processes and databases. Data preparation and interoperability with traditional data sources are essential factors to consider.
- Quantum Hardware: While quantum-inspired machine learning does not require actual quantum computers, improvements in quantum hardware can assist the discipline. Access to quantum computing resources is still restricted.
- Interpretability: As with traditional machine learning, assuring the interpretability of outcomes in quantum-inspired techniques remains a difficulty.
- Education and Skill Development: The use of quantum-inspired machine learning in bioinformatics needs the training of a workforce in both quantum computing and bioinformatics.

Quantum-inspired machine learning in bioinformatics is an innovative technique that has the potential to revolutionize data processing in the biological sciences. As the area develops, it promises to provide more efficient, accurate, and quick solutions for analyzing biological data and expanding our understanding of genomes, proteomics, and drug development. Researchers and practitioners are ready to push bioinformatics forward by leveraging the capabilities of quantum-inspired machine learning algorithms [10].

15.2.5 Challenges and Limitations

Quantum computing has issues such as error correction, hardware stability, and requiring for specialized quantum software. Overcoming these constraints is critical for the widespread use of quantum computing in the biological sciences [2].

- Limitations of Quantum Hardware: The current status of quantum hardware is one of the foremost critical obstacles in quantum computing for bioinformatics. Quantum computers are still in their early phases of development, with a limited amount of power and qubit count. This can make it difficult to efficiently manage vast and complicated biological datasets.
- Error Rates: Because of issues such as decoherence and noise, quantum computers are prone to mistakes. Error mitigation is a serious difficulty in bioinformatics, where accuracy is important. Quantum error correcting algorithms are still in the works and can add a large amount of overhead.
- Algorithm Development: Designing quantum algorithms for bioinformatics applications necessitates knowledge of both quantum computing and bioinformatics. These algorithms are still in their early stages and must be adapted to the specific peculiarities of biological systems.
- Quantum Computing and Classical Systems: Quantum computing is frequently utilized in combination with classical systems. It can be difficult to ensure smooth integration of quantum and conventional components, and data flow between the two types of systems might bring latency and compatibility issues.
- Data Encoding: Quantum computers necessitate particular data encoding methods. It can be difficult to adapt biological data to various encoding techniques and efficiently decode the findings back into traditional data formats.
- Scalability: As the area of bioinformatics works with more and larger datasets, the scalability of quantum algorithms and technology becomes increasingly important. It is a huge

difficulty to ensure that quantum systems can manage rising data volumes.

- Quantum Computer Access and Cost: Quantum computers are not as widely available as traditional computing resources. Researchers frequently require access to specialized quantum gear or cloud-based quantum services, which can be costly and have usage restrictions.
- Interpretability: Quantum algorithms can give results that are difficult to comprehend or explain, particularly for individuals unfamiliar with quantum computing. It is a constant struggle to ensure that the insights generated from quantum-based investigations are intelligible and useful.
- Complexity of Quantum Simulation: While quantum computers excel at modeling quantum systems, translating complicated biological systems into a quantum-representable format can be extremely difficult. Some biological challenges may be less amenable to quantum simulation by definition. Given the constraints and costs of quantum computing, resource allocation and job prioritization in bioinformatics must be carefully handled to establish a balance of quantum and conventional computing resources.
- Quantum Variational Algorithms: Quantum variational algorithms, which are frequently employed in quantum computing for optimization issues in bioinformatics, may have limits in locating global minima and may not always provide optimum solutions.

While quantum computing has immense potential for enhancing bioinformatics, it also has a number of hurdles and constraints. Addressing these difficulties will be crucial as the field advances for the effective integration of quantum computing into bioinformatics applications, ultimately leading to more efficient and accurate analysis in genomes, proteomics, drug development, and other fields of life sciences.

15.3 Conclusion

The incorporation of quantum computing into bioinformatics and medicinal research is a frontier highlighted by enormous potential as well as inherent limitations. On the path to harnessing the power of quantum technologies, it is obvious that quantum computing provides innovative and unparalleled capabilities that have the potential to revolutionize data processing, modeling, and problem-solving in the health sciences. With its capacity to handle massive information and solve complicated problems at quantum speeds, quantum computers promise to greatly accelerate important activities in genomics, proteomics, drug development, and illness prediction. The possible uses range from optimizing molecular simulations to unraveling protein folding mysteries and developing customized medicinal compounds with pinpoint precision.

However, the way towards fully realizing these advantages is not without challenges. Quantum hardware is still in its early stages, with practical constraints like as error rates and qubit count to overcome. The creation of algorithms in quantum bioinformatics is an interdisciplinary task that necessitates the collaboration of quantum physicists, computer scientists, and life science experts. Data encoding, integrating with traditional systems, and attaining interpretability are all important but difficult components of the trip. Nonetheless, the path is obvious. In bioinformatics and biomedical research, quantum computing is more than a potential route; it is a transformational catalyst.

As quantum technology advances and quantum-inspired algorithms grow more complex, the life sciences stand to acquire unprecedented computational capacity, which will open new insights, streamline research methods, and expedite the pace of discovery. Despite difficulties, the use of quantum computing into bioinformatics and biological research holds the possibility of unraveling the mysteries of life at an unparalleled rate. The convergence of quantum computing and the biological sciences is set to transform our knowledge of biology, unearth fresh treatment methods, and propel healthcare to new heights as we continue to study this intriguing frontier. This integration is more than a possibility; it is a daring step towards a future in which the secrets of life itself are unraveled and the frontiers of what is possible in biomedical research and bioinformatics are constantly pushed.

15.4 The Future of Quantum Computing in Bioinformatics and Biomedical Research

The use of quantum computing into bioinformatics and biomedical research holds the prospect of game-changing advances in the life sciences. As we look ahead, some significant themes and possibilities emerge that give us a taste of what is to come in this intriguing junction of quantum technology and the biological sciences:

- Improved Drug Discovery: Quantum computing will revolutionize drug discovery by allowing for quick and exact simulations of molecular interactions. The capacity to accurately anticipate drug-protein binding will lead to the creation of more effective and personalized medications.
- Personalized Medicine: Quantum computing will be critical in realizing personalized medicine. Healthcare practitioners will be able to analyze a patient's genetic and proteomic data at quantum rates.
- Accelerated Genomic Analysis: Due to the exponential expansion of genomic data, strong computational techniques are required. Sequence alignment, variant calling, and metagenomics analysis will be accelerated by quantum computers, making genomics more accessible and informative.
- Precision Protein Folding: Quantum-inspired algorithms and quantum annealers will help us better understand protein folding, a complicated process with important consequences for both health and illness. This understanding will allow for the creation of novel medicines and tailored interventions.
- Quantum Machine Learning: Algorithms for quantum machine learning will acquire significance in bioinformatics, increasing tasks such as biomarker discovery, illness categorization, and treatment response prediction. These algorithms will extract more information from large biological datasets.
- Quantum-Supervised Learning: Researchers will be able to solve issues such as de novo drug creation, bimolecular characterization, and the discovery of genetic markers for illnesses using supervised learning on quantum computers.
- Quantum Cloud Services: Cloud-based services will make access to quantum computing resources more widely available, boosting cooperation and innovation in the health sciences community.
- Quantum Databases: Quantum databases are expected to develop as a new frontier, allowing for the efficient storing and retrieval of quantum-encoded biological data while also

meeting the particular data handling requirements of quantum computing in bioinformatics.

- Interdisciplinary Collaboration: The quantum bioinformatics area will continue to flourish on interdisciplinary cooperation amongst quantum physicists, computer scientists, biologists, and physicians. New educational programs will arise to cultivate this talent pool.
- Quantum Hardware Evolution: Quantum hardware will grow more complex, with higher qubit counts and lower error rates. This advancement will increase the variety of challenges that quantum computing can handle.
- Ethical and Regulatory Frameworks: As quantum computing becomes more prevalent in healthcare and drug research, ethical considerations and regulatory frameworks will evolve to address privacy, transparency, and security concerns connected with quantum-powered bioinformatics.

The integration of quantum computing with bioinformatics and medicinal research has limitless potential. It is a future in which illnesses are recognized and treated with unprecedented accuracy, medication development grows faster and more effective, and genetic data is quickly analyzed to reveal the mysteries of life. While problems remain, the path forward is clear: quantum computing is poised to rewrite the limits of what humans can do in the living sciences, ushering in a period of extraordinary creativity and discovery.

References

1. Pyrkov, A., Aliper, A., Bezrukov, D., Lin, Y.-C., Polykovskiy, D., Kamya, P., Ren, F., Zhavoronkov, A., Quantum computing for near-term applications in generative chemistry and drug discovery. *Drug Discov. Today*, 28, 8, 103675, 2023, ISSN 1359-6446, https://doi.org/10.1016/j.drudis.2023.103675.
2. Alsubai, S., Alqahtani, A., Binbusayyis, A., Sha, M., Gumaei, A., Wang, S., Quantum Computing Meets Deep Learning: A Promising Approach for Diabetic Retinopathy Classification. *Mathematics*, 11, 9, 2008, 2023, https://doi.org/10.3390/math11092008.
3. Avramouli, M., Savvas, I.K., Vasilaki, A., Garani, G., Unlocking the Potential of Quantum Machine Learning to Advance Drug Discovery. *Electronics*, 12, 11, 2402, 2023, https://doi.org/10.3390/electronics12112402.

4. Balgani, S. and Sangeetha, S., An Efficient Approach to Improve Response Time in Multibiometric Patterns Retrieval from Large Database. *Int. J. Comput. Sci. Netw. Secur. (IJCSNS)*, 14, 5, 102, 2014.
5. Lau, B., Emani, P.S., Chapman, J., Yao, L., Lam, T., Merrill, P., Warrell, J., Gerstein, M.B., Lam, H.Y.K., Insights from incorporating quantum computing into drug design workflows. *Bioinformatics*, 39, 1, btac789, January 2023, https://doi.org/10.1093/bioinformatics/btac789.
6. Selvaraj, C., Elakkiya, E., Prabhu, P., Velmurugan, D., Singh, S.K., Chapter 9 - Advances in QSAR through artificial intelligence and machine learning methods, in: *QSAR in Safety Evaluation and Risk Assessment*, H. Hong (Ed.), pp. 101–116, Academic Press, 2023, ISBN 9780443153396, https://doi.org/10.1016/B978-0-443-15339-6.00033-3.
7. Emani, P.S., Warrell, J., Anticevic, A., Bekiranov, S., Gandal, M., McConnell, M.J., Sapiro, G., Aspuru-Guzik, A., Baker, J.T., Bastiani, M., Murray, J.D., Sotiropoulos, S.N., Taylor, J., Senthil, G., Lehner, T., Gerstein, M.B., Harrow, A.W., Quantum computing at the frontiers of biological sciences. *Nat. Methods*, 18, 7, 701–709, 2021 Jul, doi: 10.1038/s41592-020-01004-3, PMID: 33398186, PMCID: PMC8254820.
8. Weidner, F.M., Schwab, J.D., Wölk, S., Rupprecht, F., Ikonomi, N., Werle, S.D., Hoffmann, S., Kühl, M., Kestler, H.A., Leveraging quantum computing for dynamic analyses of logical networks in systems biology. *Patterns*, 4, 3, 100705, 2023, ISSN 2666-3899, https://doi.org/10.1016/j.patter.2023.100705.
9. Kanamori, Y. and Yoo, S.-M., Quantum Computing: Principles and Applications. *J. Int. Technol. Inf. Manage.*, 29, 2, Article 3, 43–71, 2020, DOI: https://doi.org/10.58729/1941-6679.1410.
10. Zinner, M., Dahlhausen, F., Boehme, P., Ehlers, J., Bieske, L., Fehring, L., Quantum computing's potential for drug discovery: early stage industry dynamics. *Drug Discov. Today*, 26, 7, 1680–1688, 2021.
11. Nałęcz-Charkiewicz, K. and Nowak, R.M., Algorithm for DNA sequence assembly by quantum annealing. *BMC Bioinf.*, 23, 122, 2022, https://doi.org/10.1186/s12859-022-04661-7.
12. Orengo, C., Velankar, S., Wodak, S. *et al.*, A community proposal to integrate structural bioinformatics activities in ELIXIR (3D-Bioinfo Community). *F1000Research*, 9, ELIXIR, 278, 2020.
13. Pal, S., Bhattacharya, M., Lee, S.S. *et al.*, Quantum Computing in the Next-Generation Computational Biology Landscape: From Protein Folding to Molecular Dynamics. *Mol. Biotechnol.*, 66, 163–178, 2023, https://doi.org/10.1007/s12033-023-00765-4.
14. Li, R.Y., Gujja, S., Bajaj, S.R., Gamel, O.E., Cilfone, N., Gulcher, J.R., Lidar, D.A., Chittenden, T.W., Quantum processor-inspired machine learning in the biomedical sciences. *Patterns*, 2, 6, 100246, 2021, ISSN 2666-3899.
15. Sangeetha, S., Baskar, K., Kalaivaani, P.C.D., Kumaravel, T., Deep Learning-based Early Parkinson's Disease Detection from Brain MRI Image. *2023 7th International Conference on Intelligent Computing and Control*

Systems (ICICCS), Madurai, India, pp. 490–495, 2023, doi: 10.1109/ICICCS56967.2023.10142754.
16. Ur Rasool, R., Ahmad, H.F., Rafique, W., Qayyum, A., Qadir, J., Anwar, Z., Quantum Computing for Healthcare: A Review. *Future Internet*, 15, 3, 94, 2023, https://doi.org/10.3390/fi15030094.
17. Wang, S., Pei, Z., Wang, C. *et al.*, Shaping the future of the application of quantum computing in intelligent transportation system. *Intell. Converged Netw.*, 2, 4, 259–276, 2021, https://doi.org/10.23919/ICN.2021.0019.
18. Wang, Y., When Quantum Computation Meets Data Science: Making Data Science Quantum. *Harv. Data Sci. Rev.*, 4, 1, 2022, https://doi.org/10.1162/99608f92.ef5d8928.

16

Future Perspective and Emerging Trends in Computational Intelligence

Chander Prabha

Chitkara University Institute of Engineering and Technology, Chitkara University, Punjab, India

Abstract

An emerging discipline leading the bioinformatics and biomedical system is Computational Intelligence (CI). To solve the toughest challenges in disease understanding and healthcare, the cutting-edge CI integrates biological disciplines. In the field of bioinformatics, there has been a lot of progress in the prediction of genetic analysis, protein structure, and the decoding of intricate networks of cells. The reason is due to the synchronization of CI techniques together (viz. Neural Networks (NN), Deep Learning (DL), and Evolutionary Algorithms, Machine Learning (ML)). Additionally, CI is discovering and inventing treatment approaches, patient care, and diagnostics in biomedical systems. More precise ML models are being used for each patient to understand medical imaging, predict the course of illness, and enhance therapy regimens customized. The focus on ethical Artificial intelligence (AI) is a main component of CI's future in biomedical and bioinformatics systems. Making sure AI is used ethically by taking into account problems viz. permission, bias, and privacy, will be crucial as CI applications become integrated into healthcare and biological studies. Developing strong ethical standards and frameworks will be necessary to maximize the impact of CI while minimizing dangers and guaranteeing fair access to innovations. The chapter delves into exploring CI's growing trends and prospective views. It emphasizes how it can revolutionize the biomedical and bioinformatics fields.

Keywords: Bioinformatics, biomedical systems, genetic analysis, machine learning (ML), Artificial intelligence (AI), cells, quantum computing (QC), ethics

Email: prabhanice@gmail.com

Neha Sharma, Korhan Cengiz and Prasenjit Chatterjee (eds.) Intelligent Data Analytics for Bioinformatics and Biomedical Systems, (381–396) © 2024 Scrivener Publishing LLC

16.1 Introduction

The CI is a subfield of AI. It uses a variety of strategies for computation and solves challenging real-world issues that can't be solved by using conventional methods of modeling. It draws motivation from the surrounding environment of biological systems. It integrates ideas and methods from numerous fields including psychology, neurology, and evolution. Evolutionary Computation (EC), Neural Networks (NN), Swarm Intelligence (SI), Fuzzy Systems (FS), and Artificial Life are some of the fundamental techniques used in CI [1]. Every one of these techniques has certain advantages and works well with certain kinds of issues. A brief overview of each is shown in Table 16.1.

When it comes to problem-solving, CI varies from conventional AI in that it frequently uses heuristics, autonomy, and adaptability rather than just logic and preset algorithms. Because of this, CI is especially skilled at handling settings that are dynamic, loud, and complex. There are many different and extensive uses for CI, such as but not restricted to as shown in Figure 16.1.

CI improves bioinformatics research's precision and effectiveness; these approaches make it possible to examine biological data that was before unmanageable. The use of CI to better understand genetic illnesses, tailor treatment based on individual genetic profiles, and expedite the identification of therapeutic targets and biomarkers is what the future holds. To facilitate ongoing wellness tracking and immediate information analysis, wearable technology and Internet of Things (IoT) devices combined with CI algorithms have emerged. This has opened the door to more proactive healthcare treatments and better control of illnesses. Furthermore, the use of CI in robotically assisted operations shortens recuperation periods and is accurate [2].

The combination of Quantum Computing (QC) and CI is a prominent new trend. It promises a significant increase in computational power and processes massive biological statistics. The combination of these two technologies would open up new avenues for molecule simulation, the discovery of drugs, and systems biology modeling. This results in the advancement of understanding of disease mechanisms and the creation of innovative treatments. The cross-disciplinary collaboration will be essential to the development of CI applications for genomics and biomedical systems [3]. The amalgamation of medicine, biology, ethics, and computer science encourages creative responses to challenging medical problems and provides a comprehensive strategy for illness prevention and treatment.

Table 16.1 CI techniques.

Name	Purpose	Feature
Neural Networks	It mimics the composition and operation of neural systems in the human brain.	Applied to projections, data categorization, and recognizing patterns Deep Neural Networks (DNN), a subclass of NN has shown promising results on images and recognition of speech tasks.
Swarm Intelligence	Encompass methods viz. Particle Swarm Optimization (PSO) and Ant Colony Optimization (ACO). Inspired by the collective actions of distributed, autonomous systems, such as bird swarming or ant colonies	Helps in locating the best routes inside expansive and intricate search environments.
Evolutionary Computation	It encompasses techniques based on genetics and biological programming. Inspired from the theory of natural selection	Suited for problems with optimization, progressively altering responses through crossover, mutation, and selection.
Fuzzy Systems	Rely on fuzzy logic. Helpful in managing ambiguity and inaccuracies as fuzzy logic enables greater versatility in interpretation than classic binary logic	Employed in domains requiring intricate rule-based inference, such as systems of control and processes for making decisions.
Artificial Life	Comprises simulations of living processes to explore the creation of intricate behaviors from straightforward regulations and interactions	Applications in the fields of social science, automation, and biology studies. Helps in the development of artificial systems that resemble living things. Gains insight into the internal workings of evolutionary systems.

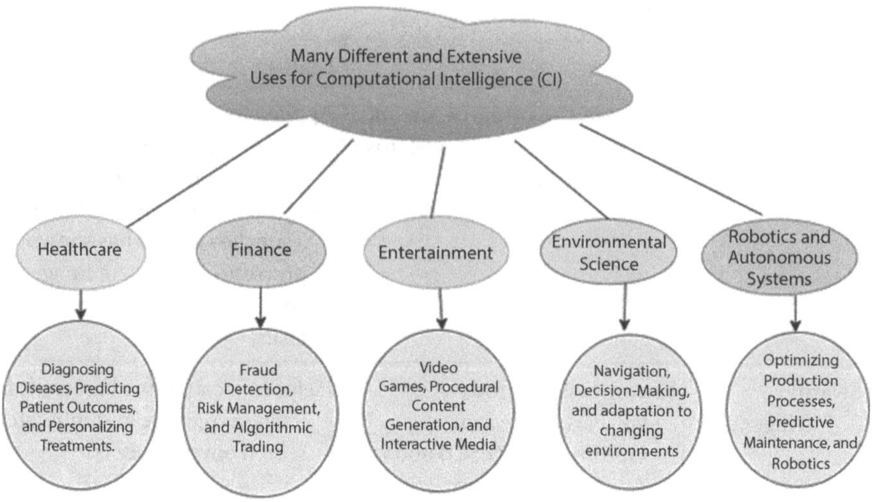

Figure 16.1 Extensive uses for CI.

In a nutshell, there is an abundance of prospects and fascinating possibilities for CI in genomics and biomedical systems going forward. Personalized medicine is going to be made possible by merging the physiological and medical sciences with cutting-edge computational methods. This will change the understanding of diseases and improve healthcare delivery. To fully realize the potential of computer-aided health (CI) in enhancing the well-being and health of people, one must prioritize ethical issues, cross-disciplinary cooperation, and the investigation of cutting-edge technologies like quantum computing, etc. [4].

Development in the field of CI is constantly expanding the realm of possible outcomes. The potential uses of CI grow as processing power rises and our understanding of the natural systems that give rise to these approaches deepens, providing creative answers for certain of the most difficult issues in a variety of fields.

16.2 Emerging Trends in CI for Bioinformatics

A combination of complex computations, enormous datasets, and computing power is altering research and applications in medicine, biology, and health. This is signaled by recent developments in CI for bioinformatics. This change is not only technological but also intellectual, bringing with it new approaches to forecasting results, tailoring treatment, and resolving intricate biological challenges [5]. The most promising trends in this area are:

1. ML and DL Enhancements: Forecasting, recognizing patterns, and data analysis in bioinformatics are just a few of the areas where ML, and especially DL, is still leading the way. Advances in the comprehension of genetic patterns, structures of proteins, and causes of illness are being made possible by improved algorithms that can handle complicated, data with high dimensions.
2. Computational Design and Synthetic (Artificial) Biology: The development of new biological elements, apparatus, and processes is being made easier by the combination of CI and biosynthesis. With increasing frequency, scientific biology is using computerized simulations and models to foresee the responses of synthetic (artificial) biological structures, which simplifies the design-build-test-learn cycle [6].
3. Integrative Omics Analysis: An emerging pattern is the synthesis of diverse 'omics' data (genetics, proteomics, metabolomics, etc.) using tools from CI. Using supportive details from several sources involving biological data, this integrated strategy seeks to construct broad models of biological events and states of disease.
4. Systems Medicine and Network Biology: With the use of CI technologies, biological systems, and networks are being analyzed to shed light on the intricate connections that occur between and within organisms. This method aids in discovering possible targets for treatment as well as helping to comprehend ailments at the systemic level.
5. Precision and Personalized Medicine: Dealing with the massive amounts of data produced by genetic material and health records requires CI. Helps in customizing medical care for every patient, resulting in better outcomes and lesser side effects.
6. Natural Language Processing (NLP) for Biomedical Text Mining: The extensive body of scientific research and clinical data is being mined for valuable information using NLP. This makes it easier to learn new information and link genetic variants to illnesses [7].
7. Blockchain: In bioinformatics research, blockchain is becoming a viable tool for guaranteeing data confidentiality,

sharing, and integrity. Authenticity and repeatability are guaranteed by providing a decentralized environment to oversee the enormous volumes of confidential information produced by biomedical research.

8. Quantum Computing: The prospective use of QC in bioinformatics is presently in its infancy, but it holds the possibility of solving intricate biological issues far more quickly than traditional computers. This involves simulating biological systems, describing molecular structures more precisely, and analyzing genetic information more quickly.

These developments demonstrate the dynamic connection between bioinformatics and CI, each of which is pushing forward the boundaries in terms of improving diagnosing illnesses, devising customized treatments, and comprehending life at the level of molecules. These technologies will surely open up novel perspectives in biomedical research and medicine as they develop further.

16.3 CI Emerging Trends for Biomedical Systems

The field of health and medicine research is changing in biomedical due to new developments in CI. These take advantage of developments in the analysis of data, computing techniques, and methods to tackle challenging issues in patient care, diagnosis, and therapy. Some of the major new developments in this area are discussed below:

1. **Wearable Health Monitoring Devices**: The gadgets with CI features are growing, thus making it easy for early identification of health issues and regular tracking of patients' conditions. These devices monitor health indicators and activity levels, and can even anticipate extreme medical occurrences viz. coronary artery disease, which can improve the patient outcome by providing active care.
2. **Genomics and Precision Medicine**: The switching to personalized medicine enables patient-specific medicines to be customized and is being speeded up by the amalgamation of genomics and CI. The ML approaches evaluate biological and medical information to anticipate illness vulnerability, drug-negative effects, and response to therapy allowing more personalized healthcare.

3. **Medical Imaging Analysis**: Deep learning and other advanced CI approaches are reforming medical imaging by increasing precision and effectiveness. Due to the high degree of precision, the instruments can identify abnormalities like malignancies or fractures. This helps radiologists to diagnose patients and cut down on the amount of time needed for analysis.
4. **Drug Development and Discovery**: AI and ML are integrating the process of drug discovery, starting from the drug compound's initial screening to predicting its success on testing. These models by examining complicated biological data can more quickly and precisely identify possible therapeutic targets than usual approaches.
5. **Robot-Assisted Surgery**: Optimization of surgical robotic systems' accuracy and capability is a prominent task for CI. By using data from before surgery, the medical records direct the surgeon's instrument instantaneously throughout procedures; these technologies lower the chances of error and can shorten recovery times for patients.
6. **Healthcare Data Analytics**: CI is extracting the abundance of healthcare data from wearables, genetics, and Electronic Health Records (EHR) to enhance healthcare delivery. Through the analysis of trends and patterns in the data, predictive modeling can pinpoint at-risk groups, maximize usage of available resources, and enhance patient outcomes.
7. **Natural Language Processing (NLP) in Clinical Decision Support**: NLP is being used to mine text and disorganized medical records for valuable pieces of information. Healthcare professionals can use the above-said data to stay updated on the most recent discoveries and available treatments that aid in clinical decision-making.
8. **Telemedicine and Virtual Health Assistants**: More effective use of telemedicine is given by CI usage. It lets medical professionals to give distant surveillance and counseling. AI-powered virtual health assistants can offer patients individualized assistance and guidance, enhancing accessibility to care and lessening the strain on medical facilities.
9. **Blockchain for Secure Medical Data Exchange**: Reliable and accurate health information sharing across stakeholders is ensured by the use of blockchain-based technologies in biomedical systems. It helps in combining data from

numerous sources for thorough analysis, thereby improving the security of information and patient privacy.

10. **Quantum Computing in Biomedical Research**: QC, however still in its infancy, has the potential to transform biomedical research by facilitating the molecular modeling of intricate biological processes and medication interactions. This could result in novel insights into disease mechanisms and therapeutic approaches [8].

These new developments show how CI is revolutionizing biomedical systems and present opportunities for profound shifts in the way we identify, treat, and control illnesses. Healthcare services will become even more efficient, more accessible, and more customized as these technologies advance.

16.4 CI Future Perspective in Bioinformatics

The field of bioinformatics is expected to witness a revolutionary expansion in the field of CI due to the swift progress of technological advances, the increasing quantity of biomedical data, and the constant demand for increasingly complex analytical instruments [9]. It is anticipated that the fusion of bioinformatics with CI would speed up the search for new medicinal targets, transform personalized healthcare, and provide fresh insights into intricate biological structures. Table 16.2 shows some important viewpoints regarding the future course of CI in bioinformatics.

Table 16.2 Important viewpoints regarding future course of CI.

S. no.	Future course of CI	Description
1	Multi-Omic Data Integration	• Future advancements in omic data integration (proteomics, genomics, metabolomics, etc.) will make it possible to comprehend biological functions and illnesses on a deeper level. • Understands the intricate relationships and interdependencies among various biological forms of information with CI • Resulting in more thorough models of cellular activity and pathology of diseases.

(*Continued*)

Table 16.2 Important viewpoints regarding future course of CI. (*Continued*)

S. no.	Future course of CI	Description
2	Advanced ML Models	• ML will find greater use in bioinformatics due to their intelligence. • Upcoming advancements in the fields of reinforcement learning, unsupervised learning, and DL will make it possible to derive more complex conclusions from biological data. • Enhance the ability to forecast the course of disease and find new biomarkers for a range of illnesses.
3	Personalized and Precision Medicine	• CI will drive the evolution of personalized medicine by enabling the analysis of individual genetic, environmental, and lifestyle factors. • This will allow for the development of highly personalized treatment plans, optimized drug dosages, and targeted therapies based on the patient's unique biological makeup, significantly improving treatment outcomes and reducing side effects.
4	Enhanced Drug Discovery and Development	• The drug discovery process becomes more efficient and less costly. • By simulating drug interactions at the molecular level and predicting the efficacy and toxicity of compounds before clinical trials, CI can greatly accelerate the pace of drug development and increase the success rate of new medications reaching the market [10].
5	Predictive Modeling of Disease Outbreaks	• Judge early detection of outbreaks. • Inform public health strategies. • CI will enhance our ability to predict and manage infectious disease outbreaks by analyzing vast amounts of data from multiple sources, including genomic data of pathogens, environmental data, and social media trends. • Mitigate the impact of infectious diseases.

(*Continued*)

Table 16.2 Important viewpoints regarding future course of CI. (*Continued*)

S. no.	Future course of CI	Description
6	Automated and Real-Time Data Analysis	• Reducing the need for manual intervention. • Allowing researchers to focus on higher-level interpretation and decision-making. • Future bioinformatics tools powered by CI (offer more automated data analysis capabilities). • Real-time data analysis will become more prevalent. • Enables immediate insights that can be critical in fast-moving fields like infectious disease research.
7	Ethical and Privacy Concerns	• Ensuring the responsible use of genetic and health-related data, protecting patient privacy, and addressing biases in data and algorithms will be crucial challenges to address. • As CI becomes more integrated into bioinformatics, ethical and privacy considerations will gain prominence.
8	Quantum Computing (QC) in Bioinformatics	• Integration of QC into bioinformatics could dramatically enhance computational capabilities. • Enabling the simulation of complex biological systems and the processing of vast datasets in ways currently unimaginable. • Lead to breakthroughs in understanding disease mechanisms, genetic interactions, and protein folding.
9	Cross-disciplinary Collaboration	• Bringing together experts from computer science, biology, mathematics, and medicine. • Tackling the complex problems of biology and medicine, leading to innovative solutions and breakthroughs [11].
10	Democratization of Bioinformatics	• Contribute to the democratization of bioinformatics. • Making powerful analytical tools more accessible to researchers and clinicians worldwide. • Enable a broader range of institutions to participate in cutting-edge research and contribute to global health initiatives.

The field of CI in bioinformatics has a promising future due to its potential to greatly expand knowledge of life at the level of the molecules, enhance healthcare outcomes, and boost human welfare [12]. As long as new CI is integrated with biological study, innovations, and discoveries will surely continue to emerge.

16.5 The Future of CI in Biomedical Systems

In the future, the CI in biomedical systems has a substantial impact on outcomes for patients, clinical studies, and the provision of healthcare [13]. Several important considerations that show how CI may affect the biomedical system are presented in Table 16.3.

Table 16.3 Important viewpoints of CI regarding biomedical systems.

S. no.	Viewpoint	Description
1	Advanced Predictive Analytics for Personalized Medicine	• More precise predictive analytics, enabling personalized medicine to reach new heights. • CI will facilitate the development of customized treatment plans that are more effective and have fewer side effects.
2	Integration of AI with IoT in Healthcare	• Deeper integration of CI with the Internet of Things (IoT) in healthcare. • Lead to an ecosystem of smart medical devices capable of continuous health monitoring and real-time data analysis. • Enable early detection of potential health issues, timely interventions, and improved management of chronic diseases.
3	Revolutionizing Drug Discovery and Development	• Transform drug discovery and development process by making it faster, cheaper, and more efficient [14]. • By the use of ML algorithms and simulation models, CI will quickly identify promising drug candidates, predict their efficacy and safety, and optimize clinical trial designs.

(Continued)

Table 16.3 Important viewpoints of CI regarding biomedical systems. (*Continued*)

S. no.	Viewpoint	Description
4	Enhanced Medical Imaging and Diagnosis	• Offer superior diagnostic capabilities. • AI-driven image analysis tools will provide more accurate and detailed interpretations of medical images, assisting healthcare professionals in making faster and more accurate diagnoses [15].
5	Breakthroughs in Genomic Medicine	• Pivotal role in advancing genomic medicine. • Enable the analysis of vast genomic datasets to uncover insights into genetic disorders. • Identify novel therapeutic targets, and contribute to the development of gene therapies. • Open new avenues for treating hereditary diseases and conditions with a genetic component [16].
6	Improvements in Surgical Robotics	• The future of surgical robotics is intertwined with advancements in CI. • Due to the evolution of AI technologies, robotic systems become more autonomous, precise, and capable of performing complex procedures with minimal human intervention. • Reduce surgical errors, and improve patient outcomes. • Make advanced surgical techniques more accessible [17].
7	Telemedicine and Remote Care	• Providing more accurate and efficient remote diagnostics, patient monitoring, and virtual health consultations. • AI-powered chatbots and virtual assistants will assist in personalized health advice and support. • Making healthcare more accessible, especially in underserved areas [18].

(*Continued*)

Table 16.3 Important viewpoints of CI regarding biomedical systems. (*Continued*)

S. no.	Viewpoint	Description
8	Ethical AI in Healthcare	• The ethical considerations will gain prominence due to the embedding of CI. • It's crucial to ensure the ethical use of AI, including transparency, fairness, and respect for patient privacy and autonomy. • Developing guidelines and standards for ethical AI in healthcare.
9	Cross-disciplinary Collaboration for Holistic Health Solutions	• Increased collaboration across disciplines. • Lead to more holistic health solutions and innovations [19].
10	Democratization of Healthcare through CI	• Contribute to the democratization of healthcare by making advanced diagnostic tools and personalized treatment options more widely available. • This will help to reduce health disparities and improve global health outcomes [20].

In further coming years, there is a great deal of promise and interesting possibilities for CI. Researchers anticipate significant developments that will revolutionize the way healthcare is delivered, improve patient care, and herald in an exciting period of medical inventiveness as continue to investigate and leverage the potential of CI.

16.6 Conclusion and Future Scope

The CI's future promises game-changing solutions as it is deemed fit with the paralleled technology developments. Its inclusion is changing real-world concerns. The latest trends in CI, defined by efficiency, accuracy, and adaptability, exhibit an entirely novel period of problem-solving capacities. The incorporation of NN, FS, EC, and SI together is changing healthcare, industry, environmental management, and society structures. It is improving the control over the digital realm.

The potential of CI to transform individual healthcare via sophisticated analysis enables therapies to be customized as per the patient's genome and lifestyle. In respect of environmental conservation, CI presents novel methods for managing natural resources and climate modeling, offering practical insights to lessen the effects of worldwide warming. Robust models for risk evaluation and systems for identifying fraud have the potential to enhance economic systems' resilience and security, hence benefiting the finance industry. In the meantime, smart automation and proactive upkeep models will drive additional procedures, asset, and management of supply chain efficiency in the production and shipping sectors.

The emerging discipline of QC holds the potential to unleash new levels of computational capability, allowing CI systems to address challenges that are presently unachievable in terms of complexity and scope. The combination of QC with CI has the potential to propel scientific advancements in the fields of biology, chemistry, and physics, leading to novel approaches in drug development and material research.

As CI's applications grow more widespread and significant, ethical issues and its proper implementation will become more crucial. To preserve public confidence and protect individual rights, AI-driven systems must guarantee privacy, equity, and openness. A major area of concentration will be the creation of moral standards and regulations for CI applications, making sure that these potent instruments are applied for the good of society at large.

To fully utilize CI, cross-disciplinary cooperation will be essential. By combining knowledge from engineering, computer science, and the biological, psychological, and social sciences, more comprehensive and practical solutions will be able to be developed, offering novel approaches to solving challenging global issues.

In conclusion, CI has a promising and bright future. Not only novel innovations are created as one keeps pushing the frontiers of CI, but also influence the course of human civilization and the planet. The road ahead is full of obstacles, but because to CI, we are more prepared than ever to overcome them. This bodes well for a time when human brilliance and technology will combine to build a better world.

References

1. Asim, M., Wang, Y., Wang, K., Huang, P.-Q., A Review on Computational Intelligence Techniques in Cloud and Edge Computing. *IEEE Trans. Emerging Top. Comput. Intell.*, 4, 6, 742–763, Dec. 2020, doi: 10.1109/TETCI.2020.3007905.

2. Shamshirband, S., Fathi, M., Chronopoulos, A.T., Montieri, A., Palumbo, F., Pescapè, A., Computational intelligence intrusion detection techniques in mobile cloud computing environments: Review, taxonomy, open research issues. *J. Inf. Secur. Appl.*, 55, 102582, 102582, 2020.
3. Thakur, A., Mishra, A.P., Panda, B., Rodríguez, D.C.S., Gaurav, I., Majhi, B., Application of artificial intelligence in pharmaceutical and biomedical studies. *Curr. Pharm. Des.*, 26, 29, 3569–3578, 2020.
4. Shahid, A.H. and Singh, M.P., Computational intelligence techniques for medical diagnosis and prognosis: Problems and current developments. *Biocybern. Biomed. Eng.*, 39, 3, 638–672, 2019.
5. Athanasopoulou, K., Daneva, G.N., Adamopoulos, P.G., Scorilas, A., Artificial Intelligence: The milestone in Modern Biomedical research. *BioMedInformatics*, 2, 4, 727–744, 2022.
6. Guo, K. *et al.*, Artificial intelligence-driven biomedical genomics. *Knowl. Based Syst.*, 279, 110937, 110937, 2023.
7. Banyal, S., Mehra, D., Amartya, Banyal, S., Sharma, D.K., Ghosh, U., Computational intelligence in healthcare with special emphasis on bioinformatics and internet of medical things, in: *Internet of Things*, pp. 145–170, Springer International Publishing, Cham, 2022.
8. Matschinske, J. *et al.*, The AIMe registry for artificial intelligence in biomedical research. *Nat. Methods*, 18, 10, 1128–1131, 2021.
9. Hulsen, T., Literature analysis of artificial intelligence in biomedicine. *Ann. Transl. Med.*, 10, 23, 1284–1284, 2022.
10. Malik, A. *et al.*, Ten simple rules for engaging with artificial intelligence in biomedicine. *PLoS Comput. Biol.*, 17, 2, e1008531, 2021.
11. Prabha, C., Singh, J., Agarwal, S., Verma, A., Sharma, N., Introduction to computational intelligence in healthcare, in: *Computational Intelligence in Healthcare*, pp. 1–15, CRC Press, Boca Raton, 2022.
12. Sharma, N. and Prabha, C., Computing paradigms: An overview, in: *2021 Asian Conference on Innovation in Technology (ASIANCON)*, pp. 1–6, 2021.
13. Singh, J., Prabha, C., Singh, G., Muskan, Verma, A., Addressing role of ambient intelligence and pervasive computing in today's world, in: *Lecture Notes in Electrical Engineering*, pp. 257–269, Springer Nature Singapore, Singapore, 2023.
14. Prabha, C., Mittal, P., Gahlot, K., Phul, V., Smart healthcare system based on AIoT emerging technologies: A brief review, in: *Lecture Notes in Electrical Engineering*, pp. 299–311, Springer Nature Singapore, Singapore, 2023.
15. dos Santos, Á.O., da Silva, E.S., Couto, L.M., Reis, G.V.L., Belo, V.S., The use of artificial intelligence for automating or semi-automating biomedical literature analyses: A scoping review. *J. Biomed. Inform.*, 142, 104389, 104389, 2023.
16. Bhardwaj, K.K., Banyal, S., Sharma, D.K., Artificial intelligence based diagnostics, therapeutics and applications in biomedical engineering and

bioinformatics, in: *Internet of Things in Biomedical Engineering*, pp. 161–187, Elsevier, 2019, https://doi.org/10.1016/B978-0-12-817356-5.00009-7

17. Chouhan, S.S., Kaul, A., Singh, U.P., Image segmentation using computational intelligence techniques: Review. *Arch. Comput. Methods Eng.*, 26, 3, 533–596, 2019.
18. Yang, Q., Wang, Z., Guo, K., Cai, C., Qu, X., Physics-Driven Synthetic Data Learning for Biomedical Magnetic Resonance: The imaging physics-based data synthesis paradigm for artificial intelligence. *IEEE Signal Process. Mag.*, 40, 2, 129–140, March 2023, doi: 10.1109/MSP.2022.3183809.
19. Kaushal, C., Islam, M.K., Singla, A., Al Amin, M., An IoMT-based smart remote monitoring system for healthcare, in: *IoT-Enabled Smart Healthcare Systems, Services and Applications*, pp. 177–198, Wiley, 10-Jan-2022. doi: 10.1002/9781119816829.ch8.
20. Vashisht, S., Sharma, B., Lamba, S., Using Support Vector Machine and Generative Adversarial Network for Multi-Classification of Pneumonia Disease, in: *2023 4th International Conference for Emerging Technology (INCET)*, IEEE, pp. 1–6, 2023.

Index

Also of Interest

Check out these published and forthcoming titles in "Sustainable Computing and Optimization" series from Scrivener Publishing

Intelligent Data Analytics for Bioinformatics and Biomedical Systems
Edited By Neha Sharma, Korhan Cengiz and Prasenjit Chatterjee
Published 2024. ISBN 978-1-394-27088-0

Optimization Techniques in Engineering
Advances and Applications
Edited by Anita Khosla, Prasenjit Chatterjee, Ikbal Ali and Dheeraj Joshi
Published 2023. ISBN 978-1-119-90627-8

Computational Intelligence in Sustainable Reliability Engineering
Edited by S. C. Malik, Deepak Sinwar, Ashish Kumar, S. R. Gadde, Prasenjit Chatterjee and Bui Thanh Hung
Published 2023. ISBN 978-1-119-86501-8

Decision Support Systems for Smart City Applications
Edited by: Loveleen Gaur, Vernika Agarwal and Prasenjit Chatterjee
Published 2023. ISBN 978-1-119-89643-2

Fuzzy Computing in Data Science
Applications and Challenges
Editors: Sachi Nandan Mohanty, Prasenjit Chatterjee and Bui Thanh Hung
Published 2022. ISBN: 978-1-119-86492-9

Handbook of Intelligent Computing and Optimization for Sustainable Development
Edited by: Mukhdeep Singh Manshahia, Valeriy Kharchenko, Elias Munapo, J. Joshua Thomas and Pandian Vasant
Published 2022. ISBN 978-1-119-79182-9

Machine Learning Algorithms and Applications
Edited by Mettu Srinivas, G. Sucharitha and Anjanna Matta
Published 2021. ISBN 978-1-119-76885-2

Smart Sustainable Intelligent Systems
Edited by Namita Gupta, Prasenjit Chatterjee and Tanupriya Choudhury
Published 2021. ISBN 978-1-119-75058-1

www.scrivenerpublishing.com

Printed in the USA/Agawam, MA
September 16, 2026

910661.141